CARDIAC REHABILITATION: EXERCISE TESTING AND PRESCRIPTION

VOLUME II

Edited by

Linda K. Hall, PhD
The Christ Hospital

G. Curt Meyer, MS
Lee Memorial Hospital

Life Enhancement Publications
Champaign, Illinois

Library of Congress Cataloging-in-Publication Data
(Revised for vol. 2)

Cardiac rehabilitation.

(La Crosse exercise and health series)
Vol. 2 edited by Linda K. Hall and G. Curt Meyer.
Reprint. Originally published: New York: SP Medical
& Scientific Books, c1984. Originally published in
series: Sports medicine and health science.
Includes bibliographies and index.
I. Coronary heart disease—Patients—Rehabilitation.
2. Exercise tests. 3. Exercise therapy. 4. Heart—
Diseases—Patients—Rehabilitation. I. Hall, Linda K.
II. Meyer, G. Curt. III. Hellerstein, Herman K.,
1916-   . IV. Series. [DNLM: 1. Exercise Therapy.
2. Heart Diseases—rehabilitation. WG 200 C2635 1984a]

RC685.C6C27 1988   616.1′23   87-22622
ISBN 0-87322-909-6 (v. 1)
ISBN 0-87322-910-X (v. 2)

Developmental Editor: Sue Wilmoth, PhD
Production Director: Ernie Noa
Projects Manager: Lezli Harris
Copy Editor: Peter Nelson
Assistant Editor: Julie Anderson
Typesetters: Brad Colson and Sonnie Bowman
Text Design: Keith Blomberg
Text Layout: The Admakers
Printed By: Braun-Brumfield

ISSN: 0894-4261
ISBN: 0-87322-910-X

Printed in the United States of America

10 9 8 7 6 5 4 3 2 1

Life Enhancement Publications
A Division of Human Kinetics Publishers, Inc.
Box 5076, Champaign, IL 61820
1-800-342-5457
1-800-334-3665 (in Illinois)

Contributors

R. Anne Abbott, PhD   President, Abbott-Jeffers & Associates, Stevens Point, Wisconsin. Associate Professor, Health Promotion, University of Wisconsin–Stevens Point

Ruth M. Anderson, MS, MPH   Administrative Director, Health Institute, St. Paul Medical Center, Dallas, Texas

Michael J. Asken, PhD   Clinical/Health Psychologist, Cowley Associates Medical Group, Camp Hill, Pennsylvania; Department of Behavioral Science, College of Medicine, Pennsylvania State University, Hershey, Pennsylvania

Steven N. Blair   Director of Epidemiology, Institute for Aerobics Research, Dallas, Texas

Wendy Dion, RN   Mount Sinai Medical Center Cardiac Rehabilitation Program, Milwaukee, Wisconsin

Carl Foster, PhD   Assistant Professor of Medicine, University of Wisconsin Medical School, Milwaukee Clinical Campus, Mt. Sinai Medical Center, Milwaukee, Wisconsin

Thomas T. Gushiken, PhD   Director, Workshops/Symposium Unit, La Crosse Exercise Program, Parks and Recreation Department, University of Wisconsin–La Crosse

Linda K. Hall, PhD   Director, Cardiac Rehabilitation, The Christ Hospital, Cincinnati, Ohio

Patricia L. Hutchinson, EdD   La Crosse Exercise and Health Program, University of Wisconsin–La Crosse

Charles P. Lucas, MD   Clinical Nutrition Unit, Wayne State University School of Medicine, Detroit, Michigan

Janet A. Lunn, MA   Exercise Physiologist, Division of Diabetes and Endocrinology, Scripps Clinic and Research Foundation, La Jolla, California

Patrick McBride, MD, MPH   Associate Director, Preventive Cardiology Program, Department of Family Medicine and Practice, University of Wisconsin Medical School, Madison, Wisconsin

G. Curt Meyer, MS   Wellness Center, Lee Memorial Hospital, Ft. Myers, Florida

Miriam Miller, RN, MS   Associate Director of Nursing Education, Cardiac Treatment Centers, Inc., Camp Hill, Pennsylvania

Catherine Reith Murphy, MS   Exercise Physiologist, American Rehab, Camp Hill, Pennsylvania

Glen H. Porter, PhD   Director, Rehabilitation Services, Seton Medical Center, Daly City, California

Daniel R. Timmons, MS   Exercise Physiology Education Advisor, Cardiac Treatment Centers, Camp Hill, Pennsylvania

Janet Treftz, MS   Health Promotion Coordinator, St. Luke's Hospital, Davenport, Iowa

K. Zirkel, PhD   Counseling Psychologist, Counseling and Testing Center, University of Wisconsin–La Crosse

Contents

Series Preface

On behalf of the chapter authors and editors and Human Kinetics Publishers, it is my pleasure to welcome you to this book. *Cardiac Rehabilitation: Exercise Testing and Prescription, Volume II* is one of a collection of eight books of the La Crosse Exercise and Health Series, offered by Life Enhancement Publications of Human Kinetics Publishers. The series is an outgrowth of various topics of the annual symposiums of the La Crosse Exercise and Health Program of the University of Wisconsin-La Crosse. Offered by the program's Educational Services Unit, these symposiums are directed to professionals in athletic training and rehabilitation, cardiac rehabilitation, corporate and hospital-based fitness and wellness programs, nutrition, and sports medicine. The individual editors of each book in the series were initially responsible for developing the topics and presenters for that specific symposium.

We intend for these books to provide readers with both theoretical and practical information specific to their fields of interest. Symposium topics and speakers, and consequently authors, have been chosen to provide "hands-on" information to assist practitioners. The symposiums and the resulting books are intended to truly assist you in the everyday practice of your profession. Cognitive knowledge applied in both theory and practice to daily problems and concerns is the ultimate goal of the La Crosse symposiums and book series. It is truly the hope of the symposium presenters and chapter authors, of the book editors, and of myself that each reader finds that the information provided appropriately serves their daily professional needs.

On behalf of the chapter authors and book editors, I thank Human Kinetics Publishers of Champaign, Illinois, for its involvement as the La Crosse Series publisher. Over the past 10 years Human Kinetics has become a leading publisher in the field of health and physical fitness, and we are pleased and appreciative for its commitment to this book series.

Philip K. Wilson, EdD
Series Editor

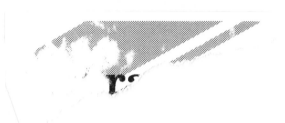

CARDIAC REHABILITATION: EXERCISE TESTING AND PRESCRIPTION

VOLUME II

Contributors

R. Anne Abbott, PhD   President, Abbott-Jeffers & Associates, Stevens Point, Wisconsin. Associate Professor, Health Promotion, University of Wisconsin–Stevens Point

Ruth M. Anderson, MS, MPH   Administrative Director, Health Institute, St. Paul Medical Center, Dallas, Texas

Michael J. Asken, PhD   Clinical/Health Psychologist, Cowley Associates Medical Group, Camp Hill, Pennsylvania; Department of Behavioral Science, College of Medicine, Pennsylvania State University, Hershey, Pennsylvania

Steven N. Blair   Director of Epidemiology, Institute for Aerobics Research, Dallas, Texas

Wendy Dion, RN   Mount Sinai Medical Center Cardiac Rehabilitation Program, Milwaukee, Wisconsin

Carl Foster, PhD   Assistant Professor of Medicine, University of Wisconsin Medical School, Milwaukee Clinical Campus, Mt. Sinai Medical Center, Milwaukee, Wisconsin

Thomas T. Gushiken, PhD   Director, Workshops/Symposium Unit, La Crosse Exercise Program, Parks and Recreation Department, University of Wisconsin–La Crosse

Linda K. Hall, PhD   Director, Cardiac Rehabilitation, The Christ Hospital, Cincinnati, Ohio

Patricia L. Hutchinson, EdD   La Crosse Exercise and Health Program, University of Wisconsin–La Crosse

Charles P. Lucas, MD   Clinical Nutrition Unit, Wayne State University School of Medicine, Detroit, Michigan

Janet A. Lunn, MA   Exercise Physiologist, Division of Diabetes and Endocrinology, Scripps Clinic and Research Foundation, La Jolla, California

Patrick McBride, MD, MPH   Associate Director, Preventive Cardiology Program, Department of Family Medicine and Practice, University of Wisconsin Medical School, Madison, Wisconsin

G. Curt Meyer, MS   Wellness Center, Lee Memorial Hospital, Ft. Myers, Florida

Miriam Miller, RN, MS   Associate Director of Nursing Education, Cardiac Treatment Centers, Inc., Camp Hill, Pennsylvania

Catherine Reith Murphy, MS   Exercise Physiologist, American Rehab, Camp Hill, Pennsylvania

Glen H. Porter, PhD   Director, Rehabilitation Services, Seton Medical Center, Daly City, California

Daniel R. Timmons, MS   Exercise Physiology Education Advisor, Cardiac Treatment Centers, Camp Hill, Pennsylvania

Janet Treftz, MS   Health Promotion Coordinator, St. Luke's Hospital, Davenport, Iowa

K. Zirkel, PhD   Counseling Psychologist, Counseling and Testing Center, University of Wisconsin–La Crosse

Contents

Preface

It is with much pride and satisfaction that we present to you *Cardiac Rehabilitation: Exercise Testing and Prescription, Volume II*. Within, one will find presented much information that can only be shared by authors who have functioned in the clinical arena of cardiac rehabilitation. Each section of this book presents information that is essential for the clinician or administrator who constantly seeks to achieve excellence in delivery of service to patients, while working closely with physicians and other allied health professionals.

Several new topics are presented in Volume II. Section I, on administrative concerns, encompasses information that is applicable both to the persons just completing formal education and to those who have worked for years in the field. All chapters are authored by professionals who have dealt with such concerns as physician involvement, equipment selection, program administration, and payment for services.

Sections II and III present applied physiological principles balanced against the reality of patient care in a clinical environment. These sections expand upon the first volume of *Cardiac Rehabilitation: Exercise Testing and Prescription* to include medical problems associated with early intervention, prescribing exercise for the well-conditioned patient, upper extremity exercise, energy cost of occupational work, counseling for leisure activity, the importance of behavioral intervention, and the multifaceted approaches to exercise testing.

Section IV addresses the choice of care for patients with coronary heart disease. Use of medications and of therapeutic intervention and the balance of providing both are well outlined. Long-standing philosophic discussion of this issue will continue as new indications and therapeutic interventions are researched and developed.

Cardiac Rehabilitation: Exercise Testing and Prescription: Volume II represents decades of medical experience. Its authors and editors have helped rehabilitate over 12,000 patients with coronary artery disease. Each author has contributed information relevant to the discipline of cardiovascular rehabilitation as it is practiced in the 1980s. Using this text as a resource, the reader will find many valuable lessons as well as be reminded of the basics of the field.

G. Curt Meyer, MS
Linda K. Hall, PhD

Part I

Administrative Concerns

Chapter 1

Who Should Administer the Cardiac Rehabilitation Program: Exercise Physiologist, Nurse, Physical Therapist, Physician?

R. Anne Abbott

Over the past decade cardiac patients have received a higher quality of health care than ever before. This is due, in part, to incorporating the use of exercise, nutrition, and behavior modification techniques with medical treatment and surgical interventions. The field of cardiac rehabilitation has emerged from several multidisciplinary professions, which have formed its scientific basis. In the multidisciplinary approach the *result* is defined as the sum total of efforts of each discipline working side by side (Wilson, 1984). Not only has this approach become an accepted practice, but recent research has indicated that the multifactorial approach provides for more effective rehabilitation (Kallio, Hamalainen, Hakkila, et al., 1979; Kallio, 1982).

It has been recognized that each of the multidiscipline professionals—physicians, exercise physiologists, nurses, physical and respiratory therapists, psychologists, nutritionists, and related allied health professionals—has made significant scientific contributions to advancing the field. In addition, each of these contributions has been maximized as the profession of cardiac rehabilitation has become interdisciplinary. Each discipline works synergistically: The result, produced as a whole (i.e., patient care), is more than the scientific disciplines might accomplish separately or working side by side (Wilson, 1984). The professional, regardless of specialty, must be prepared to reinforce or refer to the knowledge base and clinical practice of the other disciplines that contribute to the field. All of the disciplines within the cardiac rehabilitation profession subscribe to the common goal of quality patient care. Acceptance of the field as interdisciplinary, as well as multidisciplinary, emphasizes that although this field has emerged from the other professional disciplines, cardiac rehabilitation now represents a new and separate body of knowledge.

As the field of cardiac rehabilitation has grown philosophically, the approach has come to concern not only rehabilitation, but also wellness and health promotion, or how to keep patients well and improve their quality of life. The programmatic goal of the cardiac rehabilitation professional is to return the patient to normal by finding an acceptable balance of activity, nutritional status, stress, relaxation, work, and play (see Table 1.1). Although the professional must accomplish this within the physiological limitations imposed by the disease process, the real challenge is how to practice the art of the profession. The cardiac rehabilitation professional must become a facilitator who interacts with and assists the patient in establishing realistic, achievable goals. The ability to put this art into practice depends on the professional's ability to combine the scientific principles of exercise, nutrition, and behavioral change and the medical or surgical treatment outcomes with the patient's state of psychological readiness, attitudes, and values. Recognizing that all of these components are necessary for behavior change, practicing professionals in cardiac rehabilitation have become cross-trained, which allows them to be ready to facilitate the patient's behavior change at that critical moment of the patient's psychological state of readiness, as opposed to the patient's having to wait for the appearance of the appropriate professional, who performs only one specific discipline (e.g., nurse who only educates, physical therapist who only exercises the patient, etc.).

Conceptualizing cardiac rehabilitation as a behavioral model allows each of the factors influencing the patient's cognitive restructuring to be considered (see Figure 1.1). This is much less restrictive to the patient's care than considering merely the individual components. In the past cardiac rehabilitation programs have been ineffective in making an impact on returning to work, decreasing mortality and morbidity, and changing patients behavior (Kallio, Hamalainen, Hakkila, et al., 1979; Sivarajan et al., 1983). Perhaps this is because even though education alone does not sufficiently change behavior, it is difficult for professionals, who themselves so highly value education, not to retain the expectation that education will suffice. A behavioral approach offers a broader, more realistic program in which patients may make lifestyle changes. By amplifying the philosophy of rehabilitation to include specific *quality of life* outcomes, professionals will be able to elude routinization (e.g., merely prescribing exercise) and respect the inherent inertia of patients that leads to danger-ous nonadherence. Such an approach creates with the patient a new con-tract and a deeper and different spirit under which cardiac rehabilitation may be mutually pursued. This approach allows for the *art of practice*, the essential ingredient setting the profession apart from the scientific fields upon which it is based.

Credentials/Knowledge Base

Many sources are presently available to describe the knowledge base re-quired of a professional working in cardiac rehabilitation (American Col-lege of Sports Medicine [ACSM], 1986; Cardiopulmonary Section of the American Physical Therapy Association [APTA], 1983; Subcommittee on Rehabilitation, 1979). Although program specific, job descriptions gener-ally fall into the specific areas of program director, medical consultant/ director, clinical psychologist, clinical exercise specialist, and exercise specialist (Appendixes 1A, 1B, 1C, 1D, & 1E). Size limitations of the insti-tution and lack of resources increase the necessity of the interdisciplinary approach to professional training. Equally as important, multidisciplinary teams in larger institutions can increase efficiency and productivity when each member is cross-trained in each of the professional disciplines. In the context of the broader approach to cardiac rehabilitation, the use of an exercise specialist over a nurse, exercise physiologist, or physical thera-pist becomes more effective.

The job descriptions of the clinical exercise specialist and the exercise specialist allow for cross-fertilization of the various specialties. These two job titles draw upon expertise from exercise physiology, nursing, physical therapy, clinical psychology, behavioral medicine, and health education. However, the exercise specialist position is considered an entry-level posi-tion. Credentials in any one of these aforementioned disciplines gives the new cardiac rehabilitation professional the required background knowledge upon entering the field. The clinical exercise specialist is an experienced professional who has worked specifically in cardiac rehabilita-tion for a minimum of 2-3 years. These professionals generally have clinical experience in both inpatient and outpatient programs. A minimum of a masters degree, supervisory skills, and clinical experience specific to cardiac rehabilitation blends the multidisciplinary backgrounds into an interdisciplinary specialty. Fortunately, the American College of Sports Medicine (ACSM, 1986) and medicare (Cardiac Rehabilitation Programs, 1983) have begun to recognize the emerging cardiac rehabilitation profes-sional and have not specified licensure requirements. Evaluations of professional proficiencies have also become readily available through ACSM (1986) and the American Physical Therapy Association (APTA; Cardiopulmonary Section, 1983). Unfortunately, the APTA has chosen not to recognize the other important professional disciplines and has excluded them from taking part in their proficiency testing. Proficiencies of staff may be evaluated by use of a performance appraisal (see Appendix 1C). Productivity measures and documentation of attending professional conferences may also add an important dimension to staff evaluations (Appendix 1G).

Transition of a Professional

Inherent to this new view of cardiac rehabilitation (i.e., that it is not only an exercise program but also an interdisciplinary approach concerned with improving quality of life) is obtaining an appreciation of the patient's perspective. This requires that professionals new to the field take the time to observe their patients and listen to what they have to teach them. This perspective can come only with experience as one learns the art of practicing the profession. If professionals are made more aware of the patient's perspective, the ability to practice the art may be escalated. To some degree this can be achieved through visualization and integration of the cardiac patient's experiences.

Table 1.1   Cardiac Rehabilitation Program Objectives

I. Developing an *awareness* of desired behavior changes
 • PHASE I (inpatient): Awareness through
   • crisis intervention
   • evaluating and/or developing a knowledge base
   • setting the stage for attitude change by patient goal orientation
II. Providing programs to bring about *lifestyle change*
 • PHASE II (outpatient): Lifestyle Change through
   • self-assessment and risk factor modification
   • revisions of patient goals for long-term compliance
   • incorporation of techniques to modify behavior (i.e., smoking cessation, weight and lipid reduction, stress reduction, physical fitness, emotional wellness, etc.)
III. Providing a *supportive environment* for continuing and maintaining desired health behaviors
 • PHASE III (outpatient, extended): Supportive Environment created by professional staff and peers for
   • long-term follow-up and gradual behavior changes
   • restructuring life priorities realistically within physiological limitations

Professionals who take the time to understand the patient's perspective of the experiences surrounding the cardiac event will find that three important questions surface: "Am I going to die?" "What if I only have x-amount of time to live?" and "What if I live?" Recognizing the impact of these questions on the patient's perspective will help the professional understand not only that the patient may be unable to verbalize these concerns aloud but also that the patient's priorities will change quickly as they move from the situation of crisis to routine care, convalescence, and the complete rehabilitation process. Until they recognize the powerful impact of these questions on the patient's priorities, professionals' priorities for their patients may be inappropriate. Although the professional's scientific knowledge may create a perception of knowing what is good for the patient, until the patient arrives at the "What if I live?" stage of recovery, information may be irrelevant (e.g., teaching risk factor modification while the patient is still in a stage of crisis or denial). In a review of the literature, it appears that, in fact, this may be happening (Sivarajan et al., 1983). Incorporation of the patient's priorities (questions) within the behavior model (see Figure 1.1) may bring about more realistic, achievable objectives for the cardiac rehabilitation program.

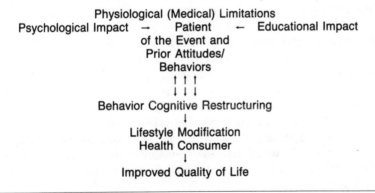

Figure 1.1. Cardiac rehabilitation behavior model.

Personal and Professional Transitions

Professionals new to the area of cardiac rehabilitation may find themselves evolving through a three-step transition which allows them to practice the art as well as the science of their profession. The faster these personal and professional transitions are acknowledged the quicker the professional can handle patient concerns.

The first step for the professional new to cardiac rehabilitation is to accept the personal implications of assuming the role of *caretaker*. This role is a nurturing one which typically draws people to the health care field, in that it is personally rewarding to provide care for those who are sick. Once immersed in the caretaker role, people begin to pursue how to become a *careprovider* as they enter their chosen academic careers. Once out of school and into initial stages of their career, professionals are eager to impart all of the scientific knowledge they have acquired over the years of study. Unsuspecting patients may receive an unproductive and burdensome oversupply of scientific information in an unknown language with a pat for reassurance that everything is going to be OK. In the meantime, the patient may be thinking: "What if I only have x-amount of time to live?" "I want to eat more of what I like, not less!" and so forth.

The second stage of the professional transition comes when the professional realizes that not everyone responds positively to the reassuring pat or to acquiring scientific knowledge of why they should change their behavior. Although patients may be able to recite what they should or should not do, very little behavior change occurs. Sometimes the "pat" approach only reinforces the patient's helplessness and depressing plight of becoming a cardiac cripple. At this point, the cardiac rehabilitation professional's transition includes learning to use a confrontational approach, which, rather than being aggressive, is assertive nurturing requiring enormous tact, subtlety, and titration. Being confrontational in nature assists patients in dealing with the seriousness of their disease. Until patients face their denial that coronary artery disease is a life-threatening event, little behavioral change may take place. The cardiac rehabilitation professional facilitates patients in giving themselves consent to allow entry of the grieving stages associated with crisis. Without assessing where the patients are in relation to their own questions, the cardiac rehabilitation professional may not be effective because of inappropriate timing in applying the art.

The third transition for cardiac rehabilitation professionals is to recognize their own personal and professional limitations. This stage is exemplified by the following scenario. A patient becomes totally dependent upon a cardiac rehabilitation program for social support, but continues to make little or no behavioral changes. The professional's excessive interaction with the patient is to no avail. Typically, the cardiac rehabilitation professional might give up on the patient. Seasoned professionals, however, might recognize that the patient is asking for more than they are capable of giving. Although patients are indirectly expressing a desire to seek help, the behavior change they are seeking may go beyond the normal commitment to diet, exercise, or stress management techniques. The professional should be able to recognize this as a nonverbal request for professional counseling or more specific medical or psychiatric diagnosis or treatment. Cardiac rehabilitation professionals, recognizing their own limitations, will interact with the patient to facilitate a referral to the appropriate professional discipline.

Internal Makeup of the Cardiac Rehabilitation Professional

Criteria to determine if one has the internal makeup to become a cardiac rehabilitation professional transcend what generally can be evaluated by objective techniques. Whether one has the philosophical makeup to provide the essence of cardiac rehabilitation by example (i.e., health role model, and/or applying the art) might be evaluated by applying the "Cardiac Rehabilitation Professional Quiz." This quiz is designed to evaluate the cardiac rehabilitation professional's ability to understand the dynamics of the personal commitment to this type of work. Ability to pursue personally an improved quality of life contributes to understanding the patient's perspective of the cardiac rehabilitation program.

Briefly, the "Cardiac Rehabilitation Professional Quiz" works like this. Question 1 identifies whether staff can relate to the patient's having been faced with the crisis of possible death. If the answer to Question 1 is "no," one might employ the following descriptive imagery to create an experience analogous to the process that the cardiac patient might undergo when faced with a cardiac crisis and questions, "Am I going to die?" Write down the five most important things in your life. With your list in front of you, use each of the following descriptive imagery situations to arrange your list in order of priority from least important to most important.

SITUATION #1—You have just become alert after having passed out. You see a startled look on your loved ones' faces, paramedics are quickly moving you from your environment to an ambulance. Mark the thing of least importance from your list of five items.

SITUATION #2—You have just arrived at the emergency room of your local hospital—paramedics are replaced by emergency room personnel. Your body is wired for monitoring, people hustle about you, their faces are unfamiliar, and you are groggy and unable to talk. Mark the second least important item from your list.

SITUATION #3—You've been stabilized, so they say, although you are still in the emergency room. Your personal physician has been notified, but is unavailable. You still haven't seen any member of your family and feel disoriented. You've seen this situation on TV but you have never been in a hospital as a patient yourself. You suddenly experience lightheadedness and slight nausea; you hear the nurse say that your pressure has dropped and to notify the physician. Mark the third least important item from your list.

SITUATION #4—You wake up in the intensive care unit, groggy. You feel you are in and out of reality; vaguely you remember your loved ones being there in between the revolving doctors, nurses, and others in white uniforms. You realize there is a constant heart monitor above your head; everyone glues their eyes on it as they come in and out of the room to check your status. You sense you have no control over your body functions as you lie among IV lines, catheter, oxygen tubes, and so on. You wait. An alarm sounds, bodies begin to swarm around you. Mark the fourth least important item from your list.

There should be only one item left on your list, which is probably not exercise, nutrition, or work. This mental exercise demonstrates why the patient's priorities may be very different from those of the cardiac rehabilitation professional and stresses how important it is to meet the patient at his or her own particular stage of readiness.

Now that it is better understood how the patient's priorities may develop, we can move on to Question 2. Questions 2 through 4 and Question 7 have to do with being in control of one's own self. It is often easier and less complicated to answer these questions about personal priorities by first asking: "How would I answer these questions if I had only 6 months to live?" To make these questions less self-centered, they might be tempered by adding, "But what if I live?" These questions attempt to make us aware, as we must make our patients, of what is truly important to us. In other words, what is the individual's perception of quality of life, and how might we, as professionals, use the patient's priorities to bring about positive behavior changes?

Questions 5 and 6 have to do with how the cardiac rehabilitation professional interacts with the patient. What are the professional and personal expectations for the patient? In answering Question 5, the professional must remember that it is not human to be perfect. The patient may find it difficult to conform to all of the suggested risk factor modifications. The objective for the patient and professional at the outset is to achieve in practice a balance that supports an improved quality of life. Imbalances often occur when patients as well as professionals become obsessed with the compulsion to be perfect. For example, if patients become so obsessed with lipid restrictions that their children avoid taking meals with them, the quality of life modification demanded may be counter-productive.

Question 6 cautions the professional about seeking self-validation from the patient. If the professional seeks the patient's approval to the extent that the professional is unable to use a confrontational approach, as is sometimes appropriate, that person may be failing to meet the patient's needs.

Question 8 points out the necessity of being a healthy role model. How can professionals ask patients to modify their behaviors if the professionals are not willing to make the same modifications (e.g., smoking cessation). In addition, professionals must know how to temper what they believe; that is, to avoid giving the impression that their having chosen to pursue a healthy lifestyle makes them one of the chosen few (i.e., placing the professional above the patient's ability to achieve similar goals). Professionals must be aware of how humbling the experience of making significant lifestyle changes can be.

Question 9 identifies an important element of accepting the variation in professional expertise and cross-training necessary within the cardiac rehabilitation profession. This question addresses the check-and-balance system essential to protecting quality care for patients (e.g., the physician or nurse may intervene by providing safety standards whereas the exercise physiologist may intervene by reducing an overly protective environment for patients). In other words, everyone on the cardiac rehabilitation team takes individual responsibility for implementing proficient, safe, and quality patient care.

Question 10 recognizes that cardiac rehabilitation is a relatively new profession, which has drawn upon many scientific disciplines as well as clinical experience with patients to develop a new knowledge base. Professionals will continue to learn from each other, their patients, and themselves to be dreamers and risk takers. This will allow professionals to find new solutions and innovations for improving the future care of cardiac patients.

The "Cardiac Rehabilitation Professional Quiz" is a subjective method of determining whether one has the internal makeup to become a cardiac rehabilitation professional and reflects my own philosophy. The correct score, therefore, may be biased. However, the correct score is considered a balance of "yes" and "no" responses.

Summary

Combining credentials, scientific knowledge, and a philosophy of cardiac rehabilitation is the challenge as the art of cardiac rehabilitation comes of age. The question, "Are you ready to accept such a challenge?" may evoke more revealing answers than "Who should administer the cardiac rehabilitation program?"

REFERENCES

American College of Sports Medicine. (1986). *Guidelines for graded exercise testing and exercise prescription* (3rd ed.). Philadelphia: Lea & Febiger.

Cardiac Rehabilitation Programs. (1983, September 15). In *New developments, Medicare, Medicaid guide* (Paragraph 27201). Chicago: Commerce Clearing House.

Cardiopulmonary Section of the American Physical Therapy Association. (1983). *Specialty competencies in physical therapy: Cardiopulmonary.* Manhattan Beach, CA: Cardiopulmonary Specialty Council.

Kallio, V., Hamalainen, H., Hakkila, J., et al. (1979). Reduction of sudden death by a multifactorial intervention program after acute myocardial infarction. *Lancet, 2,* 1091-1094.

Kallio, V. (1982). Rehabilitation programs as secondary prevention: A community approach. *Advances in Cardiology, 31,* 120-128.

Sivarajan, E.S., Newton, K.M., Almes, M.J., Kempf, T.M., Mansfield, L.W., & Bruce, R.A. (1983). Limited effects of outpatient teaching and counseling after myocardial infarction: A controlled study. *Heart & Lung, 12*(1), 65-73.

The Subcommittee on Rehabilitation Target Activity Group. (1979). *The exercise standards book: Standards for adult exercise testing laboratories; specifications for exercise testing equipment; standards for cardiovascular exercise treatment programs; standards for supervised cardiovascular maintenance programs.* Dallas: American Heart Association.

Wilson, J.A. (1984). How to deliver comprehensive rehabilitation using a matrix organization model. *Hospital Topics, 62*(1), 29-32.

JOB DESCRIPTION

Director
Cardiopulmonary Rehabilitation

BASIC PURPOSE

The director is responsible for all day-to-day operations, quality of patient care, and long-range planning of the cardiopulmonary prevention/ rehabilitation laboratory, including all existing programs (behavior modification, education, evaluation, research) and future programs. In conjunction with the associate vice president, the medical director, and the director, is administratively responsible for the cardiopulmonary prevention/ rehabilitation laboratory and its personnel and functions.

MAJOR ACTIVITIES

1. Responsible for development and implementation of all program protocol and operating policies as well as expanding services of the development of cardiopulmonary prevention/rehabilitation. This includes the authority to issue orders and request services (test, protocols, procedures, etc.) for patients and clients within the program under a one time blanket authority of the medical director/ consultant/cardiologist/referring physician.
2. Responsible for developing, supervising, and administration of all program components for open heart surgery and post myocardial infarction inpatients and outpatients. These duties also include expanding services to other patient populations as well as area corporations desiring exercise testing, cardiac rehabilitation, and/or wellness programs.
3. Coordinates services between the cardiopulmonary prevention/ rehabilitation lab and other hospital departments by interphasing the program with hospital administration, physicians, and other health-related personnel.
4. Supervises a cardiopulmonary rehabilitation team consisting of a clinical psychologist, clinical specialists, exercise specialists, nutritionist, clerical staff, and student interns.
5. Responsible for implementing teaching, training, and research to provide for continued professional development of the staff.

6. Supervises all cardiopulmonary rehabilitation staff, authorizes and negotiates all hiring and firing and periodic evaluation of personnel to work within the cardiopulmonary prevention/rehabilitation laboratory.
7. Administratively responsible for the graded exercise testing evaluation unit. In conjunction with the medical consultant, supervises the graded exercise testing, assesses functional capacity of patients and their ability to return to work, and devises an exercise prescription for each patient as appropriate.
8. On an on-call basis, the director provides individualized counseling to patients in Phase I, II, and III, as requested by the cardiopulmonary team or on an appointment basis to any patient not entering the CPR program through the Phase I program. This counseling may include crisis intervention, risk factor analysis, assessing patient's understanding of CAD, assisting the patient and spouse in setting goals for accepting the disease process, behavior modification (stress management, nutrition, exercise, and smoking cessation), or returninng to work.
9. Responsible for budget development and expenditure control over an approved annual budget. Capital investments are under the direction of the director with hospital board approval.
10. In consultation with the medical consultant/director and associate vice president, is responsible for facility planning and expansion necessary for program growth.
11. Responsible for final approval on all public relations endeavors, advertising or marketing plans, to be implemented by the hospital for services or programs provided by the cardiopulmonary/ rehabilitation laboratory.
12. May design and coordinate research efforts that evolve from cardiopulmonary/rehabilitation testing, behavior modification, or education programs. Research may also be initiated in order to update programs and/or develop new programs.
13. Responsible for recommending policy to limit legal liability of the cardiopulmonary prevention/rehabilitation laboratory.

QUALIFICATIONS

Minimum of PhD with emphasis in exercise physiology, behavior psychology or epidemiology. A minimum of three years experience in cardiac rehabilitation including inpatient and outpatient services. Current American College of Sports Medicine certification as a program director. Current American Heart Association certification in advanced cardiac life support.

Minimum of 2 years experience in supervision and interpretation of graded exercise testing and prescription. Minimum of 2 years experience in teaching/counseling adults and in administration.

JOB DESCRIPTION

Medical Consultant
Cardiopulmonary Rehabilitation

BASIC PURPOSE

The medical consultant is responsible for the proper medical evaluation, quality of care, and safety of patients participating in all the cardiopulmonary prevention/rehabilitation programs. The medical consultant is responsible for implementing medical policies and procedures and standards for quality care as specified by the medical director. The medical consultant is responsible for training and supervising personnel participating in the implementation of such policies. The medical consultant is responsible to the director, division of cardiology and the director, cardiopulmonary prevention/rehabilitation.

MAJOR ACTIVITIES

1. Responsible for day-to-day operation of the graded exercise testing, including: screening applications for contraindications to exercise; examining patients prior to the exercise test to detect recent changes in cardiovascular status; supervising the graded exercise test; medical interpretation and reporting of test results; and interacting with referring physician and/or CPR staff when medical findings or recommendations require immediate or follow-up care.
2. In conjunction with the exercise physiologist, assesses functional capacity and ability of participants to return to work, designs individualized exercise prescriptions for each patient, and participates in ongoing assessment (e.g., adequate medication regime, etc.) of patient's treatment plan and rehabilitation goals.
3. On an on-call basis or by case review, acts as a medical advisor to the CPR staff during day-to-day operation of all phases of the program.
4. Acts as a liaison between the cardiopulmonary prevention/rehabilitation lab and hospital physicians and administrators, other health-related personnel, and referring physicians. The medical

consultant is expected to educate the medical staff regarding patient selection, expected benefits, and limitations of graded exercise testing and rehabilitation programs. Specifically, the medical consultant will make residents and cardiology fellows aware of the services provided by cardiopulmonary rehabilitation.

5. Directly responsible for implementing policies, procedures and personnel regarding emergency situations. This includes implementation of standing orders, training personnel in advanced life support, selection and operation of emergency equipment, and management of on-call system for physician coverage and transport of patients in emergencies.

6. Responsible for implementing teaching, training, and research to provide for continued professional development of the staff.

QUALIFICATIONS

A minimum of board certification/board eligibility in internal medicine (licensure to practice within the state). Minimum of 2 years of experience in supervision and interpretation of graded exercise testing and/or cardiac rehabilitation/exercise prescription. Minimum certification by the American Heart Association in Advance Life Support or its equivalent. Desire to work within a comprehensive health care team approach and ability to promote a healthy lifestyle change in participants of the program.

JOB DESCRIPTION

Clinical Psychologist Consultant
Cardiopulmonary Rehabilitation

BASIC PURPOSE

The clinical psychologist will provide as requested by the cardiopulmonary rehabilitation team individualized patient psychological evaluation and psycho-therapy as necessary. Acts as moderator and coordinator for the patient and spouse education and behavior modification programs. Participates in staff developmental projects and publication of research data and acts as liaison person between the cardiac rehabilitation program and medical staff, health-related staff, the patient, and family members.

MAJOR ACTIVITIES

1. Provides individualized psychological evaluation and follow-up therapy consisting of the following items 2–7.
2. Assesses the personality coping mechanisms, communication abilities, and work style of each patient referred to CPR by means of a clinical interview in psychometrics.
3. Identifies immediate patient needs and coordinates with the cardiopulmonary rehabilitation team for inpatient, outpatient, or home care follow-up services. Identifies any major problems that might interfere with hospitalization or with cardiac rehabilitation of the patient during the patient's participation in CPR programs (Phase I, II, III) or may cause major problems upon discharge from Phase I.
4. Prepares a written psychological report on each patient, documenting the evaluation, interview, and follow-up.
5. Orients the patient and, wherever possible, the spouse, to the implications of the psychological assessment and the optimal coping methods conducive to rehabilitation and recovery.
6. Recommends and initiates treatment procedures or makes the appropriate referrals for specific psychological treatment needs of the patient.
7. Consults with the staff on patient management and records specific guidelines for staff follow-up.

QUALIFICATIONS

Minimum of 2 years of experience in behavioral medicine and clinical psychotherapy. A desire to work with a comprehensive health care team and ability to promote a healthy lifestyle change in participants of the program. A minimum of licensure to practice clinical psychology within the state.

JOB DESCRIPTION

Clinical Exercise Specialist
Cardiopulmonary Rehabilitation

BASIC PURPOSE

The clinical specialist is responsible for day-to-day supervision of the cardiopulmonary rehabilitation (CPR) team, implementing inpatient and/or outpatient programs and coordinating the efforts of the team with the director, the medical consultant, and/or other necessary health care professionals (e.g., social services, home care, vocational rehabilitation). This person is responsible for keeping current with the medical status of all inpatients and/or outpatients. This person, in collaboration with the director, is responsible for providing inservice training and continuing education for the CPR team and other health care professionals in order to expedite all CPR services.

The clinical specialist is responsible for obtaining, developing, and updating all programmatic materials for Phase I (inpatient consultation, patient risk factor education/counseling, exercise and nutrition prescriptions, and appropriate follow-up), Phase II (outpatient educational/counseling sessions), and Phase III (outpatient monitored and unmonitored exercise prescriptions), and developing new programs. The clinical specialist, in conjunction with the director and medical consultant, is responsible for maintaining the crash cart, training the CPR staff in cardiopulmonary resuscitation, and implementing emergency protocol.

MAJOR ACTIVITIES

1. Responsible for day-to-day operation of Phase I, II, and III programs and the exercise testing services offered by the cardiopulmonary prevention/rehabilitation laboratory. This includes coordinating the CPR team efforts and organizing, delegating, and supervising day-to-day operations. Making staff assignments, implementing policies and procedures for screening patients, electrocardiograph (ECG) monitoring, recording and determining appropriate patient progression, implementing inpatient and/or outpatient testing and behavior modification programs are all included in these duties as well as

reporting relevant data to the director, medical consultant, and referring physician.

2. Responsible for implementation and follow-up of policies and procedures for effective program growth, safety, and quality assurance.
3. In conjunction with the director, develops new program areas for improved patient services and develops product-related services to be marketed to health consumers and new clinical populations (renal, diabetic, etc.).
4. Assists the director in developing research pertinent to the cardiac rehab program. This will include reviewing literature, developing the hypothesis, methods, and protocol, and supervising implementation of the projects for publication and/or incorporation of relevant findings into clinical practice.
5. Acts as a liaison for the CPR program and patient/spouse-family, doctor, hospital staff, home care, social services, vocational rehabilitation, and the community.
6. In conjunction with the director, assists in hiring, orienting, training, and evaluating the cardiac rehabilitation staff (exercise specialists).
7. With assistance from the director and medical consultant, responsible for updating the emergency protocol. The person designates or coordinates staff/patient training in cardiopulmonary resuscitation, monthly emergency drills (including evacuation and ambulance services), and up-to-date maintenance of emergency equipment and supplies. In the absence of the medical consultant, the clinical specialist initiates and supervises the emergency code as specified in the medical director's standing orders.
8. Assists with all phases of the CPR program including Phase I, Phase II, and Phase III, and exercise testing including data processing, devising the exercise prescription, reporting patient progress, and scheduling appropriate patient follow-up.
9. Develops, obtains, and updates patient education materials for Phase I, II, and III outpatient programs as well as for new programs (e.g., wellness, corporate fitness, lifestyle awareness, diabetic, pulmonary, renal, etc.).
10. Trains and supervises volunteer and/or student interns from participating university educational programs.

NATURE AND SCOPE OF POSITION

A. The clinical specialist's work may be assigned by the director or may be self-generated in an attempt to meet programmatic and increased productivity goals.
B. The clinical specialist participates in developing program policy and management goals with the final approval of such plans resting with

the director of cardiopulmonary rehabilitation. The clinical specialist may be requested by the director to participate in hiring and evaluating employees. The incumbent may make recommendations for staffing ratio, time off, and personnel scheduling for efficient use of human resources. The clinical specialist is responsible for day-to-day decisions concerning patient care in his or her specific clinical areas and follow-up including seeking input from the director or medical consultant. In the absence of the director, the clinical specialist may intervene appropriately to give direction to staff in critical or emergency situations and to clarify policy and procedures.

C. The clinical specialist acts as liaison for the CPR program and patient/spouse-family, doctor, hospital staff, home care, social services, vocational rehabilitation, and the community.

D. The clinical specialist supervises the exercise specialist staff who provide day-to-day services of cardiopulmonary rehabilitation. These include medical screening and monitoring of behavioral modification programs including patient/spouse education and behavioral change techniques for prescribed exercise, smoking cessation, weight and lipid reduction, stress management, and other risk factor modifications. Duties also include providing technical expertise for stress testing and interpretation of data for functional capacity return to work and exercise prescription.

QUALIFICATIONS

A. Minimum qualifications: MA/MS in nursing, exercise physiology, physical therapy, or behavioral medicine; advanced cardiac life support and 2 years of experience in cardiac rehabilitation. Nurses, in addition, should have a minimum of 2 years of critical care experience and hold current state licensure. Physical therapists, exercise physiologists, and behavioralists should have a minimum of 2 years experience in general practice. Physical therapists are required to hold a current state license. Applicants should be willing to apply for and attain ACSM Exercise Specialist Certification.

B. Good knowledge base and clinical skills in cardiovascular, exercise physiology, and cardiac rehabilitation are critical; experience, judgment, ability to follow up and complete projects, and high energy are necessary.

POSITION DESCRIPTION

Exercise Specialist
Cardiopulmonary Rehabilitation

BASIC PURPOSE

The exercise specialist is responsible for performing day-to-day implementation and follow-up care for patients in all phases of the cardiopulmonary rehabilitation program. This consists of direct caseload responsibility for 8-12 patients in the Phase I program, in which the exercise specialist works independently and/or in conjunction with other cardiac rehabilitation team members to provide an individualized program tailored to each patient's particular needs. In addition, the exercise specialist assists in all phases of the cardiac rehabilitation program by having rotating assigned duties in teaching/counseling, providing staff inservices, exercise stress testing, and other special programs sponsored by the cardiopulmonary prevention/ rehabilitation lab.

MAJOR ACTIVITIES

1. Directly responsible by caseload assignment for 8-12 patients in the Phase I program. This consists of obtaining appropriate medical records, reviewing the patient's present medical status, assessing coronary risk factors, leisure time, and work-related activities, evaluating socio-economic factors, and developing a program tailored to the patient's individual goals and set within the physiological limitations imposed by the disease. In conjunction with the director/clinical specialist/physical therapist/clinical psychologist, the exercise specialist provides the patient with a plan for crisis intervention, education, counseling, appropriate exercise, and behavior modification programs. Reviews discharge instructions with the patient and family. Conclusion of the Phase I service includes scheduling the patient for follow-up and writing a discharge summary to be sent to the referring physician.

2. In conjunction with the clinical specialist/clinical psychologist, implements and supervises educational programs for individuals and small groups of patients/spouse/family or employees.

3. In conjunction with the clinical specialist, assists in implementation of the Phase III exercise program. This includes screening patients, assessing vital signs and symptoms, ECG monitoring to determine the appropriate progression of the exercise prescription as well as recording and reporting relevant data.
4. Participates in periodic emergency procedures including initiating emergency treatment and transport. In the absence of a physician, initiates and carries out the emergency code as specified in the medical consultant's standing orders.
5. In conjunction with the clinical specialist, prepares reports on the individual participant's progress to be distributed to the referring physician and the patient.
6. Assists with graded exercise stress testing, including data analysis, preparation of reports, and follow-up patient consultations.
7. Participates in implementation of special programs sponsored by the cardiopulmonary rehabilitation lab for patients and employees as deemed necessary for program growth.
8. Participates in staff developmental projects and collecting and publishing of research data.
9. Assists the clinical specialist in the development of motivational techniques to increase patient compliance to all programs sponsored by the cardiac rehabilitation lab.
10. The exercise specialist will assist the clinical specialist in training, supervising, and evaluating student interns from participating university educational programs.
11. Performs other duties as assigned by the director.

NATURE AND SCOPE OF POSITION

A. The exercise specialist's work may be assigned by the director or the clinical specialist, or may be self-generated in an attempt to meet programmatic and increased productivity goals.
B. The exercise specialist participates in implementation of policy, programmatic, and management goals. The exercise specialist may be invited by the director and/or the clinical specialist to participate in developing policy, programmatic, and management goals with the final approval of such plans resting with the director. The exercise specialist is responsible for day-to-day treatment decisions and recognizing his or her own clinical limitations concerning caseload assignment. The exercise specialist, in conjunction with the referring physician, may intervene as appropriate to give directions to patients concerning appropriate rehabilitation treatment. However, questionable patient treatment should be reported and discussed with the clinical specialist and/or director and the medical consultant.

C. The exercise specialist acts as a liaison for the CPR program and patient/spouse-family, doctor, hospital staff, home care, social services, and vocational rehabilitation.
D. The exercise specialists are staff personnel who provide day-to-day services of the cardiac rehabilitation laboratory as part of a multidisciplinary team. As such, they are not concerned with day-to-day supervision other than patient care.

QUALIFICATIONS

A. Minimum qualifications: BS in nursing, exercise physiology, physical therapy, or behavioral medicine; current basic and advanced cardiac life support certification and 2 years of critical care nursing experience, or 2 years of general experience in physical therapy, or a masters degree in exercise physiology or behavioral medicine, and an internship in cardiac rehabilitation or corporate wellness. Physical therapists and nurses are required to hold a current state licensure. Applicants should be willing to apply for and attain ACSM exercise specialist certification.
B. Good technical/clinical skills in cardiovascular nursing, physical therapy, or exercise physiology and cardiac rehabilitation. Ability to develop a good knowledge base in clinical medicine and cardiovascular and exercise physiology. Ability to work independently and with a multidisciplinary team. Must be able to develop good rapport with patients/staff and physicians.

PERFORMANCE APPRAISAL

Employee Name: Job Title:

Date of Review: Evaluator:

TESTING PERFORMANCE **Factors**	LOW 1	 2	AVERAGE 3	 4	HIGH 5
I. Test Preparation					
A. Familiarize with ECG recorder, calibrate equipment, check scope	___	___	___	___	___
B. Review emergency procedure, turn on/test defribrillator, check drug cart; successful completion of ACLS	___	___	___	___	___
C. Review patient records, medical history	___	___	___	___	___
D. Patient Interview	___	___	___	___	___
1. Screen patient appropriately for contraindications to testing (medications, orthopedic problems, etc.)	___	___	___	___	___
2. Evaluate home activity routine	___	___	___	___	___
3. Review risk factor assessment	___	___	___	___	___
E. Review consent form and have patient sign it (explain purpose of the test, answer questions, etc.)	___	___	___	___	___

    F. Report pertinent information
       to physician/decide on appro-
       priate test protocol   ___ ___ ___ ___ ___

II. Technical Skills

    A. Measure height, body weight   ___ ___ ___ ___ ___

    B. Locate anatomical sites, prep
       skin, attach electrodes   ___ ___ ___ ___ ___

    C. Locate brachial sites, measure
       supine blood pressure (BP)   ___ ___ ___ ___ ___

    D. Record supine ECG, mark
       leads, note significant ECG
       changes   ___ ___ ___ ___ ___

    E. Measure standing preexercise
       BP and record ECG   ___ ___ ___ ___ ___

    F. Familiarize patient with exer-
       cise mode and RPE scale
       (where appropriate, also
       review four-point anginal
       scale)   ___ ___ ___ ___ ___

    G. Operate exercise mode,
       recording all pertinent data
       (HR, BP, ECG change, RPE
       responses, symptoms, etc.)   ___ ___ ___ ___ ___

    H. Observe participant, question
       for signs and symptoms of
       intolerance   ___ ___ ___ ___ ___

    I. Terminate test according to
       ACSM criteria, or on decision
       of attending physician   ___ ___ ___ ___ ___

    J. Record immediate postexercise
       12-lead ECG and BP; note
       significant changes   ___ ___ ___ ___ ___

    K. Record supine recovery data
       (ECG, BP, sign/symptoms) at
       appropriate times   ___ ___ ___ ___ ___

    L. Discharge patient and explain
       postexercise procedures (e.g.,
       showering, eating, resting)   ___ ___ ___ ___ ___

III. Posttest Responsibilities

    A. Label ECGs and organize   ___ ___ ___ ___ ___

B. Write first draft of physician's
letter   ___ ___ ___ ___ ___

C. Plot HR and BP responses on
graph   ___ ___ ___ ___ ___

D. Develop tentative exercise
prescription   ___ ___ ___ ___ ___

PHASE I PERFORMANCE FACTORS

I. Patient Screening

  A. Accurately clarifies physician's orders for patient's
admission into the cardiac
rehabilitation program   ___ ___ ___ ___ ___

  B. Adequately assesses the physical needs of Phase I participants through an initial and
ongoing assessment of relevant clinical parameters as
established through the
department's procedure
guidelines   ___ ___ ___ ___ ___

II. Assess the psychological needs
of Phase I participants, including
the following:

  A. Assessment of patient's cogni-
tive capacity   ___ ___ ___ ___ ___

  B. Psychological/emotional impact
imposed by the disease state
and/or hospitalization   ___ ___ ___ ___ ___

III. Assess the learning needs of
Phase I participants   ___ ___ ___ ___ ___

  A. Assessment of risk factors   ___ ___ ___ ___ ___

  B. Assessment of physical/
vocational activity   ___ ___ ___ ___ ___

  C. Assessment of patient's knowledge base in reference to the
disease state   ___ ___ ___ ___ ___

IV. Follow-Up Activities

  A. Accurately completes and
files historical/medical records

reviewed during the consultation process   ___ ___ ___ ___ ___

B. Completes and files the "request for consultation" form in the medical record immediately after the patient's consultation is completed   ___ ___ ___ ___ ___

C. Develops, initiates, supervises, surveys, and adjusts physical activity program for Phase I participants in accordance with assessed alternatives in the patient's clinical status   ___ ___ ___ ___ ___

   1. Accurately assesses the apical rate and regularity of the patient's heart rhythm before, during, and after each exercise session as established through the department's procedural guidelines   ___ ___ ___ ___ ___

   2. Accurately assesses the patient's blood pressure before, during, and after each exercise session as established through the department's procedural guidelines   ___ ___ ___ ___ ___

   3. Demonstrates the correct operating procedure when utilizing the portable Lifepak monitor   ___ ___ ___ ___ ___

   4. Demonstrates the correct operating procedure when utilizing the telemetry monitoring system on the nursing unit   ___ ___ ___ ___ ___

   5. Demonstrates the correct use of the exercycle for appropriate patients on

the cardio-throracic nursing units ___ ___ ___ ___ ___

6. Demonstrates the correct
stair climbing procedure
for selected cardiac
patients as established
through the department's
procedure guidelines ___ ___ ___ ___ ___

7. Correctly demonstrates
the sitting/standing range-
of-motion exercises as established through the
department's procedure
guidelines ___ ___ ___ ___ ___

D. Effectively provides the
patient and family members
with a means by which they
will be able to adapt to the
coronary event or disease
state ___ ___ ___ ___ ___

1. Provision of psychological
support for enhancing the
recovery process ___ ___ ___ ___ ___

2. Referral to staff psychologist when appropriate ___ ___ ___ ___ ___

3. Enhanced individualized/
group instruction for
patients/family ___ ___ ___ ___ ___

a. Provision of
individualized/group
instruction based on
assessment of learning
needs ___ ___ ___ ___ ___

b. Provides patients as-
sistance in developing
treatment goals and
selecting appropriate
lifestyle modifications.

c. Assisting the indivi-
dual in the develop-
ment of realistic

attitudes concerning
physical capacity   ____ ____ ____ ____ ____

   d. Promotion of the
patient's and family's
awareness of need for
their responsible com-
mitment to continued
formal outpatient
rehabilitation   ____ ____ ____ ____ ____

E. Discharge planning and
instruction   ____ ____ ____ ____ ____

   1. Accurately completes and
files the designated areas
on the "Discharge Sum-
mary" in the medical
record as the patient is
transferred out of the
specialty care unit to the
general cardio-thoracic
nursing units   ____ ____ ____ ____ ____

   2. Consistently updates the
patient rehabilitation
progress through daily
entries in the medical
record   ____ ____ ____ ____ ____

   3. Promotes liaison communication with patient's family
and health care team
from admission through
discharge   ____ ____ ____ ____ ____

   4. Upon discharge, accurately
completes a written dis-
charge summary to the
patient's primary physician
regarding the participant's
inpatient progress   ____ ____ ____ ____ ____

   5. Contributes to the promotion of a better
understanding concerning
the purpose, goals, and
procedures of the cardiac
rehabilitation program   ____ ____ ____ ____ ____

PHASE II EDUCATION/COUNSELING SESSIONS, PERFORMANCE FACTORS

I. Phase II Organization and Follow-up

   A. Collects and reviews patient's chart prior to start of Phase II   ____ ____ ____ ____ ____

   B. Mails out Phase II reminder letter prior to start of Phase II   ____ ____ ____ ____ ____

   C. Follows up each session with a phone call to absentees   ____ ____ ____ ____ ____

   D. At the end of Phase II, promptly completes report on patient's participation and returns file to central filing   ____ ____ ____ ____ ____

   E. Expedites patient's progress from Phase II to Phase III by promptly providing patient with Phase III medical prescription form   ____ ____ ____ ____ ____

II. Preparation and Delivery

   A. Displays adequate knowledge in all major teaching areas   ____ ____ ____ ____ ____

   B. Communicates knowledge in an informative, creative manner   ____ ____ ____ ____ ____

   C. Provides patients with appropriate handouts and self-assessments each week   ____ ____ ____ ____ ____

III. Individual Counseling and Triage

   A. Recognizes common physical and psychological problems encountered in the home recovery period   ____ ____ ____ ____ ____

   B. Meets with patient and spouse on an individual basis to further assess problems described above   ____ ____ ____ ____ ____

   C. Promptly and effectively triages patient to other cardiac

rehab team members or referring physician group when
necessary ___ ___ ___ ___ ___

D. Provides patient with access
to appropriate cardiac rehab
team member when adjust-
ment in home exercise or
dietary programs is necessary ___ ___ ___ ___ ___

IV. Communication

A. Develops rapport with patient
and spouse within group
and/or individual basis ___ ___ ___ ___ ___

B. Promptly provides physician
groups with information
regarding untoward changes
in the patient's physical
status ___ ___ ___ ___ ___

C. Provides testing and Phase III
staff with important information regarding patient's
physical and psychological
status ___ ___ ___ ___ ___

V. Motivation

A. Provides the patient with a
positive health professional
role model ___ ___ ___ ___ ___

B. Creates atmosphere where
the patients are able to communicate openly and freely
with each other and the staff ___ ___ ___ ___ ___

C. Encourages patient to enter
appropriate outpatient program for exercise reconditioning ___ ___ ___ ___ ___

D. Nurtures realistic attitudes
toward resumption of activities of daily living, sexual
activity, and return to work ___ ___ ___ ___ ___

PHASE III EXERCISE SESSION PERFORMANCE FACTORS

I. Supervision-Warm-up

   A. Screens patients appropriately prior to exercise and reports significant findings to supervisor   ____ ____ ____ ____ ____

   B. Demonstrates creativity, innovation, improvisation   ____ ____ ____ ____ ____

   C. Utilizes activities that encourage flexibility, muscle tone, coordination   ____ ____ ____ ____ ____

   D. Discourages competition and encourages fun during group activities   ____ ____ ____ ____ ____

   E. Demonstrates group control   ____ ____ ____ ____ ____

II. Supervision-Aerobic Phase

   A. Ability to recognize participant's visible signs of physiological stress   ____ ____ ____ ____ ____

   B. Knowledge and control of individual participant's intensity, duration, and mode of exercise   ____ ____ ____ ____ ____

   C. Demonstrates and conveys to participants sound knowledge of the principles of physical conditioning   ____ ____ ____ ____ ____

   D. Responds appropriately to participant's questions   ____ ____ ____ ____ ____

   E. Teaches pulse taking and when appropriate self-monitoring techniques   ____ ____ ____ ____ ____

III. Supervision-Cool-down

   A. Monitors participant's visible signs and symptoms of fatigue during cool-down   ____ ____ ____ ____ ____

   B. Instructs patient regarding postexercise activity (showering, checking with staff before leaving exercise site, etc.)   ____ ____ ____ ____ ____

IV. Exercise Leadership Techniques
   A. Voice projection/clarity of
      instructions   ___ ___ ___ ___ ___
   B. Organization/maintains group
      control   ___ ___ ___ ___ ___
   C. Rapport/responsiveness to in-
      dividual participant needs   ___ ___ ___ ___ ___
   D. Attitude   ___ ___ ___ ___ ___
   E. Appearance   ___ ___ ___ ___ ___
   F. Shows reliability and respon-
      sibility in following directions
      and carrying out supervisor's
      instructions completely and
      accurately   ___ ___ ___ ___ ___
   G. Demonstrates an understand-
      ing of and ability to imple-
      ment emergency procedures   ___ ___ ___ ___ ___
   H. Demonstrates ability to moti-
      vate individual participants to
      achieve personal goals   ___ ___ ___ ___ ___

CLINICAL SUPERVISORS PERFORMANCE FACTORS
   I. Planning and Organizational Skills
   A. Flexibility; able to forecast or
      adapt to peak workloads; ad-
      justs priorities without loss of
      maintaining ongoing
      operation   ___ ___ ___ ___ ___
   B. Problem solving; recognizes
      potential problems, seeks im-
      mediate and long-term so-
      lutions   ___ ___ ___ ___ ___
   C. Follows through; assures suc-
      cess of completing assign-
      ments or develops alternate
      solutions/strategies   ___ ___ ___ ___ ___
   D. Time management; organizes
      work/projects effectively and
      efficiently   ___ ___ ___ ___ ___

II. Supervisory Effectiveness
   A. Humble; recognizes limita-
      tions, seeks input from
      manager/subordinates prior
      to creating/implementing
      policy changes   ___ ___ ___ ___ ___
   B. Communication; effective in
      finding objective solutions to
      problems while respecting
      subordinates' personality and
      strengths/weaknesses. Effec-
      tively acts as a means of com-
      munication between staff and
      management   ___ ___ ___ ___ ___
   C. Team leader; seeks subor-
      dinates' ideas, opinions,
      suggestions to accomplish
      program goals   ___ ___ ___ ___ ___
   D. Delegates; effectively
      delegates and obtains results
      in a timely manner   ___ ___ ___ ___ ___
   E. Example; provides a personal
      example of proficient perfor-
      mance, expertise of theo-
      retical knowledge base, and
      clinical skills; provides model
      for healthy life-style   ___ ___ ___ ___ ___
   F. Resourceful; makes appropri-
      ate, creative use of available
      resources; puts program goals
      ahead of personal goals   ___ ___ ___ ___ ___

PERFORMANCE APPRAISAL: PERSONAL/PROFESSIONAL/ PRODUCTIVITY

Employee Name: Job Title:

Date of Review: Evaluator:

Certifications Completed/Updated   Continuing Education

BLS _____   Inservice Credits for Year _____
                                                      (maximum 25)

ALS _____   Productivity Credits for Year _____

                                 CEC for Professional Conferences
                                 Attended _____

ACSM _____   Productivity Scale:

                                 % Treatment/Standard _____

                                 % Patients initially seen who

                                 complete:

                                 Phase II _____
Other: Phase III _____

STRENGTHS

WEAKNESSES

ACHIEVABLE GOALS PRIOR TO NEXT EVALUATION

Evaluation Completed By: _____   Employee Signature _____

Cardiac Rehabilitation Professional Quiz

	Yes	No
1. Have you ever had a personal life-threatening event?	_____	_____
2. Do you find yourself wishing it were some other day/time than it currently is?	_____	_____
3. Do you plan at least one thing per day you would like to do?	_____	_____
4. Do you find you say *should* a lot?	_____	_____
5. Do you find a compulsion to make people or events be the way you want them, usually perfect?	_____	_____
6. Do you strive to be loved/approved by practically every significant person in your life, including your patients?	_____	_____
7. Are the most important things in life achievement, money, control, retirement?	_____	_____
8. Do you believe in what you are doing strongly enough to become a role model, a leader? Can you temper what you believe so as not to preach or become ego involved?	_____	_____
9. Do you believe in what you are doing strongly enough to quit based on violation of a personal/ professional principle?	_____	_____
10. Are you a listener, dreamer, risk taker?	_____	_____
TOTAL	_____	_____

Chapter 2

A Framework for Enhancing Physician Involvement in the Rehabilitation Continuum

Miriam Miller

Before physician involvement can be enhanced, those directing cardiac rehabilitation programs need to take a detailed and critical look at the system. Knowing how to read physicians within their surroundings will determine what strategies are best to employ for enhancing their involvement. This is not a simple task. It requires the use of a framework to facilitate this search for ways to improve a physician's involvement in the rehabilitation continuum. A logical way to approach this topic is to turn to the literature on planned change. Bennis, Benne, Chin, and Corey (1976) define *planned change* as "the conscious, deliberate and collaborative effort to improve the operations of a human system . . . through the utilization of valid knowledge." When observations are made within a conceptual framework they become facts.

The model of planned change is built on the premise of the importance of knowing the person, the physician in this situation, and knowing the environment, the hospital. This system assessment of both the person and the environment entails a thorough exploration of a set of variables unique to each one of them. These unique variables, as determined by cardiac rehabilitation, will be discussed in more detail within the appropriate sections. Based upon the knowledge acquired while observing the system, the strategies most appropriate to effect the planned change (i.e., physician involvement) will evolve. A more definitive discussion of specific strategies to apply to cardiac rehabilitation will be presented later in this chapter. The person (or persons) responsible for planning the change and coordinating the implementation of various strategies for effecting change is the *change agent*. The following pages discuss how the

43

framework of planned change can be used by the director of a cardiac rehabilitation program to maximize the potential of enhancing physician involvement in the rehabilitation continuum.

Assessment of the Physician

The factors that are discussed in this section all pertain to variables that evolve around the physician as the person in this model of planned change. The key issues that need to be assessed, in order to have a better insight into the physician, are motives, philosophy, orientation, and knowledge base. How amenable the physician is to becoming involved in a structured cardiac rehabilitation program depends on the combination of the aforementioned factors. The lack of information in any of these areas may reduce the ability of the program director to effect change.

Physician's Motives

The first concern is, what motivates physicians to incorporate a controversial medical approach, such as structured cardiac rehabilitation, into their practice? The reasons why a physician would incorporate cardiac rehabilitation into the management of CAD clients originate from either an intrinsic or extrinsic rationale. Possible intrinsic factors could be dissatisfaction with the current method of treating clients with CAD (low adherence rates, no time for teaching), curiosity, desire to be state of the art in this field, or perhaps a genuine commitment to and belief in this approach as having real and necessary benefits (surveillance capabilities, improvement in functional capacity, reduction in depression, etc.). The extrinsic motives might be financial incentives, clients asserting their demands for it, strong opinions of colleagues who support it, authoritative professionals reporting its benefits in respected journals, or the lack of an alternative approach (tried everything else).

Before proceeding, I want to elaborate on two of these motives because it has been my experience that the surveillance capabilities and the profit incentive are the two most frequently observed issues affecting physician involvement in organized rehabilitation programs. In addressing the issue of the importance of the surveillance capabilities, I will use the detection of dysrhythmias as an example of how their identification and subsequent management can benefit the participant and the primary care physician; however, this is not to imply that this is the only benefit the monitoring capability fulfills (other examples are amount of angina, change in mood, degree of blood pressure control, response to increasing workloads).

Table 2.1 Occurrence of Symptoms Associated With Significant Dysrhythmias

N	Type of dysrhythmia	% with symptoms	% without symptoms
20	Unifocal PVCs	20.0	80.0
9	Multifocal PVCs	22.0	78.0
22	Ventricular tachycardia	13.6	86.4
18	Ventricular couplets	22.0	78.0
10	Paroxysmal atrial tachycardia	40.0	60.0
79	Total Average	23.6	76.4

In a retrospective study conducted at eight outpatient rehabilitation centers, it was found that of the 79 subjects who had dysrhythmias requiring medical intervention, 76% were without symptoms at the time of the rhythm disturbance. Table 2.1 presents the types of dysrhythmias and the percentage with or without symptoms. The prevalence of asymptomatic ventricular tachycardia is quite alarming considering its life-threatening potential. The medical interventions that were prompted as a result of identifying these dysrhythmias consisted of changing, adding, or adjusting medications; defibrillation; a physician office visit; or hospitalization. The subsequent intervention in each case led to better medical management of the subjects—a result of the monitoring process available from a structured cardiac rehabilitation program.

The surveillance capabilities of an inpatient program were also shown in a study by Dion (1982). During the monitored inpatient exercise program, patients were shown to have problems associated with ventricular dysrhythmia, hypotension, and angina pectoris. The added surveillance during this phase of cardiac rehabilitation also appeared to improve patient care and management.

The second issue, which many physicians are curious to know yet reluctant to admit, is how profitable is it for them to be involved in a cardiac rehabilitation program? The financial incentives may not be a prime factor when experimenting with a cardiac rehabilitation program, but if physicians are to remain consistently involved in such programs, these incentives will become a more important issue. The amount of time that is consumed or freed up by being involved in a cardiac rehabilitation program is a concern (e.g., additional paperwork vs. reduction in the constant interruptions from a demanding client). The indirect revenue either taken from or returned to the physician's practice because of involvement becomes another concern (Are the required exercise tolerance tests [ETTs] done by his or her office or by the cardiac rehabilitation program? Do the surveillance capabilities reduce or enhance office visits?). At the present time, there are no direct financial incentives for physicians to be involved in a cardiac rehabilitation program unless they own their own rehabilitation program. A review of several programs that are physician operated reveals that monetary incentives do motivate many physicians to become more involved. Perhaps hospitals could learn from the physician-operated centers, which are profitable (in light of the fact that so many hospital-based programs are suffering financial hardship). If creative arrangements could be made to subsidize physicians financially for their involvement in a cardiac rehabilitation program, while at the same time not violating the ethics of medicine, then this would be mutually beneficial for the hospital and the physicians. Physicians could add to their practice incomes without the exceptional burden of adding to their practice demands by owning their own programs. At the same time, this approach could reduce the competitive market that hospital-operated programs are facing as more and more physicians are setting up their own programs.

Along the same lines, the opposite thinking should be applied. What would prevent physicians from getting involved in cardiac rehabilitation? Some plausible explanations might be

1. misconceptions about what cardiac rehabilitation is, which result in a mismatch in expectations;
2. fear of losing control over managing the client;
3. the need to be all things to their clients so outside assistance is not wanted; "their way is just fine";
4. belief that genuine physical (sudden death), psychological (increased dependency), and/or social (financial burdens) harm could come from cardiac rehabilitation, which outweighs the benefits;
5. hospital politics (personality conflict with a medical advisor);
6. previous reputation of the program (safety record, price, personnel); or
7. the merit of secondary prevention from cardiac rehabilitation versus surgery and/or pharmacologic agents.

To substantiate my projections about what motivates physicians to employ cardiac rehabilitation services in their management of CAD clients, I conducted a phone survey (Miller, 1983) involving fifteen hospital-based cardiac rehabilitation programs throughout the United States. The program coordinators were asked open-endedly to identify the motives for why physicians had or had not used the program in their hospital. Free-standing, physician-owned centers were not included in the survey for obvious reasons. The most prevalent reasons reported (see Table 2.2) as to why physicians used cardiac rehabilitation services were for its surveillance capabilities (better client management), its ability to improve the client's functional capacity, its psychological benefits, and its being requested by the participant. The reasons repeatedly given (see Table 2.3) for why it was not used were the cost, the belief that his or her method of managing the client was satisfactory, the credibility of exercise, and the fear of losing the client to another doctor.

Table 2.2   Physicians' Reasons for Using a Cardiac Rehabilitation Program

Rationale	N = 15
Surveillance capabilities	11
Improvement in functional capacity	9
Psychological benefits	9
Participant requested it	6
Routine practice	5
Education	4
Improves the quality of life	3

Table 2.3   Physicians' Reasons for Not Using a Cardiac Rehabilitation Program

Rationale	N = 15
Cost	9
Satisfied with own method of managing clients	8
Credibility of physical conditioning and rehabilitation	6
Losing control in managing client	5
Distance	4
Too much extra work	2
Disliked the medical advisor	2

Physician's Philosophy

In addition to identifying a physician's motives, being able to identify a physician's philosophy of cardiac rehabilitation is equally relevant. Included in physicians' philosophies are the recognition of their responsibilities, their perceptions of what they are responsible for, and the period of responsibility. Wenger (1981) states that "the responsibility for restoration of the coronary patient to productive life or independent living, and therefore the initiation and coordination of all rehabilitative efforts, is the responsibility of the patient's primary physician."

An issue that relates closely to the scope of responsibility is how the physician defines cardiac rehabilitation. Just how the term is delineated (which is open to a broad range of interpretations) determines how responsible physicians will be for meeting their clients' rehabilitative needs. If cardiac rehabilitation is not viewed as the blending of exercise therapy, health teaching, and psychological support to assist individuals with ischemic heart disease to obtain or reestablish their *optimal physical, psychological, occupational, social,* and *recreational status,* then how much this definition varies will determine the degree of acceptance and utilization of a cardiac rehabilitation program by each physician.

Equally as subjective as the definition of cardiac rehabilitation is the time commitment the physicians acknowledge for this responsibility. It is from their own definition of cardiac rehabilitation that this timetable of involvement will develop. By understanding when physicians believe they are responsible, the program director is capable of determining the phase or phases in the cardiac rehabilitation continuum most amenable to the physicians' involvement. It is much better to encourage physician support at a level they are ready for, than to try to promote a level that the physicians do not even recognize as their domain of responsibility.

Physician's Orientation

The physician's practice orientation is of critical importance relative to whether physician involvement will be made possible. A physician who strictly practices from the biomedical model will have difficulty relinquishing it for a model that is at the root of cardiac rehabilitation and in opposition to the biomedical practice model. The openness of physicians to a new perspective in managing clients will have a great impact on whether they can involve themselves in cardiac rehabilitation. The biopsychosocial model has as its elements of practice a self-care, health-promotion, and multidisciplinary philosophy. Contrary to this is the biomedical model, which encourages dependency, focuses on acute illness, and prescribes only medical or surgical approaches to treat symptoms.

Although the biopsychosocial approach to health care has become common parlance (especially to many other health care disciplines), resistance to dealing with psychological and social issues of the client is still prevalent among physicians (Williamson, Beitman, & Katon, 1981). The reasons for this avoidance are complex; however, a central issue is that most of the physicians practicing were educated when the biomedical model was the major paradigm. Physicians who are to become involved voluntarily in cardiac rehabilitation are certainly required to rethink or reframe their practice in order to consciously integrate an approach contrary to the biomedical model.

Physician's Lifestyle

Another concern that needs to be addressed is, how oriented are the physicians in their own lives to practicing the health promotional behaviors espoused in cardiac rehabilitation programs? A study conducted by Glanz, Fiel, Walker, and Levy (1982) surveyed the preventive health behavior of 296 physicians (46.5% response rate; median age 38 years) at a university medical center and compared these data with information from two large surveys that examined the health practices among American adults. The results showed that there were no marked consistent differences between the physicians and the general public. Another study by Wechsler (1983), surveyed a group of primary care practitioners' beliefs about health promotion and found that there was a lack of consensus among them as to the relative importance of various health behaviors (see Table 2.4); many of the behaviors are recognized risk factors to CAD. Moreover, in a third study (David & Boldt, 1980), it was found that, irrespective of socioeconomic status, respondents ranked physicians as the most frequent source of health care information. Is it any wonder that physicians are having a difficult time seeing the need for cardiac rehabilitation when they themselves can't agree on what is healthy behavior and whether to practice it themselves? It is disconcerting to think that they are so influential in determining the health care choices of the general public and specifically those inflicted with CAD.

Degree of Collaboration.   The final concern of the physician's orientation is, how comfortable is the physician in a collaborative relationship with health care disciplines other than medicine? Collaboration develops from a voluntary relationship in which a joint effort is made to determine mutual goals (Bennis et al., 1976). It is essential in this relationship for each discipline to have some knowledge and understanding of the training and function of the other, and for each to respect and have a readiness to learn from the other (Jacobsen, 1974). Ross and Schour (1954) state, "Further, not only must each discipline know its own functions and limitations, but it must be ready to see these in relation to that of the others."

Table 2.4   Percentage of Physicians Perceiving Health-Promoting Behaviors as Important

Behavior	GP* N = 82	FP N = 72	Internists** N = 273	All physicians N = 427
Eliminate cigarette smoking	85	94	94	93
Avoid excess calories	74	82	65	70
Drink alcohol moderately	35	45	49	46
Decrease salt consumption	52	49	31	40
Avoid undue stress	44	42	24	30
Engage in aerobic activity (3x/ week)	19	31	27	27
Avoid foods high in cholesterol	32	39	30	25

*Oldest Practicing Group
**Youngest Practicing Group
GP = General Practitioners
FP = Family Practitioners
Note. From " The Physician's Role in Health Promotion: A Survey of Primary Care Practitioners" by H. Wechsler et al., 1983, *New England Journal of Medicine,* **308**(2). Copyright 1983 by *New England Journal of Medicine.* Reprinted by permission.

Table 2.5   Attitudes Physicians Have About Outpatient Cardiac Rehabilitation

Outpatient program N = 50	Increase	Decrease	No change	Unknown
Mortality	0	28	19	3
Morbidity	1	36	10	3
Reinfarction	0	25	21	4
Dysrhythmias	2	11	29	8
Contractility	26	1	15	8
CAD progression	0	24	14	12
Health costs	11	28	4	7
Physician control	26	5	14	5
Return to work	38	0	6	6

Note. From "Cardiac Rehabilitation: Current Physician Attitudes" by C.K. Frances, 1981, in L. Cohen, M. Mock, and I. Ringquist (Eds.), *Physical Conditioning and Cardiovascular Rehabilitation,* New York: John Wiley and Sons. Copyright 1981 by John Wiley and Sons. Reprinted by permission.

In a cardiac rehabilitation program the focus is on a collaborative, multidisciplinary approach. Wenger (1981) supports such an approach when she suggests that "the physician may and *often should* use the knowledge, skills, techniques and services of various medical consultants, health care professionals and community resources for the implementation of rehabilitation." Physicians who are not able to deal with this sudden involvement of others in the collaborative care of their clients may cope by labeling this as "losing control." Their perceived loss of control convinces them that support of any kind to such a program is not warranted.

Physician's Knowledge

An important concern is what expectations, realistic or unrealistic, does a physician have about cardiac rehabilitation? Despite how much has been printed on this topic, the prevailing question that seems to engulf most physicians is, Does cardiac rehabilitation reduce morbidity and mortality? Because cardiac rehabilitation has not been able to show consistently that it does reduce morbidity (except NEHDP study) and mortality (except Kallio's study) (Naughton, 1982), physicians with the biomedical mentality are convinced that their lack of involvement in such programs is justified. How many of these same physicians have readily accepted an alternative surgical or pharmacological approach with equal or less guarantees than cardiac rehabilitation? The Council on Scientific Affairs of the American Medical Association (AMA) announced publicly that "cardiac rehabilitation should be considered one of the treatments for coronary heart disease complimentary to drug therapy or surgery."

Shepard (1982), in his article "Are We Asking the Right Questions?" comments that perhaps individuals with CAD are seeking an "attainment of happiness" for their remaining years rather than an increase in longevity. If so, then research that measures the effect of cardiac rehabilitation on mood, return to work, resumption of sexual activity, and so on (although more difficult to measure) would be more relevant than statistics on longevity or reinfarction.

What a physician comprehends and believes about cardiac rehabilitation can be beneficial for the program director to know because it will help establish where to begin the education process of the physician. An example of how this can be evaluated was demonstrated by Frances (1981) who conducted a survey that involved a questionnaire's being sent to a group of physicians affiliated with Hartford's American Heart Association. Of the 50 physicians who responded to the questionnaire, Table 2.5 reports the findings of the physicians' attitudes about outpatient cardiac rehabilitation programs. Although the results from this study are enlightening, the more important reason for mentioning it here is the fact that such an approach to the question of a physician's knowledge and attitude is an objective way to collect the data and is more insightful than any hunches or projections the program director might provide. Another factor in this area is identifying who can influence physicians most in their quest for learning and change—peers, authoritative authors in the field, participatory learning experiences, or client testimonials (Geertsma, Parker, & Whitbourne, 1982).

Assessment of the Environment

Knowledge of physicians without knowledge of their environment is only a portion of the information needed if planned change is to occur. It is the environment that contributes to much of who the physician becomes and provides the context in which the change will take place. If the environment is not understood neither will be the change. It is from the environment that the resources will come that will be used to effect the change.

There are three levels in the environment: the system, the subsystem, and the suprasystem. For the purposes of this discussion the system is the hospital organization, the subsystem is the cardiac rehabilitation program, and the suprasystem is the community in which the hospital resides.

The degree to which each level of the environment impacts on the physician varies for each physician and for each location. The same environment will affect two physicians differently, and the same physician will respond differently in two separate environments. It is because of the uniqueness of each situation that there is no universal solution to the problem of enhancing physician involvement. However, by analyzing the elements (the physician and the environment) in a logical and organized way, as suggested by the planned change model, the likelihood of a more successful outcome for enhancing physician involvement is possible. A thorough discussion of each level will follow in order to provide the framework for assessing the environment for planned change.

The Hospital as System

The organizational factors within a hospital can determine how nurturing the environment is for cardiac rehabilitation. The type of hospital it is— medical center (research or teaching based), community, or rural—has much to do with determining the physician's openness to the concept of structured cardiac rehabilitation. Whether residents and interns are practicing at the hospital is another factor. What medical committees are there? The level of segregation of specialists and generalists needs to be considered. The previous impact that a physician's peers have had on him or her in selecting new approaches for the management of various health care problems, specifically CAD, is a further concern.

The physician mix on staff in a hospital should be examined because it has much to do with who is or is not likely to get involved in the referral process to a program. Wenger, Hellerstein, Blackburn, and Castranova (1982) found, in a study on physician practices in managing myocardial infarction (MI) patients, that on the average a cardiologist manages 45 MI patients a year, an internist 20, and a family practitioner 13. During the poll I conducted by phone of 15 cardiac rehabilitation programs (Miller, 1983), it was found that on the average fewer than 15% of family practitioners on staff refer, compared to 35-50% of the internists and more than 75% of the cardiologists. Despite the smaller number of potential referrals from each family practitioner and internist, the ratio of these two groups on staff is considerably greater than the cardiology service. Their potential for being a powerful referral base comes from their collective strength. In addition, the fact remains that consulting cardiologists generally refrain from following the client after discharge from the hospital.

Whether the hospital is a primary or tertiary health care provider will have impact on whether the clients are later accessible candidates for a cardiac rehabilitation program. In the survey, distance was the fifth most frequent reason given for a physician's not referring to a program (Miller, 1983). If clients receive bypass surgery at a hospital which is in or near their hometown they are more likely to be rehabilitated in a structured program. However, if they are referred back to their hometown, they are likely to be a lost referral. Only 2 of the 15 centers had cardiac surgeons directly referring into the outpatient phase of the program. The responsibility for the rehabilitative process of clients who have been seen by consulting cardiologists and cardiac surgeons still rests with the primary physician.

Physician loyalties to a particular hospital or hospitals may have an impact on whether they feel they can involve themselves in a partisan service like cardiac rehabilitation, particularly if hospitals are competitors of one another. The internal politics of the medical staff may do much to undermine physicians from getting involved especially if the program is used as a pivotal point in the power struggle. The number of physicians on staff, the size of the catchment area, and the potential number of clients do much to determine how vigorous the competition is for clients as well as the security a physician will have for making referrals to another physician, service, or agency. Who originally supported the concept of a cardiac rehabilitation program and when staff physicians become involved in its planning have a lot to do with how involvement will proceed postprogram development. If the program is associated so strongly with one person or group, it may be plagued by partisan politics that are difficult to rectify.

The administrator of the hospital may either enhance or deter physician involvement simply by his or her commitment to the program and awareness of its ongoing need for support. The location of the program in the hospital and its operational budget provide the physician with a commitment statement from the hospital administrator. The location of the program in the hospital can provide its rating in terms of its priority with administration. The way budgetary concerns are handled for the program speaks of the administrator's ongoing support. How an administrator views the worth of a cardiac rehabilitation program can determine how accessible the services of the community relations department are for promoting the program. The marketing tone that the administrator sets for the program can either attract or detract physician involvement depending on whether the services are promoted for the program's community image, revenue producing capability, or competitive service ability.

In addition to this, the department to which the program is assigned has its influence on physicians. Physicians are aware of which departments can be respected, which ones hold some consequence with administration, and which departments have a charismatic leader for its department head.

In addition to meeting the educational needs of physicians in order to promote their involvement, often the knowledge and confidence of others less directly involved in the program (hospital staff personnel) have a lot to do with reinforcing the message to the physician. If physicians are skeptical about cardiac rehabilitation, they will try to find other supporters of their opinions. Involving as many in the hospital as possible as a support network may be advantageous from the standpoint of shaking the convictions of those who resist cardiac rehabilitation.

Finally, the degree to which a hospital promotes wellness and employee health programs is a subtle force that can slowly influence physicians to become involved in cardiac rehabilitation and health promotion. The degree to which no smoking signs, low-fat menus in the cafeteria, fitness trails, or promotions to walk the steps are encouraged has an indirect bearing on getting physicians to view health care from a perspective that is in line with the thinking of cardiac rehabilitation.

The Cardiac Rehabilitation Program as Subsystem

This section will concern itself with all those features of the program that could have an influence on a physician's decision to get involved in a cardiac rehabilitation program. One concern is, what are the component parts of the cardiac rehabilitation program based upon the program's philosophy and objectives? Will the program consist of exercise therapy, stress management, nutrition counseling, and/or behavioral programs for modifying the client's recognized risk factors? In a recent study conducted by Wechsler et al. (1983), a group of primary care physicians were asked how successful they thought they had been in helping their clients change selected behaviors. The physicians reported that they were most optimistic about being able to help their clients change their exercise patterns and were progressively less successful with each of the following: changing their diet, eliminating cigarettes, and managing stress. The physician who finds a cardiac rehabilitation program that contains components which he or she has not been able to manage successfully will be more inclined at least to experiment with the program as an alternative option. If exercise therapy is the component that is primarily used to attract physicians to the program, but is viewed as an area that the physician has been successful at changing, it is doubtful that this will enhance his or her involvement.

In the study previously mentioned by Wenger et al. (1982) that looked at physician practices, 95% of the physicians reported that they recommended progressive physical activity upon discharge. Of these, 45% recommended home exercise programs with another 45% recommending physician-supervised programs. Those who refer to a supervised program probably need specific help with the exercise component because of the client's age, special needs (handicapped or other concomitant diseases), or high risk for sudden death (low-ejection fractions, high-grade ventricular ectopy).

The Council on Scientific Affairs (1981) has implied the need for an integrated approach by this statement:

Cardiac rehabilitation should include much more than an exercise program. However, it is the exercise program that frequently serves as the main focus of the rehabilitation program and sets it apart from a simple counseling service.

It is for this reason that programs have been encouraged to adopt a structured approach to their education style. Programs that only utilize an informal approach have a difficult time demonstrating to a physician what the program can accomplish. Because the acquisition of information through health education does not ensure that behavior will be changed, more programs have begun to incorporate behavioral medicine programs. Such programs assist clients more intensely in modifying their overt behavior by applying behavioral science to the medical problem (CAD) (Blumenthal, Califf, Williams, & Hindman, 1982).

An important question is, how do those directing cardiac rehabilitation programs define *involvement*? It is difficult to enhance involvement if it has not been clearly identified. Are physicians involved if they make a referral to a cardiac rehabilitation program? If this is how involvement is defined then a program is in for a long, uphill battle. A physician's referral without his or her commitment to cardiac rehabilitation is certain to be a power struggle approach.

- The program suffers because physicians see requests for their involvement as being beyond what they bargained for (signing papers, repeating ETTs, receiving phone calls about client's problems, etc.), which is eventually going to undermine the staff's enthusiasm and work efficiency.
- Participants suffer because their doctors will neither give the reassurance they need about the program nor openly criticize facets of the program, which is certain to make the participants question the benefits versus the costs (time, money, energy, changes they have to make). This will undermine the participants' confidence and ability to adhere to the program (especially if they are motivated to attend for extrinsic reasons).
- Physicians suffer because they are never likely to change their attitude or behavior about cardiac rehabilitation. Also, a number of physicians, because of a limited cardiac population in their practice, will be overlooked because they are not good potential referrants; however, they may be able to strengthen the atmosphere of support by their indirect involvement.
- If involvement is equated only with the number of participants in a program, then the available options for enhancing that kind of involvement are self-limiting. But if involvement is expanded to mean direct and indirect support of the program then the available options are self-perpetuating and likely to have an impact on all sectors.

Physicians are usually concerned about how affordable the program is for their clients. The costs to the participant need to be in line with the recognized benefits; otherwise, this can become the most frequently used reason for boycotting a cardiac rehabilitation program. The costs incurred go beyond the fees charged, but include the distance, time, energy, and lifestyle adjustments required of the participant. The physician's critique of the program (which includes all phases of cardiac rehabilitation) gets more stringent as the amount of third party coverage declines. Related to this issue of affordability is the history of insurance reimbursement (chapter 3), which has been established for this service in each particular part of the country, because it does vary. The code numbers and terminology that will expedite the process most easily should be known in advance. Participants who will have financial difficulties should be identified early, and alternative methods for subsidizing the program when possible should be determined. One disgruntled consumer can do more to undermine the services of a cardiac rehabilitation program than 10 recommendations if a physician's involvement is not substantially based.

The next factor that may be of concern is the entry requirements. If the criteria are nebulous then physicians will be confused and unsure of whom to refer. However, if the guidelines are excessively demanding and stringent, physicians may believe their control in decision making is lost. A flexible approach is important if the program is to have a broad base of support. The entry criteria should guide selection to enhance safety yet not restrict it to accommodate the elite or to avoid getting the "toughies." This is not to say that standards should not be established; but if the standards keep physicians away then perhaps they are being viewed as the law, and revisions might be in order. Some concerns are, What tests are needed prior to entry and how often are they repeated? Who performs and interprets the ETT or writes the exercise prescription? Whatever the current guidelines for entry into the cardiac rehabilitation program may be, these should be reviewed annually because the changing economy and health care policies of the country may influence how physicians can practice relative to how they are reimbursed.

The safety record of the program may be the reason why a physician chooses a monitored program over an unmonitored or unsupervised program. Haskell (1978) has reported that the complication rates (fatal and nonfatal combined) of a monitored program are 1/117,333 participant-hr versus 1/22,028 participant-hr for an unmonitored program. If the program has a lower rating than this, it is reasonable for the physician to question using such a program. If the program guidelines are based upon American College of Sports Medicine (ACSM) and American Heart Association (AHA) standards, and if mock codes and emergency equipment checks are performed regularly, then the probability of preventing and managing emergencies is much improved.

Closely related to this issue of safety are the credentials of the personnel. The preparation and training of the staff to manage the acute, convalescing, and fit cardiac through the unique problems of each phase have much to do with maintaining safety. Also, if the physician has had a prior working relationship somewhere else in the hospital with the staff members in the program that was mutually gratifying, this can reinforce his or her confidence in the program. A low turnover of staff helps the physician become familiar with its members and emphasizes the satisfaction the staff reaps from working in a program. Whether the staff members practice in their own lives what they are requesting of participants further reinforces their dedication to the principles of lifestyle modification and their ability to serve as role models at a point in time when the physician may or may not be able to. The personalities of the staff members working in cardiac rehabilitation need to be dynamic. They should be assertive and enthusiastic without being overpowering or offensive.

The choice of a medical advisor(s) should be carefully considered because that person is the representative to the medical staff. The decision as to whether he or she is a cardiologist should be weighed. The benefits of the expertise at the expense of alienating the generalists need to be considered. How the advisor is selected and the term of the position should be decided. Rotating rather than fixed appointments to rejuvenate new thinking and policies might be advantageous. A decision also needs to be made as to whether the position is a paid one, and whether there are to be contractual expectations. Many medical advisors lose incentive after a year or two if not financially recognized. Even if they are paid an honorarium, unless the duties are clearly delineated they can become figureheads and a budgetary expense item to the program.

The title used to describe this position can be equally suggestive to physicians as to how influential this medical person might be in their client's care. For instance, titles like *medical director* or *chief of cardiac services* might be more intimidating to attracting physician involvement than a title like *medical advisor*. The politics surrounding this person and his or her history (e.g., whether he or she is respected, has cardiac rehabilitation expertise, has held positions that have prepared him or her for the job) can be decisive factors concerning whether the medical advisor reduces or enhances the following to a program.

The phases that are and are not included in a cardiac rehabilitation program's continuum may influence the level of involvement of the physicians. Like most, unless a service is kept at the forefront of a physician's mind it is forgotten. So it is with cardiac rehabilitation. If a program lacks a Phase I component then there is likely to be a less direct reminder to the physician. Also, if the staff rotates through the various phases physicians may be able to become more confident and familiar with the Phase II operations and staff through the security they gain from their Phase I involvement. The development of the Phase I inpatient exercise center, like the prototype at Mt. Sinai Medical Center in Milwaukee, has helped bridge the gap between supervised routine activity on the unit only and monitored exercise therapy in a center. This concept allows the physician to have an initial exposure to the exercise equipment during Phase I and to the surveillance capabilities in subsequent phases of cardiac rehabilitation. Phase III keeps the community and physician in touch with the special ways that health maintenance needs of cardiac patients can be met once they return to work and recreational pursuits. Programs that lack such a continuity only perpetuate the concept of cardiac rehabilitation as a 12-week stint rather than a continuum with important resources to offer at each facet of recovery.

Another concern is the location of the program phases. The visibility of Phase II can determine physician involvement as well as prompt clients' curiosity as they pass it in the corridor. The amount of space available for the program to enhance its aesthetic appeal is a concern for all phases but more so with Phase II and Phase III because the participant is footing a portion of the bill. The accessibility of the sites of the Phase II and Phase III programs can determine whether a physician would recommend these programs.

The ongoing communication maintained between the staff in the program and the primary physician has much to do with how the physician views the program. A mechanism must be established that provides continual involvement of the primary physician (organizational flowchart) and ongoing status updates of the referred client (Wilson, Edgett, & Porter, 1979). The physician needs to be convinced that, due to the information gained from his or her client's participation in the program (from discharge summaries and activity record sheets in Phase I and progress notes in Phases II and III), the physician's management of care is improved through a better understanding of the client. Wilson, Fardy, and Froelicher (1981) reiterated this point: "The physician must feel that involvement of the client in the program will supplement physician care, not replace it."

Finally, the advertising and marketing approach (both past and present) can have an impact on the image of the program. This will effect both the physicians on staff and the community. The following questions are especially relevant to this issue. Whose responsibility is it to market the program: staff, medical advisor, hospital's public relation's department, administrator, or a special marketing team; or is it a joint effort? How prepared and capable are those responsible? When will it be done: at the opening of the program, as new services are added, in response to a crisis in census, at anniversaries, or as an ongoing, regular feature of the program? What phases will be the focus of such promotional and awareness campaigns: Phase I, II, or III? What mediums are appropriate for disseminating information about the program: brochures, radio, newspapers (hospital and/or community), TV spots, posters, appearances at health fairs, tours of the program, public speaking engagements, or a hospital- or community-sponsored function (walkathon, open house, golf tournament, etc.)? Who will be the target(s) of such campaigns: physicians, public, hospital staff, individuals with recognized disease, local heart clubs, community service groups (Lions, Kiwanis, etc.), schools, churches, local industries, or physician office nurses? How much time will be afforded to this task? What amount of time will be given to the target group(s)? How much has been budgeted for it? What is the competition in the area? How does the competition compare with your program (better/ worse, similar/different)? And finally, how will the effects or results of such public relations endeavors be measured?

The Community as Suprasystem

The hospital's reputation in the community can influence the physician's level of involvement in the services within the hospital. In addition, once a referral is made, whether or not a client will follow up on it will depend upon the location of the hospital, accessible parking, and previous experience with that particular hospital.

The size and character of the community (metropolitan or rural) can influence the type of physicians who practice there, how they practice, how responsive they are to changing trends, and how assertive their clients are in making suggestions about their own care. The type of hospital that the community can support, the kinds of services offered (e.g., coronary artery bypass surgery, CABS), and the degree of competition are also related to demographic size.

The economics of the community will affect the physicians' decisions on what type of care they will offer to clients. During the recent recession with high employment and reduction in health care benefits, physicians became more aware of the need to cut health care costs. Once physicians become inclined to think of a cardiac rehabilitation program as an unnecessary service, even after the economy begins to recover it is not easy for them to change their opinion of this service.

How industries view the benefits of a program can also influence a physician's thinking. In many cities where a significant amount of the population is employed by one or two industries, whether or not a program is active will depend on the insurance benefit package the industries provide.

How oriented the community is to health care issues can be quite important to the field of cardiac rehabilitation in general. How these issues are covered by the media can either excite interest or create boredom. Whether individuals on staff in the program are active in local government (city council) or organizations (e.g., AHA) will also effect attitudes that may indirectly affect the program.

What about the medical community at large? How many physicians are there? How cohesive a group are they? How involved are the physicians on staff with other practicing physicians in the community? How powerful a force is the medical group in shaping this community? What organizations do they support? What offices do they hold? How respected are they in the community?

Strategies for Effecting Change

Once the knowledge has been collected about the physician and the environment, the program director (or change agent) is ready to select the most appropriate strategy for effecting change in a physician's involvement. There are three types of strategies: empirical-rational, normative-reeducative, and power-coercive (Bennis et al., 1976).

The empirical-rational approach assumes that humans are rational and motivated by self-interest. A proposed change that is based upon self-interest is likely to be adopted if it can be shown that the person will gain by the change. In the case of cardiac rehabilitation, physicians might be moved to use a program if it made them better practitioners, provided them with financial rewards, gave them recognition, fulfilled a service they could not provide, or uncomplicated their lives. Below is a list of a variety of ideas with regard to how this type of strategy could be implemented for each of these aspects of self-interest.

Empirical-Rational Approach

1. Appeal to the physician's desire to be a better practitioner
   - Extend office care by providing
     — progress notes
     — notification as problems develop or adjustments are needed
   - Collect statistics on various facets which would reflect better client management
   - Record participant testimonials
2. Provide financial incentives
   - Indicate that office visits may increase
   - Include ETT interpretation fees
   - Give free memberships to health clubs and salaries for participating in Phase III
   - Create contracts with physicians to prevent them from starting their own programs
   - Have a supporter bring a nonsupporter as a guest to a meeting or luncheon and provide a complimentary gift or memento
3. Give more clout, more recognition
   - Conduct research and have the physician co-author
   - Have the physician serve on an advisory board or panel
   - Have him or her serve as the medical expert for a question/answer column
   - Co-present a case with the physician who made the referral at grand rounds
4. Provide a service the physician wants but can't offer or is not successful at providing, including
   - work assessments for determining readiness to return to work
   - behavioral medicine programs for weight loss, stress management, smoking cessation
   - education programs

- CPR classes
- exercise guidelines for the atypical client (COPD, angina, PVD, elderly, DM)

5. Provide easy process for entry (this uncomplicates the physician's life)
   - Provide a prescription pad
   - Combine forms
   - Attend ETT to screen referrals
   - Use stickers for reminders
   - Obtain a list of referrals from the admitting office and the office nurse

The second approach that might be used is the normative-reeducative. This approach assumes that a change in a practice occurs only as the person involved is brought to change the normative orientations to old patterns and develops commitments to new ones. The changes in normative orientations involve changes in not only knowledge but also attitudes, skills, and significant relationships. Below is a list of specific ways to implement this strategy by changing attitudes, skills, and significant relationships as applied to a cardiac rehabilitation program (CRP).

Normative-Reeducative Approach

1. Change attitudes/knowledge
   - Audit an education series
   - Report CRP functions in a hospital newsletter
   - Relocate center to become more visible
   - Record participant testimonials
   - Establish a multidisciplinary panel to encourage collaboration
   - Have a learning lunch
   - Develop Phase I (standing orders, visibility serve on ICU committee)
   - Send out mailings of
     —supportive literature
     —new services
     —yearly statistics
   - Encourage as many wellness projects in the hospital as possible

2. Change skills/knowledge
   - Offer complimentary exercise sessions (Phase II)
   - Assist at LLETT and SLETT (technique and screening process)
   - Encourage participation in the Phase III program

3. Change significant relationships/knowledge
   - Visit each physician to address individual needs and concerns
   - Invite nonreferring physicians to an advisory panel meeting
   - Encourage supporters of program to bring a nonsupporter to a CRP function

The last approach is the power-coercive. This strategy is based on the application of power in some form (political or otherwise). Because the physician is one of the most powerful forces in the hospital and perhaps the community, this strategy usually entails getting administrative backing to effect the change. Because of a physician's need for clients, assertive clients, if aware of their options for rehabilitation, may be a persuasive force in convincing a physician to become involved in the services of a cardiac rehabilitation program. The list below consists of several concrete suggestions for using various avenues of power to effect the change in physician involvement.

Power-Coercive Approach

1. Affiliate the program with a department that has more clout or is more respected
2. Obtain media coverage to heighten public awareness of the program
   - Develop a coronary club
   - Conduct program tours for community groups (senior citizens, schools)
   - During National Heart Month, feature the cardiac rehabilitation program
   - Have health fairs
   - Provide participant testimonials
   - Sponsor time-predicted walk/jogs, walkathons, and golf tournaments
   - Have an open house at the anniversary of the program
   - Volunteer to speak at professional and community organizations
   - Develop a hypertension clinic for exposure of the program
3. Send a list of potential referrals from the Phase I CRP including the primary physician responsible for the care to the medical advisor and/or administrator
4. Invite an authority in the field to speak, and provide CME credits
5. Develop a regional cardiac rehabilitation organization or a network of support with all disciplines participating (including physicians)
6. Participate in local community group meetings or local government forums at which health care issues will be discussed

Although this may seem obvious, another concern is deciding who is to be the target of the planned change. The target may be an individual, a group, or a community (Bennis et al., 1976). The change agent may decide to approach one physician, a group of them, or the entire medical community in the area depending on the strategy used. The target may not be physicians at all, but others who could influence them indirectly such as a physician's client, the nursing staff on a progressive coronary care unit, or a community group with clout.

In addition to the above concern, an equally pressing decision is who is going to be the change agent? The person (or persons) who assumes this role must have an appreciation of organizational theory, an understanding of the impact that systems have on planned change, and the leadership ability to direct the available resources effectively to enhance change in physician involvement. In most cases, this will be the director of the cardiac rehabilitation program, but often the collaborative efforts of others within the program staff, hospital, or community may be needed. How capable this person or group is at motivating enthusiasm for these change strategies can make the difference between success and failure.

Conclusion

The problem of how to enhance physician involvement in a cardiac rehabilitation program is approached logically by applying the model of planned change. The practitioner in cardiac rehabilitation, faced with this situation, is taken step by step through this framework. The variables to include in the detailed assessment of the physician and the environment are explained. Through the knowledge acquired from this assessment, the practitioner is shown how to apply these facts to the various planned-change strategies. The available options for implementing change are explained along with numerous suggestions to help make the model pragmatic for use in existing cardiac rehabilitation programs needing to enhance physician involvement.

References

Bennis, W., Benne, K., Chin, R., & Corey, K. (1976). *The planning of change* (3rd ed.). New York: Holt, Rinehart and Winston.

Blumenthal, J., Califf, R., Williams, S., & Hindman, M. (1983). Cardiac rehabilitation: A new frontier for behavioral medicine. *Journal of Cardiac Rehabilitation, 3*(9), 637-656.

Council on Scientific Affairs. (1981). Physician-supervised exercise programs in rehabilitation of patients with coronary heart disease. *Journal of the American Medical Association,* **245**(14), 1463-1466.

David, A., & Boldt, J. (1980). A study of preventive health attitudes and behaviors in a family practice setting. *Journal of Family Practice,* **11**(1), 77-84.

Dion, W., Grevenow, P., & Pollack, M. (1982). Medical problems and physiologic responses during supervised inpatient cardiac rehabilitation. *Heart and Lung,* **11**(3), 248-254.

Frances, C.K. (1981). Cardiac rehabilitation: Current physician attitudes. In L. Cohen, M. Mock, & I. Ringquist (Eds.), *Physical conditioning and cardiovascular rehabilitation.* New York: John Wiley and Sons.

Geertsma, R., Parker, R., & Whitbourne, S. (1982). How physicians view the process of change in their practice behavior. *Journal of Medical Education,* **57**(10), 752-760.

Glanz, K., Fiel, S., Walker, L., & Levy, M. (1982). Preventive health behaviors of physicians. *Journal of Medical Education,* **57**(8), 637-639.

Haskell, W.L. (1978). Cardiovascular complications during exercise training of cardiac patients. *Circulation,* **57**(5), 920-924.

Jacobsen, S. (1974). A study of inter-professional collaboration. *Nursing Outlook,* **22**(12), 751-755.

Miller, M. (1983). [Progressive coronary care survey report]. Unpublished raw data.

Miller, M. (1982). Unpublished raw data, Cardiac Treatment Centers.

Naughton, J. (1982). Physical activity for myocardial infarction patients. *Cardiovascular Reviews and Reports,* **3**(2), 237-242.

Ross, H., & Schour, E. (1954). An experiment in interdisciplinary education. *American Journal of Orthopsychiatry,* **24**, 549.

Shepard, R.J. (1982). Are we asking the right questions? *Journal of Cardiac Rehabilitation,* **2**(1), 21-26.

Weschsler, H. (1983). The physician's role in health promotion: A survey of primary care practitioners. *New England Journal of Medicine,* **308**(2), 97-100.

Wenger, N.K. (1981). Rehabilitation of the coronary patients: Scope of the problem and responsibility of the primary care physician. *Cardiovascular Reviews and Reports,* **2**(12), 1249-1261.

Wenger, N., Hellerstein, H., Blackburn, H., & Castranova, S. (1982). Physician practice in the management of patients with uncomplicated myocardial infarction: Changes in the past decade. *Circulation,* **65**(3), 421-427.

Williamson, P., Beitman, B., & Katon, W. (1981). Beliefs that foster physician avoidance of psychosocial aspects of health care. *Journal of Family Practice,* **13**(7), 999-1003.

Wilson, P., Edgett, J., & Porter, G. (1979). Rehabilitation of the cardiac patient: Program organization. In M. Pollack & D. Schmidt (Eds.), *Heart disease and rehabilitation*. New York: John Wiley & Sons.

Wilson, P., Fardy, P., & Froelicher, V. (1981). *Cardiac rehabilitation, adult fitness, and exercise testing*. Philadelphia: Lea and Febiger.

Chapter 3

Overview of Insurance— Obtaining and Maintaining Coverage in Cardiovascular Rehabilitation

G. Curt Meyer

Currently, there are more than 1,000 private insurance companies in the United States that write individual and/or group health contracts. There are also 188 million Americans who are protected by one or more forms of health insurance. These insurance companies collect a given amount of money (premiums) from individuals and/or corporations to cover health-related expenses (claims) for those subscribers who require diagnosis or treatment of their condition (List of Benefits). The financial aspects of insurance investments are beyond the scope of this chapter; however, a basic understanding is necessary of how the insurance companies use the premiums paid for the individual.

Insurance companies collect a relatively small amount of money from each subscriber to pay for the large amount of money required when these subscribers come in need of medical attention. Although this seems very simple, there is a great amount of financial consideration made by the insurance company when determining the type of medical intervention covered and the amount of coverage for that specific diagnosis and/or treatment.

Insurance companies do make money by insuring groups and/or individual subscribers. In 1981, for example, Health Insurance premiums collected for all types of health insurance companies totaled $48.998 billion. During the same year, insurance companies paid $41.622 billion in benefit payments (Health Insurance Association of America [HIAA], 1984). Although basic math illustrates that there is a $7.376 billion difference, the cost of processing the claims and personnel time must be considered along with all of the other related expenses common to any business.

In order to stay in business, insurance companies rely primarily on statistics to determine the cost for each type of coverage. One resource used by insurance companies is the *Source Book of Health Insurance Data*, prepared by the Health Insurance Association of America. An example of data useful to companies in determining their fee schedules is the fact that the per capita expenditure for health care at the national level in 1985 is projected to be $1,882 as opposed to the 1981 figure of $1,225. With knowledge of figures such as these and others, the companies can determine their fees and adjust revenues accordingly to meet the higher cost of medical care.

History of Insurance Reimbursement

There are numerous historic dates associated with the development of insurance reimbursement to the levels that exist today. The following are some of the highlights in insurance coverage. The Massachusetts Health Insurance Company of Boston was the first to cover sickness in 1847. In the 1850s, individual accident insurance became available in the United States with the chartering of the Franklin Health Assurance Company in Massachusetts. Montgomery Ward and Company, Inc. established the first group health insurance company policy for its employees in 1910. Blue Cross was organized in the 1930s, with the first experimental citywide Blue Cross plan tried out in Sacramento, California. Five years later this resulted in the organization of the Blue Cross Commission, known as the health service plan commission. Blue Shield developed and organized its commission within a decade. As of 1949, major medical expenses were introduced to supplement basic medical care expenses by the Liberty Mutual Insurance Company. Medicare was introduced in 1965. This was a social security amendment providing hospital insurance to those individuals 65 and over. Another social security amendment became effective in 1972; this law extended the health insurance benefits of Medicare to the disabled and individuals with end-stage renal disease. During the same year the Professional Standards Review Organization (PSRO) was established to research the cost of reimbursement and make appropriate cost of living adjustments in disability benefits. The Health Maintenance Organization Act assisted in the establishment and expansion of Health Maintenance Organizations in 1973. In 1977, the Medicare-Medicaid antifraud and antiabuse amendments required uniform reporting of financial data by providers. This amendment also upgraded criminal penalties for fraud under Medicare-Medicaid programs. As the cost of health care continued to increase, Congress passed the Tax Equity and Fiscal Responsibilities Act (TEFRA) in 1983, which reduced payments for physicians' services in outpatient hospital departments. Additionally, the Social Security Amendments of 1983 (SSA) established a prospective payment amount for each medicare patient discharged from the hospital. Discharged patients are to be classified into diagnoses related groups (DRG) (Kramer, 1983). This act now has a number of health care agencies concerned as a result of their inability to interpret exactly the regulations. TEFRA and the SSA were passed in order to better control hospital reimbursement under Medicare.

Classification of Insurance Companies

In order to better discuss health insurance organizations, it is best to classify health care insurance into two distinct sectors: (a) the private sector and (b) the public sector. The private sector contracts with individuals or groups and determines the benefits that it will offer to the patient. With such contracts the premiums are paid by the individual or by the employer of the individual. Blue Cross/Blue Shield, private commercial insurance companies, and some Health Maintenance Organizations (HMO) make up the private sector. The public sector, therefore, includes the other government-administered insurers such as Medicare, Medicaid, Civilian Health and Medical Program of the Uniformed Services (CHAMPUS), Indian Health Services, Workers Compensation Medical Care, and Bureau of Vocation Rehabilitation. Here is an overview of the three basic private health care plans.

Blue Cross/Blue Shield

The Blue Cross and Blue Shield association located in Chicago coordinates Blue Cross and Blue Shield plans for the nation. Last year there were 103 Blue Cross and Blue Shield plans in the United States. There is a distinct difference between Blue Cross and Blue Shield although the plans are often referred to as one entity.

Blue Cross.   Blue Cross plans provide hospital care benefits on a *service-type* basis, under which the organization, through separate contracts with member hospitals, reimburses the hospital for covered services provided to the insured (HIAA, 1984). Those hospitals that participate in Blue Cross therefore receive direct payment for services rendered in that member hospital. When the patient is admitted to a participating hospital, the admission clerk simply needs to see the Blue Cross identification card. Once the card numbers are obtained and verified the insured individual is completely covered for bed, board, special diets, and general nursing care. The following services, taken from the Subscriber Handbook (Blue Cross/ Blue Shield of New Jersey, 1980), are also covered during the hospital stay if they are consistent with the diagnosis and treatment of the illness or injury for which that person is hospitalized:

- Use of operating, delivery, and treatment rooms and equipment
- Use of recovery rooms and equipment
- X-ray examinations
- All recognized drugs and medicines for use in and customarily supplied by the hospital
- Oxygen and use of equipment for its administration
- Dressings and plaster casts
- Serums, vaccines, intravenous preparations, and visualizing dyes
- Use of cardiographic and encephalographic equipment and services of hospital employees in connection with their use
- Use of physiotherapeutic and hydrotherapeutic equipment and treatment rendered by a hospital employee using such equipment
- Anesthesia supplies and use of anesthesia equipment; administration of anesthetics by a hospital employee
- Supplies and equipment for X-ray, radium, radon, and radioactive isotope therapy; administration of such therapy by a hospital employee
- Surgically implanted cardiac pacemakers including batteries, electrodes, and replacements thereof
- Use of blood transfusion equipment, administration of blood; blood processing services provided by the hospital or provided and charged for by a nonprofit blood supplier

Blue Shield.   Blue Shield plans provide benefits for medical and surgical services performed by a physician. A physician as defined in most benefit plans must be fully licensed to practice medicine and surgery (MD or DO) including doctors of dental surgery (DDS) and doctors of podiatry (DP). In order to keep the fee structure within a given range of charges by geographical locality and degree of specialty for that physician, the Blue Shield participating doctors comply to the usual, customary, or reasonable fee program. Under such an agreement the Blue Shield plan will make direct payment to the participating doctor. The doctor will accept this payment as payment in full for the covered services. Clearly, the benefit to the insured is that there is no responsibility for paper work, and that all payments are to be accepted by the physician as payment in full; therefore, no additional money is requested of the insured.

In the case that a subscriber would receive treatment by a physician who does not participate in the Blue Shield plan, the insured usually submits the claim and is responsible for any difference between the usual, customary, or reasonable fee paid by Blue Shield and the amount of the bill.

Usual, Customary, or Reasonable Payment Mechanism.   Rather than having a uniform fee schedule for all procedures that a physician provides to the patient, Blue Shield bases each payment on three criteria:

1. usual
2. customary
3. reasonable

In 1963 Pennsylvania Blue Shield (1981) identified three facts with important ramifications in developing this fee schedule:

1. Individual doctors did not ordinarily vary their fee for the same procedure for different patients. Each charge tended to be uniform for all patients.
2. Doctors practicing in a particular specialty and in the same geographic area tended to have fees within a definable range.
3. The geographical areas needed to be much smaller than state boundaries in order to keep the fees from increasing in rural areas and decreasing in the larger cities.

Payment by Blue Shield on the basis of usual, customary, or reasonable (UCR) charges is computed in the following manner.

Usual charges (sometimes referred to as Level 1 charges) for an individual doctor are determined from those actual charges sent to Blue Shield on the doctors' service report forms. In Pennsylvania, usual charges were first determined by a confidential fee survey in 1966. Blue Shield records the charge for each procedure reported by each doctor on each claim that did not involve unusual clinical circumstances. The usual payment for that charge is then determined as being the calculated 75th percentile of the reported charges for that procedure. These charges are monitored from January 1 to December 31 to determine the usual fee for each procedure for the following year. An example of a usual fee schedule is found in Table 3.1. These usual charges for each service are always recorded and referred to as the doctor's profile of charges.

The customary range (sometimes referred to as Level 2) is the 90th percentile of the usual charges for each procedure by doctors of the same specialty in a given geographical location, weighted by the number of times the procedure is reported. This amount of money at the 90th percentile is the maximum amount paid by Blue Shield for that procedure. The

Table 3.1 Determination of Usual Fee From Blue Shield

	JAN.	FEB.	MAR.	APR.	MAY	JUNE	JULY	AUG.	SEPT.	OCT.	NOV.	DEC.

Charges $6 6 6 7 7 7 7 7 7 7 7 7 7 7 7 7 7 7 7 7 7 7 7 7 7 7 7 7 7 7 7 8 8 8 8 8 8 8 8 8 8 8 8

Service: complete blood count

Median (Medicare)   75th Percentile (UCR)

actual calculation procedure for customary (Level 2) charges for Blue Shield is illustrated in Table 3.2.

The reasonable component of the UCR payment plan is that which accounts for complications or unusual clinical situations that require a higher amount of payment for the service.

In summary, according to Pennsylvania Blue Shield (1981), the following steps are taken in determining the UCR payment for a given procedure.

1. Each reported charge is checked against the individual doctor's usual charge for that procedure. Unless unusual circumstances are reported, the usual charge is the maximum that can be paid.
2. Each reported charge is checked against the customary charge (Level 2) for the procedure in the doctors specialty and geographical location. Unless unusual circumstances are reported, the customary charge is the maximum that can be paid.
3. In the event that unusual circumstances are reported, the following steps are taken to determine if the charge is reasonable:
   a. Each form is reviewed to determine the description of unusual circumstances.
   b. Correspondence between the doctor and Blue Shield is performed to obtain additional information for the records.
   c. The procedure is reviewed by a Blue Shield medical advisor whose specialty is the same as the physician who performed the service.
   d. The procedure is forwarded to a peer review committee.

Table 3.2 The Actual Calculation Procedure for Customary (Level 2) Charges for Blue Shield

Usual charge (Level 1) (in $)	Number of times charge made	Cumulative total by specialty	Cumulative percent
$10	56	56	14
12	84	140	35
15	160	300	75 (Medicare)
20	64	364	91 (UCR)
25	24	388	97
30	12	400	100

Major Medical

Major medical expense insurance was introduced nationally in 1951 by most insurance companies. This type of health insurance was designed to finance the expense of major illness and injury. Major medical benefits pay up to $250,000 or have no limit above an initial deductible of usually $100 for all charges incurred by the hospital, doctor, private nurses, medical appliances, prescribed out-of-hospital treatment, drugs, and medicine per subscriber year. In most cases major medical pays 80% of the charge, and the insured person is responsible for paying the remainder.

There are two types of major medical plans: one supplements basic hospital-surgical-physician's expenses; the other provides comprehensive protection in which basic coverage and extended health care benefits are integrated. Either plan covers a large number of health care services.

Private Insurance Carriers

There are a great number of private insurance companies that offer individual or group health insurance policies to the public. Insurance companies such as Aetna, Metropolitan Life, and Prudential are similar to Blue Cross/Blue Shield in the way that they charge their clients. Payment, however, is usually different. Most private insurance companies do not have participating hospitals and/or physicians, as opposed to Blue Cross/ Blue Shield. Therefore, when the insured receives treatment for a given injury or illness, that person is responsible for submitting the claim to the insurance carriers. Once the claim has been submitted it is processed through the insurance company. For each type of claim, the company has a usual, customary, or reasonable fee, which sets the upper limit for the amount of money paid for that claim similar to that described under Blue Shield. As long as the charge by the provider is below this upper limit, it should be processed without any delay. In the event that the charge is above the usual, customary, and reasonable fee for that claim, the higher limit for that code and description will be reimbursed. In most cases it then becomes the responsibility of the insurance company professional relations department and the insured to pursue the correct channels to determine who is responsible for payment of the remainder of the charge. In some cases the insurance company will challenge the charge, resulting in the provider's accepting the payment from the insurance company as payment in full.

Health Maintenance Organizations

Health Maintenance Organizations (HMO) provide a wide range of comprehensive health care services for a specified group at a fixed periodic payment. Individual HMOs can be sponsored by the government, medical schools, hospitals, employers, labor unions, consumer groups, insurance companies, and hospital-medical plans. The key to HMOs is that comprehensive health care services are provided to the consumer at a fixed periodic payment. HMOs have become better accepted during the past ten years because policy holders know what amount of money must be paid each year for the provision of medical care. Another advantage of the HMO is that preventative treatment and regular office visits are usually covered, whereas most insurance companies do not pay for preventative treatment.

Public Insurance Sector

Although the public insurance sector does not contribute as much to the national health care expenditure as the private sector, the government spends a significant amount of money on health care (see Table 3.3). In 1982, the federal, state, and local government expenditure for health care was $122.5 billion, or 42.7% of the total health care expenditure during that year (HIAA, 1984). The majority of federal health spending by the government is for low-income groups, those over 65, military personnel and dependents, veterans, federal civilian employees, and native Americans. One of the most significant contributors to the governmental health care cost was the introduction of Medicare in 1967: Governmental expenditures for health care cost increased 7.5% in one year due to its implementation.

Medicare

Medicare is a federal program that provides hospital and medical insurance protection for more than 29 million people. Although it is a federal program, there are 10 regional offices of the Health Care Financing Administration (HCFA) that have the power of interpreting the guidelines emanating from the Baltimore headquarters. Those individuals who are (a) age 65 and older or (b) under age 65 but receiving cash benefits under the social security or railroad retirement program because they are disabled or have certain chronic kidney disease are covered by Medicare. Medicare consists of two parts: compulsory hospitalization insurance, also called Part A; and voluntary supplemental medical insurance (SMI) or Part B, which helps pay for physicians' services and some medical services and supplies not covered under Part A.

Medicare Part A. Part A of Medicare is usually financed by governmental taxes paid by employers and employees. In a few cases Part A coverage is voluntary, and the premiums are collected from the beneficiary. As previously mentioned there are a group of people who qualify for Medicare Part A. As a qualified receiver of Medicare, that person has coverage under Part A for the following as listed in the Medicare and Medicaid Guide (1984):

1. Accommodations
2. Nursing and related services
3. Medical social services
4. Use of hospital facilities
5. Drugs and biologicals
6. Supplies, appliances, and equipment
7. Other diagnostic or therapeutic items as services
   • Clinical laboratory services
   • Nurse anesthetists, psychologists, and physical therapists
   • Occupational therapy
   • Respiratory therapy
   • Speech pathology
   • Rehabilitative care
   • Therapeutic exercises

Part B.   Part B of Medicare is a voluntary program of supplementary medical insurance. An individual is eligible for enrollment in Part B if he or she (a) is entitled to Part A benefits or (b) has attained the age of 65 and is a resident of the United States. Premiums for Part B are financed in part by payments of the individuals enrolled in the program along with contributions from state and federal funds. The payments from those individuals can be deducted when possible from their monthly benefits such as social security or railroad retirement checks. As of July 1, 1983, the individual monthly premium was $13.50. Coverage under Part B of Medicare is fairly comprehensive. Once an individual pays the first $75.00 of health care costs each year, Medicare covers 80% of each additional charge, and the individual is responsible for the remaining 20%.

Benefits under the Part B program include medical and other health services, home health services, comprehensive outpatient rehabilitation facility services (CORF), and outpatient and ambulatory surgical services (Medicare and Medicaid Guide, 1984). Included under these general categories are the following:

1. Physicians' services
2. Services and supplies incident to physicians' services
3. Rural health clinic services
4. Outpatient hospital services
5. Physical therapy services

6. Speech pathology services
7. Diagnostic x-ray, laboratory, and other diagnostic tests
8. X-ray, radium, and radioactive isotope therapy
9. Surgical dressings and devices for reduction of fractures
10. Rental and purchase of durable medical equipment
11. Ambulance service
12. Prosthetic devices
13. Braces, trusses, and artificial limbs and eyes

Medicaid

During 1965, Title XIX of the Social Security Act provided a program of medical assistance, called Medicaid, for certain low-income individuals and families. Although Medicaid is administered by each state, the federal government provides requirements and guidelines for the state to administer the program. Almost all states participate in Medicaid with the exception of Arizona. Medicaid provides medical assistance to those persons who are eligible to receive payment under one of the cash assistant programs as outlined in the act (i.e., aid to families with dependent children and supplemental social security income). In 1981, Medicaid paid $27.3 billion in benefits to 22.1 million recipients (HIAA, 1984). In cases when individuals are aged or disabled and are also covered by Medicare, the state Medicaid programs pay for the Medicare premiums, deductibles, and co-payments as well as for services not covered by Medicare.

Civilian Health and Medical Program of the Uniformed Services (CHAMPUS)

The department of defense operates CHAMPUS to provide reimbursement for covered medical care provided in civilian facilities for wives and children of active military personnel and retired military personnel and their dependents. Primarily, the program is designed for those qualified individuals who are unable to use government medical facilities because of distance, overcrowding, or the unavailability of appropriate treatment at a military medical center. CHAMPUS spent $852 million in health care services in 1981 (HIAA, 1984).

Bureau of Vocational Rehabilitation

Each state department of labor and industry administers the Office of Vocational Rehabilitation (OVR) or Bureau of Vocational Rehabilitation (BVR). This program is available to service the physically or mentally handicapped individual who fulfills the criteria to become eligible for participation in the program. The following are some of the factors determining eligibility for BVR in the commonwealth of Pennsylvania:

- The individual must evidence a level of maturity at which it may be considered feasible to establish a vocational objective.
- The person must have a physical or mental disability or a behavioral disorder characterized by a pattern of deviant social behavior.
- The disability must create a substantial handicap to employment.
- There must be a reasonable expectation that vocational rehabilitation services will render the individual fit to engage in a gainful occupation.

Economic need for the program is also reviewed. The income assets, savings, and other available resources of the disabled individual are considered. After reviewing the above information the BVR determines what service costs will be paid.

The following services may be covered by the BVR to enhance an individual's vocational rehabilitation (according to the Pennsylvania Department of Labor and BVR, 1983).

A. Diagnostic services
a. Physical and psychiatric examinations
b. Psychologic evaluations
c. Vocational evaluations

B. Counseling and guidance
a. Case study
b. Vocational planning
c. Motivation development
d. Community resources
e. Occupational information

C. Training
a. Personal adjustment training
b. On-the-job training
c. Workshops
d. Business and trade schools
e. Tutorial services
f. College

D. Physical restoration
a. Treatment

   1. medical and surgical
   2. psychiatric
   3. dental

b. Therapy

    1. physical and occupational
    2. speech and hearing

c. Braces
d. Hearing aids and glasses
e. Prosthetic appliances

E. Selective job placement

a. Cooperative agency placement
b. Direct placement by counselors

F. Placement equipment

a. Occupational tools
b. Equipment for self-employment

G. Follow-up services

Sources of Payment for Services

As discussed in the previous sections there are three resources of payment for any incurred medical cost. Once a service has been provided to the patient, the patient, the insurance company, and/or major medical insurance is/are responsible for the payment of that charge (see Figure 3.1).

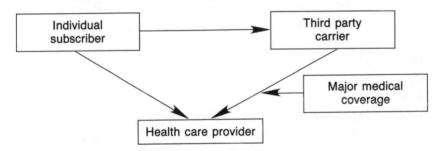

Figure 3.1.   Resources of payment for incurred medical cost.

Type of Insurance Coverage

Most insurance companies provide the consumer with a choice of two types of insurance contracts: (a) full service, and (b) indemnity. Full service contracts basically define all the benefits that are covered. Each benefit is covered 100%. An example of full service coverage would be a Blue Shield or HMO contract, which reimburses the participating physicians

for those services that are covered by the plan. Once payment is made
to the physician, the patient is not responsible for any component of that
charge.

Indemnity insurance contracts require that the insurance company
reimburse a certain amount (usually 80%) of the charge whereas the consumer is responsible for the balance of the payment. Major medical
policies are examples of indemnity insurance contracts: Once the deductible is met by the patients, major medical pays 80% of eligible charges
and the patient pays 20%.

Table 3.3 Federal, State, and Local Government Expenditures for Health and Medical Care

Year	Amount (in billions)			Total per capita	Percentage of total health care expenditure (public and private)
	Federal	State and local	Total		
1950	$ 1.6	$ 1.8	$ 3.4	$ 22	26.8
1955	2.0	2.6	4.6	27	26.0
1960	3.0	3.6	6.6	36	24.5
1965	5.5	5.2	10.8	55	25.9
1966	7.4	6.1	13.6	68	29.5
1967	11.9	7.0	19.0	94	37.0
1968	14.1	8.0	22.1	108	38.0
1969	16.1	8.8	24.9	121	37.9
1970	17.7	10.1	27.8	133	37.2
1971	20.3	11.3	31.7	150	38.1
1972	22.9	12.5	35.4	166	37.9
1973	25.2	14.1	39.3	182	38.1
1974	30.4	16.6	47.1	216	40.5
1975	37.1	19.1	56.2	255	42.4
1976	42.6	20.3	62.9	284	42.0
1977	47.4	22.7	70.1	313	41.4
1978	53.9	25.7	79.5	351	42.0
1979	61.0	29.5	90.6	395	42.1
1980	71.1	34.3	105.4	455	42.3
1981	83.9	38.6	122.5	524	42.7

Procedures for Obtaining Insurance Reimbursement for Cardiovascular Rehabilitation

Insurance reimbursement for all phases of cardiovascular rehabilitation has improved during the past years; however, to date there is no uniformity among the many insurance companies in providing this service as a benefit. Therefore, those in the discipline of cardiovascular rehabilitation must assume responsibility to expend efforts in obtaining and maintaining insurance reimbursement for such a service. In the case when third parties coverage neglect to reimburse for cardiac rehabilitation, there will be a significant decrease in participants and eventually a large number of cardiovascular rehabilitation facilities will be closed.

In attempting to obtain coverage for cardiovascular rehabilitation there are a number of steps to be taken by the administrator of the program. Each step is essential in obtaining reimbursement; however, some are more important than others. One must be cognizant of the fact that there are a number of individual circumstances to consider in applying these steps. It is beyond the scope of this chapter to discuss each of the abovementioned considerations when applying these steps; however, common sense usually prevails in determining the need for pursuing each step.

Identification of Those Insurance Companies Providing Benefits to the Population That Will Utilize Your Service

In the event that you are opening or have opened a cardiovascular rehabilitation program in a hospital or free-standing setting, it is essential to determine which companies provide benefits to those in the community. One fairly uncomplicated method of doing this is to communicate with the Chamber of Commerce. The Chamber of Commerce can, in most cases, provide information about the companies that employ the greatest number of people in that area (see Table 3.4). With such information, you can call the personnel department of each company and request the name of the insurance company and the type of contract that provides the benefits to the employees of that company.

Contact the Insurance Companies

Once those insurance companies that provide coverage for a majority of the population in the community are identified, the next step is initiation of effective communication. In order to obtain as much information as

Table 3.4 Area Insurance Survey

Company	No. of employees	Major Carriers	Reimbursement percent/per carrier deductible
Fort Howard Paper Co.	800	BC/BS United of Milwaukee, WI: MM–all employees	90%–74% ded.
Brockway Glass Co.	625	Metropolitan: MM–salaried; Basic–hourly	80%
Container Corp. of America	137	Travelers: MM–all employees	80%c ded.
Corning Glass Works	625	Self-insured: MM–all employees	80%
Coburn Industries (Revlon)	400	Self-insured: US-adm. MM–all employees	80%/c ded.
Acme Engineering & Manufacturing	465	Gave no details	
H.B. Egan	172	BC/BS: Basic; Aetna Life Surety of Tulsa: MM	80%
Fansteel Metals	130	Self-insured: MM–all employees	80%/c ded.
Funstan Nut Co.	100	Equitable of St. Louis: MM–all employees	80%/c ded.
Green County Castings	105	Benefit Trust Life, MO: MM–all employees	80%/c ded.
Griffin Grocery	150	Will not discuss insurance	
Love Bottling Co.	108	Self-insured: Aetna-adm. MM–all employees	80%/c ded.

Tubular Corp. of America	240	Travelers: MM–all employees	80%
Yaffee Iron & Metal Co., Inc.	190	Lincoln Income: adm. by 3rd party MM	80%
Zapata Industries, Inc.	152	BC/BS: MM Nat. Acc. Hbg. PA	80%
Muskogee Iron Works	289	Metropolitan: MM–all employees Subsidiary of Union Metal, Canton, Ohio	80%

BC/BS = Blue Cross/Blue Shield
MM = Major Medical
adm. = administered

possible, you should communicate with the professional relations department, which can provide you with the list of benefits that are covered under the agreement between the employer and the insurance company.

In some instances you can simply ask if cardiac rehabilitation is listed as a benefit. However, often times you will have to spend a great amount of time defining cardiac rehabilitation to the person on the other end of the phone in order to receive a "yes" or "no." In most cases, the individual in the professional relations department will forward a list of the benefits. Periodically, the company representative will not release the information to someone who does not have a provider number (i.e., hospital or physician). At that point, one of the medical directors should pursue communication with the professional relations department to obtain the list of benefits.

Determination of Code Number and Description of Service

Unless the list of benefits provides a code number and description for each phase of cardiac rehabilitation, you must ascertain what code numbers and/or description of service to use. If there is a code number and description for cardiac rehabilitation it should be used to submit claims. When the list of benefits does not include a code number or description code for cardiovascular rehabilitation, this can be explained in one of two ways. The first explanation is that cardiovascular rehabilitation is not a recognized benefit. In such circumstances the administrator should contact the director of professional services and schedule a meeting. This meeting ideally should occur at the rehabilitation center, thus enhancing the insurance company's awareness of cardiovascular rehabilitation. Procedures, protocols, charting, and qualifications of those administering the program should be presented. Questions and answers should follow. It is then the insurance representative's decision to determine whether cardiovascular rehabilitation will be a covered benefit.

The second explanation is that the service is billed as services that are part of cardiovascular rehabilitation. Oftentimes code numbers for telemetry monitoring and/or exercise therapy are utilized to describe the treatment because both are usually part of a cardiovascular rehabilitation treatment. Utilization of the current procedure terminology (CPT) (American Medical Association [AMA], 1977), the relative value schedule (RVS) (Blue Cross & Blue Shield United of Wisconsin) and the international classification of diagnostic areas (ICDA) are examples of the codes found in Table 3.5.

Table 3.5 Examples of Codes and Billing Descriptions

TOS	CPT CODE	RVG CODE	DESCRIPTION	UNIT VALUE
Cardiography				
			(For echocardiography, see 933300-93308)	
5	93000	9101	Electrocardiogram; with interpretation and report, routine ECG with at least 12 leads	3.4
5	93005	9923	Tracing only, without interpretation and report	2.0
5	93010	9924	Interpretation and report only	1.4
			(For ECG monitoring, see 99150, 99151)	
5	93015	9110	Cardiovascular stress test using maximal or submaximal treadmill or bicycle exercise; continuous electrocardiographic monitoring, with interpretation and report	14.9
5	93017	9925	Tracing only without interpretation and report	9.0
5	93018	9926	Interpretation and report only	6.0
5	93040	9102	Rythm ECG, one to three leads, with interpretation	1.7
5	93041	9927	Tracing only without interpretation and report	1.0
5	93042	9928	Interpretation and report only	0.7

TOS = Type of service
CPT = Current procedure terminology
RVG = Relative value guide

Determination of Fee Allowance

Obtaining information about the fee allowance for any service is often difficult if not impossible. As discussed earlier, the insurance company will determine the UCR fee for each benefit listed. Outpatient, hospital-based cardiovascular rehabilitation programs usually cannot determine the maximum allowable customary fee for such service. The physicians, who may run clinic-based cardiovascular rehabilitation programs, can request from Blue Shield their own profile of charges to better determine their charge for the service. Because the UCR fee usually is not released, the billing for cardiovascular rehabilitation by a hospital or physician group is often a hit-or-miss circumstance. Once the claim is forwarded to the insurance company, if the charge is above the customary fee maximum it will be denied. However, if the charge is below the customary fee maximum it will be accepted. The provider must continue to charge a fee that is within the maximum amount for customary fees in order to obtain reimbursement.

Determination of Fee Schedule

The fee schedule is as important as the UCR fee for cardiovascular rehabilitation. Because cardiovascular rehabilitation is a treatment service as opposed to a diagnostic test, most insurance companies place a limit on the frequency and number of visits each year. Most insurance companies that provide coverage for cardiovascular rehabilitation as an outpatient service limit the number of visits to 36; Medicare does the same.

Establish Communication With the Professional or Provider Relations Personnel

Whether an insurance company does or does not provide payment for cardiovascular rehabilitation, the administrator of the program should establish communication with the personnel in professional or provider relations. The objective of this communication is to enhance rapport between the cardiovascular rehabilitation department and the insurance representative. Enhanced rapport often results in fewer complications with billing. In the event that a problem does arise at a later date, the administrator of the rehabilitation program knows whom to call to correct the situation. Another advantage of this continued communication is that the representative often will contact the administrator with changes that may affect the billing procedure. Clearly, rapport with the provider relations also reduces the time involved in problems that arise with participants, resulting in a more efficient utilization of the administrator's time.

Procedures for Filing Claims

Each institution that provides services of cardiovascular rehabilitation should have a set procedure for filing claims. Prior to submitting the first claim, one must determine how much of the deductible (if applicable) has been met by that participant. This should be determined by questioning the participant or contacting the provider relations department of the insurance company that covers the individual.

Most outpatient programs submit claims on a monthly basis. To enhance payment for each claim, all information requested on the form should be completed. Examples of correct and incorrect forms are found in Figure 3.2.

	Acceptable	**Not Acceptable**
PHYSICIAN RECEIPT	Hometown, U.S.A. March 1, 1999 John Doe, M.D. To Richard Roe 2/1/99 Office visit - cold $20.00 2/10/99 Office visit - cold $20.00 2/28/99 Home - virus infection $25.00 $65.00	Hometown, U.S.A. March 1, 1999 John Doe, M.D. To Richard Roe Professional service rendered ...$65.00 **Missing:** Dates, types of services, and amount charged for each service.
NURSING RECEIPT	Hometown, U.S.A. May 4, 1999 To Mrs. Robert Doe Monday 2/7/99 8 AM - 12 AM $30.00 Tuesday 2/8/99 8 AM - 12 AM $30.00 $60.00 Service Prescribed by Emma Jones, RN John Roe, M.D. Registration No. 27595 2/4/99 **Note:** Ask your physician to give you an authorization for the nurse's services on his prescription order blank stating the date or dates that care is medically necessary.	Hometown, U.S.A. Dear Mrs. Doe, It was nice taking care of you last month, I'm glad you're feeling better. By the way, thanks for sending me your check for $60.00. Emma Jones **Missing:** Dates and shifts worked, amount charged for each shift, doctor's name, degree and registration number of nurse.
PRESCRIPTION DRUG RECEIPT	Roe Pharmacy Hometown, U.S.A. March 2, 1999 Myra Doe, Rx 976-384 ....$14.50 Dr. Smith	Receipt March 2, 1999................$14.50 Thank you Roe Pharmacy **Missing:** Pharmacy's address, patient's name, Rx number, and doctor's name.

LIST ADDITIONAL INFORMATION BELOW:

_____
_____
_____
_____
_____
_____
_____
_____
_____

Figure 3.2. Examples of insurance claims.

The participant signs the required form, which is then filled out by the appropriate person in the cardiovascular rehabilitation department, as seen in Figure 3.3.

Capital Blue Cross
Pennsylvania Blue Shield

MAJOR MEDICAL CLAIM FORM

For ______________________
Name of Patient

PLEASE PRINT:

1.
SUBSCRIBER'S NAME (Last, First, Middle) | CONTRACT NO. | GROUP NO.
PRESENT ADDRESS - STREET | CITY | STATE | ZIP CODE
EMPLOYER'S NAME | EMPLOYEE STATUS ☐ Active ☐ Retired ☐ Disabled | DATE OF RETIREMENT OR DISABILITY Month Day Year

2
PATIENT'S NAME (Last, First, Middle) | DATE OF BIRTH __/__/__ Month Day Year | SEX ☐ Male ☐ Female | RELATIONSHIP OF PATIENT ☐ Self ☐ Spouse ☐ Child
Is the patient a full time student over 19 years of age? ☐ Yes ☐ No Expected date of graduation. __/__/__ Month Day Year
Give name and address of school:

3.
DESCRIBE CONDITIONS FOR WHICH YOU ARE REQUESTING BENEFITS AT THIS TIME:
Type of Injury or Illness | Name & Degree of Doctor Treating Illness | Date First Treated
A. ______ ______ __/__/__ Month Day Year
B. ______ ______ __/__/__ Month Day Year
(Use other side if needed)

4.
IF EMPLOYED, WAS PATIENT UNABLE TO WORK DUE TO THE ILLNESS? ☐ Yes ☐ No
If yes, please list the day(s) of absence from work.
Date absence began __/__/__ Month Day Year Date returned to work __/__/__ Month Day Year

5.
WERE EXPENSES DUE TO AN ACCIDENTAL INJURY? ☐ Yes ☐ No If yes, please complete.
A. Date of Accident __/__/__ Month Day Year Type of Accident: ☐ Work ☐ Home ☐ Auto ☐ Motorcycle ☐ School ☐ Other
B. Give a brief description of accident: ______
C. Has claim been or will claim be filed under any Workmen's Compensation Act? ☐ Yes ☐ No
D. Has claim been or will claim be filed against any other person liable for the injury? ☐ Yes ☐ No

6.
INCOME: If you have Blue Shield Plan B or C, check one of the following statements:
My (our) total income for the last 12 months was:

PLAN B	PLAN C
☐ less than $4,000 for a single subscriber	☐ less than $11,000 for a single subscriber
☐ less than $6,000 total family income	☐ less than $22,000 total family income
☐ none of the above	☐ none of the above

7.
MEDICARE: Is the patient entitled to benefits under Medicare Hospital Insurance (Part A)?
☐ Yes ☐ No Effective date __/__/__ Month Day Year
Is the patient entitled to benefits under Medicare Medical Insurance (Part B)?
☐ Yes ☐ No Effective date __/__/__ Month Day Year
Health insurance number from the Medicare I.D. card ______

8.
OTHER COVERAGE: Does patient have additional health insurance through employer or other group health insurance? ☐ Yes ☐ No If yes, complete.
A. Employer's name ______ Insurance Company's name: ______
B. Policy or certificate number ______ Effective date __/__/__ Month Day Year Cancel date __/__/__ Month Day Year
C. Check type of health insurance ☐ Hospital ☐ Medical/Surgical ☐ Major Medical ☐ Drug ☐ Dental ☐ Specify others ______

I hereby authorize any person or organization furnishing services or supplies to provide the Blue Cross and Blue Shield Plans with my medical records. I certify that the information given by me in support of this claim is true and correct.

PATIENT'S SIGNATURE | DATE | (Area Code) Home Phone | (Area Code) Work Phone
X ______ | ______ | ______ | ______

Figure 3.3. Major medical claim form. *Note.* Reprinted by permission of Capital Blue Cross, 100 Pine Street, Harrisburg, Pennsylvania 17101.

Some outpatient departments request the insurance company to make direct payment to the hospital or clinic. One effective method for obtaining payment in this manner is to have the participant sign an authorization for assignment of payment form (see Figure 3.4).

For those participants who are covered by indemnity policies, the rehabilitation department may request payment of the noncovered amount on a weekly basis. Others may not request payment until the program has been completed. Each facility should determine the type of patient payment policy that works efficiently for that program.

Blue Cross/Blue Shield Major Medical Program Authorization for Assignment of Payment of Major Medical Benefits

_____   _____
(Name of Patient)   (Contract Number)

I, _____, enrolled under the Blue Cross/Blue Shield Major Medical Program, authorize and request Blue Cross/Blue Shield to pay to _____ benefits which may be due me
(Name of Provider of Services or Supplies)
under the Major Medical Program for eligible care rendered the patient identified above.

I understand that this authorization applies to those eligible charges incurred in connection with services or supplies furnished only by or through the above Provider, and does not constitute an authorization for assignment of future Major Medical payments. I further understand that this authorization does not obligate Blue Cross/Blue Shield to make payment to the above Provider.

_____   _____
(Date of Authorization)   (Signature of Employee)

(This form must accompany a completed Major Medical Claim Form, H-9)

Figure 3.4. Authorization for assignment of payment.

Maintaining Insurance Reimbursement

Once reimbursement has been obtained, there is no guarantee that it will be maintained. With the significant changes in health cost, there is always the possibility that benefits will be reduced along with fee schedules. Therefore, it is important for those in the discipline of cardiovascular rehabilitation to maintain a reasonable reimbursement for service.

Essentially there are three rules to follow in order to enhance maintenance of insurance reimbursement. First, once you have established procedure codes and descriptions that are resulting in reimbursement, continue with those codes and descriptions. When updated information, addenda, or memos are forwarded to the provider, it is extremely important to read each and ascertain whether the changes affect the codes and/or descriptions that are used in the billing for the rehabilitation treatment. One of the more common changes that occurs with cardiovascular rehabilitation is the addition of a code number for cardiovascular rehabilitation that replaces the use of one or more code numbers that describe the treatment.

One example of such a change occurred in the Medicare guidelines dated September 15, 1982 (Medicare and Medicaid Guide, 1984).

Payment for Services Rendered to Patients in Hospital-Based and Free-Standing Cardiac Rehabilitation Clinics

The guidelines in Section 35-25 of the Coverage Issues Appendix set out the circumstances that permit coverage of certain services rendered in hospital-based and free-standing cardiac rehabilitation clinics. The services these clinics usually provide have been placed in two groups. Group 1 services (continuous ECG telemetry during exercise, ECG rhythm strip with interpretation and limited examination for physician followup) are considered as one routine cardiac rehabilitation visit. The same rate per visit reimbursement should be allowed for each visit , provided at least one Group 1 service is performed. Payment should be based on the reasonable charge levels carriers have established for the procedure code which most closely approximates CPT-4 code 90060, intermediate follow-up office visit.

Group 2 services, such as new patient comprehensive evaluation including history and physical (CPT-4-90020), and ECG stress test with physician monitoring and report (CPT-4-93015) should be reimbursed on an individual basis, as should any other needed physician services.

The second rule is that inappropriate codes and/or descriptions should not be utilized in obtaining reimbursement. There have been facilities that have submitted bills to the companies for services that in fact were not performed. This is fraud. Most insurance companies and public providers periodically review claims and billing practices for isolated services. In the review process several areas are evaluated including the following:

1. Definition of service
2. Description of services that are billed as components of that primary service
3. The code numbers for each component service that is billed as part of the primary service
4. The fee schedule for each coded service
5. The frequency of the codes utilized to bill for that service

Along with the evaluation of the above, infrequently an unscheduled visit by a representative of the insurance company occurs. During this visit, charts, treatment, and qualifications of those providing the service are evaluated. Clearly, inappropriate billing procedures would be identified after such an evaluation resulting in loss of reimbursement for that facility.

The third rule is that when there are unforeseen clinical circumstances that require treatment for a period longer than permitted under the fee schedule, physician correspondence describing the necessity for that treatment should be forwarded along with the claim to the utilization review board. The more information that this review committee has for reference the less time required to determine reimbursement.

National Insurance Reimbursement Survey Results

During 1983, Cardiac Treatment Centers surveyed those facilities listed under the American Heart Association Directory of Cardiac Rehabilitation Programs to obtain information regarding insurance reimbursement for cardiovascular rehabilitation Phases I, II, and III (Miller, 1983). Specifically, the survey collected the following information:

1. Major insurance companies in the community
2. Procedure description utilized
3. Code numbers utilized
4. Amount of charge for the service
5. Amount of reimbursement for the service

As one may expect the responses for each of the above were varied. Results of this survey support the need for enhanced communication between administrators in cardiovascular rehabilitation and third party carriers.

Table 3.6 Billing Terminology and Fees Charged for Phase I

Terminology	Fee
1. Progressive cardiac care	$30 per day (visit approx. 1/2-1 hr)
2. Cardiac program under treatments	$15 fee per visit (visit approx. 1 hr.)
3. Physician-prescribed physical therapy for the cardiac patient	$19.25 fee per 2 visits/day
4. Progressive coronary care	Fee per visit, but no amount given
5. Cardiac physical therapy	$25 for hospital stay
6. Monitored progressive activity	$20 per day
7. Cardiac physical therapy and education	$30 per day
8. Cardiac treatment exercise monitored	$27.80 per visit
9. Cardiac treatment	Flat fee per hospital stay, but no amount given
10. Telemetry-monitored cardiac therapy	$20 per visit
11. Monitored progressive activity (education)	$15 per 1/2 hr visit
12. Cardiac rehab therapy	$27 per visit
13. EKG-Progressive activity	$35 per visit (visit approx. 1 hr.)
14. Monitored progressive activity and progressive coronary care consult	$20 per visit (visit approx. 30 min.)
15. Reeducation exercise	$14 per visit (visit approx. 1/2-1 hr.)
16. Occupational therapy or activities of daily living	$17.41 per visit
17. Monitored inpatient cardiac therapy	$35 per visit (visit approx. 1/2 hr.)
18. Progressive coronary care	$28 initial visit
	$14 per subsequent visit (visit approx. 1 hr.)
19. Inpatient-monitored cardiac therapy	$25 per visit (visit approx. 1 hr.)
20. Cardiac rehabilitation	fee per visit, but no amount given
21. Monitored exercise	$31.50 per visit
22. Coronary training	Flat fee, but no amount given

Phase I Reimbursement

Eighty hospital-based cardiac treatment centers were mailed a questionnaire (see Figure 3.5) requesting information about the reimbursement for Phase I of cardiovascular rehabilitation. Of the 80 centers that were mailed the survey, 56 responded resulting in a 70% response rate. Of those that responded, 53 were active in Phase I of cardiovascular rehabilitation. The diagnoses of the candidates in the programs were

1. post-myocardial infarction (100%)
2. angina pectoris (83%)
3. congestive heart failure (58%)
4. coronary artery bypass surgery (34%)
5. pacemaker (21%)

The components offered in the programs were (a) progressive activity protocol (48 centers), (b) education series (47 centers), (c) psychological support (14 centers), (d) dietary consultation (5 centers), and (e) spouse support group (2 centers). In performing these services there were only 22 centers that obtained direct third party payment for the service. The approach to reimbursement can be found in Table 3.6.

Of the 64% that obtain reimbursement for both components of Phase I, 12 (93%) filed for a combined charge, whereas 1 (7%) filed components as a separate charge. In those centers that did not receive direct reimbursement, the expense of the program was collected through an indirect charge. Three hospitals (10%) charged for a higher nursing contact hour, six (19%) charged through a telemetry charge, six others (19%) charged a higher room rate, and four (13%) were supported financially by the outpatient Phase II program.

In response to the question of why they never submitted claims for direct reimbursement, the centers cited the following reasons:

1. It was the philosophy of the institution not to charge for Phase I.
2. The history of insurance reimbursement was not good for such services.
3. The higher room charge for the diagnosis sufficed for covering the cost of the program.
4. There was no interest in filing for reimbursement.

Although the results of the survey showed varied responses for those who collected reimbursement, results indicate that there are effective means for attaining coverage for the Phase I program. Table 3.6 describes the terminology used and fees charged in those programs that obtain reimbursement.

Phase I Inpatient Cardiac Rehabilitation Insurance Coverage Survey

1. What state is your hospital in?
   _____

2. Does your hospital offer an inpatient cardiac rehabilitation program as a service?
   _____ Yes   _____ No

3. What type of candidates are ordered into the inpatient program in your hospital?
   _____ Coronary Artery Bypass
   _____ Post Myocardial Infarction
   _____ Angina
   _____ Congestive Heart Failure
   _____ Other, please specify _____
   _____

4. What components are contained in your hospital's Phase I Program?
   _____ Progressive step level activity protocol
   _____ Well-designed education series done either individually or in groups
   _____ Sessions for psychological support
   _____ Other, please specify _____
   _____

5. Does your hospital currently obtain direct reimbursement for the inpatient cardiac rehabilitation program from insurance carriers?
   _____ Yes, continue to the next question, omit answering questions number 10 and 11
   _____ No, continue to question number 10

6. What component(s) of the inpatient program is (are) reimbursed?
   _____ Only the exercise component
   _____ Only the education sessions
   _____ Both the education and exercise components; they are
      _____ filed as a combined charge
      _____ filed as separate charges

7. How is the claim for inpatient cardiac rehabilitation services processed?
   a. Terminology used _____
   _____
   b. Code numbers used _____
   _____

8. How has your hospital established charges for these services and what is the fee charged?
_____ flat fee per hospital stay $ _____
_____ fee per day $ _____
_____ fee per visit $ _____
(list amount of time per visit)
_____ other, please specify _____

9. What insurance carriers *will not* acknowledge reimbursement of your inpatient cardiac rehabilitation program? Please list them specifically.

10. If your hospital does not obtain direct reimbursement for the Phase I program, how is the expense indirectly charged to each candidate?
_____ as a higher nursing contact hour classification
_____ as a telemetry fee
_____ as a higher room charge
_____ other, please specify _____

11. Has your hospital ever attempted in the past to obtain direct reimbursement for inpatient cardiac rehabilitation?
_____ Yes, reasons why it failed. _____

_____ No, reasons why it was not attempted. _____

12. How many potential candidates for the inpatient program are admitted to your hospital every year? _____

13. How many actual candidates are ordered into the Phase I program each year? _____

14. Is your Phase I cardiac rehabilitation program a standing order on the CCU/ICU order sheet?
_____ Yes
_____ No

Comments:

Figure 3.5. Reimbursement questionnaire.

Phase II

The outpatient phase of cardiovascular rehabilitation has historically received the greatest amount of attention from the insurance industry. Efforts from several sources have resulted in coverage for outpatient Phase II cardiovascular rehabilitation by a majority of major medical policies for both Blue Cross and Blue Shield and the private insurance companies. Medicare also covers Phase II.

Medicare has reimbursed for outpatient cardiovascular rehabilitation programs in hospitals since 1980. Part B provided coverage for individually prescribed physical exercise programs and continuous telemetric ECG monitoring. In 1982, Medicare coverage expanded to include programs conducted in free-standing, physician-directed clinics. As of 1983, further guidelines have been released addressing cardiac rehabilitation in either an outpatient hospital facility or a physician-directed clinic. To receive reimbursement the following guidelines need to be fulfilled (Medicare and Medicaid Guide, 1984):

1. There must be a physician on the premises during the period of operation.
2. Each patient must be under the care of the hospital or clinic physician.
3. Cardiopulmonary emergency equipment such as a defibrillator and crash cart must be immediately available.
4. Programs must be staffed by personnel trained in basic life support and cardiac exercise therapy.
5. A physician must supervise the nonphysician personnel.

Reimbursement for cardiac rehabilitation is equated with a CPT-4 code 90060 (intermediate office visit). In most cases depending on the physician's usual fee, the amount of reimbursement is $42 per visit. Unfortunately, Medicare has neglected to consider the specialized equipment, training, and length of time for a comprehensive cardiac rehabilitation visit as compared to a much less specialized intermediate office visit.

In September 1983, a cardiac rehabilitation reimbursement questionnaire originating from the HCFA Baltimore office was circulated to the nations' Medicare intermediaries. The HCFA headquarters was "seeking information about claims and billing practices for cardiac rehabilitation services furnished by carriers to both Medicare and non-Medicare patients" (Holland, 1983). The purpose of the questionnaire as presented in the letter was to gain an understanding of the consistency or lack of it in the methodologies for paying of cardiac rehabilitation services and to provide information for deciding whether any changes were needed in the Medicare policy.

Within this questionnaire there are 10 questions put to the intermediaries.

1. How would you define the broad area of cardiac rehabilitation services?
2. What specific services do you pay for that fall under the main category of cardiac rehabilitation services? Please list these services.
3. Do you code these services separately for reimbursement purposes, or do you group them under one or more codes?
4. If you group-code these services, please list the specific services in each group.
5. How much do you pay for each cardiac rehabilitation service or group of services under each code?
6. How did you arrive at the particular prices you pay for the cardiac rehabilitation services for which you reimburse?
7. What criteria did you use in arriving at the codes you have adopted?
8. Please list the codes you use in order of the frequency of use— most used to least used.
9. Are there any services under these codes that you consider to be routine? If so, which ones?
10. How many cardiac rehabilitation facilities are there in your Medicare service area?

Although Phase II generally is covered, sometimes there is difficulty in the determination of the proper codes and descriptions to use in order to obtain or maintain coverage. It is also often difficult to determine the cost for service.

Cardiac Treatment Centers conducted a phone survey to determine the coverage for Phase II with Blue Cross/Blue Shield Major Medical plans across the country. Results of this survey are found in Table 3.7. Private insurers were also surveyed; these results are found in Table 3.8. Although coverage for Phase II service was fairly consistent, the codes, procedure descriptions, and fees charged were not. The most common procedure code number was 97200 for Phase II cardiac rehabilitation; however, a review of Tables 3.7 and 3.8 indicates that many other codes were utilized effectively.

The procedure description also varied substantially; however, there were some key words that did show up consistently:

1. Supervised
2. Monitored
3. Physician prescribed
4. Exercise therapy

The allowable charges varied significantly according to the survey results. The range for charges was $14 to $48 for a given procedure. There were some plans that paid $67 for a combination of charges performed during each visit. The mean charge for the Blue Cross/Blue Shield major medical coverage was $30. It is important to consider the program's geographical location when comparing its fee to the mean. Another consideration in a comparison of fees charged for the Phase II session is the amount of service provided for that fee. Those programs that charged above the mean fee of $30 usually provided very good programs in education, behavior modification, and dietary counseling. Other programs with an above average charge usually graduated their participants in less than 12 weeks by utilizing specific exit criteria.

Phase II outpatient cardiovascular rehabilitation continues to be the phase that most often receives 80% reimbursement from the major medical carriers and Medicare. In order to assure continued coverage for this portion of rehabilitation, more research needs to be completed in the area of return to work and morbidity with and without intervention in Phase II.

Table 3.7   Cardiac Treatment Centers Survey of Blue Cross/Blue Shield Phase II Reimbursement at 80%

CODE	Description	Fee (in dollars)
93040	Rhythm ECG 1–3 leads with interpretation	29.30
97200	Cardiac therapy visit with ECG, BP	24.00–30.00
97100	Office visit including any combination of any modality and procedure	30.00
—	Phase II–prescribed telemetry exercise	23.00
—	Cardiac rehabilitation exercise program	10.95
97200	Cardiac exercise therapy	32.50–45.00
93271	EKG-monitored service	28.00
97542	Cardiac therapy	28.00
93279	Unlisted cardiologic procedures	
97200	Cardiac exercise therapy	15.00
93040	Single lead EKG tracing	15.00
80120	Phase II–cardiac rehabilitation	35.00
93040	Rhythm strips	13.60
99961	Physical evaluation	19.40
99962	EKG-monitored service—entry	17.60
99963	EKG-monitored service—evaluation	13.60

99964	EKG-monitored symptomatic patients undergoing cardiac rehabilitation program	19.60
93040	Phase II–EKG rhythm strip with interpretation	25.00
93799	Phase II–Physician-prescribed, monitored exercise therapy	35.00
9300	Phase II–exercise visit	27.00
—	Phase II–exercise visit	21.00
97200	PT	
—	Phase II–mini stress test	31.65
—	Phase II–exercise visit	36.75
9104	Phase II–exercise visit	18.00
93270	Phase II–holter monitoring of activity session	25.00
	Phase II–telemetry-monitored C.V. treatment	28.00
	Phase II–exercise visit	14.00
	Phase II–cardiac therapy	30.00
9104	Phase II–exercise visit	28.00
	Physician prescibed non-C.V. therapy	37.50
12001	Phase II–medically-monitored exercise therapy visit	24.50
97100	Phase II–office visit	30.00
	Phase II–exercise visit	28.50

PHASE III

Historically, Phase III (or the Phase after the outpatient Phase II program) has not been covered by insurance, primarily because of the facility at which the program takes place or because often these programs are called maintenance programs. However, during the past 4 years there has been a change in insurance reimbursement toward the Phase III programs.

One significant change that has enhanced reimbursement for Phase III is the education of the insurance companies about the equipment proce-dures and qualifications of the staff members who administer the pro-grams. The state of North Carolina has the best insurance coverage for Phase III due to the efforts of program administrators to educate the insur-ance companies. In most programs in North Carolina there is 80% reim-bursement for Phase III at an average charge of $10 per session. In reviewing 17 programs throughout the country it was found that the average charge for a Phase III session was approximately $7. Of those who have attempted to receive reimbursement only 41% have been successful. Those who were denied coverage for Phase III often were told it was classified as self-help.

Table 3.8 Private Insurance Companies Reimbursement for Phase II of Cardiac Rehabilitation

Insurance Company	Procedure Code	Description of Procedure	Reimbursement
1. Aetna Life & Casualty	none used	description accepted if signed by a recognized provider (e.g., MD, DO, PT)	80%
2. American General Life	none used	accept billing description	80%
3. American Postal Workers Union	none used	accept billing description	80%
4. Bankers Life Insurance Co.	none used	detailed description of procedure	80%
5. Connecticut General	none used	accept billing description	80%
6. Educators Mutual	none used	accept billing description	80%
7. Employers Insurance of Wausau	CPT code	accept billing description	80%
8. Great Western Life Assurance Co.	RVS and CPT codes	accept billing description	80–100%
9. Gulf Life Insurance Co.	none used	individually approved	80%
10. Home life Insurance Co.	(converting)	accept billing description	80–100%
11. Independent Life	RVS codes	cardiac rehabilitation prescribed by physician	80%
12. Mutual of Omaha	RVS codes	accept billing description	80%
13. New York Life	none used	accept billing description	80%
14. Pilot Life Insurance Co.	ICDA & CPT	accept billing description	80%
15. Provident Life and Accident	none used	accept billing description	80%

In a review of the information from this survey, the evidence suggests that reimbursement potential is much greater when the billing description includes *Phase III* and *supervised, monitored exercise therapy*. If the word *maintenance* is used often there will not be any coverage for the program. In the event that the program is not covered you should follow the procedures described earlier for obtaining insurance reimbursement.

Summary

Insurance reimbursement is a very complex and interesting aspect of medical care. Billions of dollars are spent each year by employees, employers, tax payers, and individuals to provide health care reimbursement for themselves as well as others. Due to the continued increase in health care costs, both public and private insurance companies are constantly evaluating their benefits list to keep the cost of premiums at a reasonable level.

Those working in the field of cardiovascular rehabilitation need to communicate effectively with the third party carriers. The objective of this chapter has been to provide an overview of how insurance affects health care, specifically the discipline of cardiovascular rehabilitation. With the knowledge gained from an understanding of the insurance companies, better communication and reimbursement should result for those who receive cardiovascular rehabilitation therapy.

References

American Medical Association. (1977). *Physician's current procedural terminology*. Chicago: Author.

Blue Cross and Blue Shield United of Wisconsin. *Relative value guide*. Milwaukee, WI: Author.

Blue Cross/Blue Shield of New Jersey. (1980). Hospital-surgical-medical program subscriber handbook. NJ: Author.

Health Insurance Association of America. (1984). *Source book of health insurance data 1982-93*. Washington, DC: Author.

Holland, G.R. (1983, August 30). Letter to N. Oplinger, Medicare Part B, and Blue Cross and Blue Shield of Florida.

Kramer, J. (1983). New laws change medicare. *The Cardiac Output, 3*, 3.

Medicare and Medicaid Guide. (1984). Chicago: Commerce Clearing House.

Miller, M. (1983). [Progressive coronary care survey report]. Unpublished raw data, Cardiac Treatment Centers.

Pennsylvania Blue Shield. (1981). *Procedure terminology and manual with fee schedule allowances.* Camp Hill, PA: Author.

Pennsylvania Department of Labor and Industry Bureau of Vocational Rehabilitation. (1983). PA: Author.

Chapter 4

Cardiac Rehabilitation Equipment

Patricia L. Hutchinson

Since the early seventies, rehabilitation of the cardiac patient has become standard medical practice in most hospitals (Wenger, 1979). Earlier rehabilitation procedures primarily involved ambulation and self-care of the cardiac patient (Harrison, 1944). With the advancement of medical knowledge and research, cardiac rehabilitation has developed into three phases aimed at cardiac function restoration and general physical reconditioning. All three phases of rehabilitation involve graded exercise testing and active supervised exercise, which is often telemetered (Wilson, Edgett, & Porter, 1979). The progress and change in viewpoints of cardiac rehabilitation programs have resulted in extreme technological advancements in all rehabilitation equipment. The following chapter is an attempt to examine various types of cardiac rehabilitation equipment. Special attention is given to equipment cost relative to program needs and ways in which to determine the cost effectiveness of the equipment purchased.

State of the Art

Many of the early cardiac rehabilitation programs were established with two or three basic pieces of equipment—treadmill, electrocardiograph machine or telemetry, and bicycle ergometer. The equipment was sufficient at that time for effective rehabilitation and testing of a very small number of patients. However, with the goal changes of cardiac rehabilitation programs and increases in patient volume, program equipment needs have expanded tremendously. In addition, the functions now provided by cardiac rehabilitation machinery are numerous. For example, much of the exercise testing equipment on the market today provides the option of manual as well as highly computerized operation.

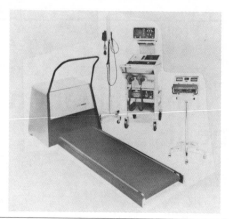

Figure 4.1. Treadmill testing system.

The earlier treadmill testing systems were large, noisy, and primarily manually operated. The state of the art in treadmill testing systems now offer space-saving, quiet, and computer-assisted operation. Most treadmills can be linked with complementary electrocardiograph (ECG) machines for simultaneous treadmill and ECG operation (see Figure 4.1).

Computer-linked treadmill testing systems generally offer a number of automatic protocol options as well as a manual option. In addition, computerized summary reports of the exercise test and patient history (see Figure 4.2) can be provided on the electrocardiogram by many systems.

The problems reported with the new computerized systems are frequently minor computer problems and not major equipment failures. In most cases, the computers have circuit boards that can easily be replaced if a problem arises. The computerized systems range in cost from approximately $15,000 to $35,000 depending on the options offered by the equipment.

State of the art in electrocardiograph machines includes mobility of the machinery, choice of number of channels, delay option, screen freeze, upper and lower heart rate limits set by a tone, visible heart rate by LED, ST-segment evaluation, warning tones for various arrhythmias, and detailed summary reports for the physician. Program directors need to examine closely the options provided by the equipment and determine which ones are needed for their program. Addition of one or more options can increase the cost of the equipment by several hundred dollars. Two common problems associated with ECG machines are cable repairs and pen replacements. Electrocardiograph machines range in cost from $500 to $6000.

Bicycle ergometers are becoming more popular with the public, and are being produced such that they are more affordable. The resistance is provided on the different ergometers by means of wind resistance (fans),

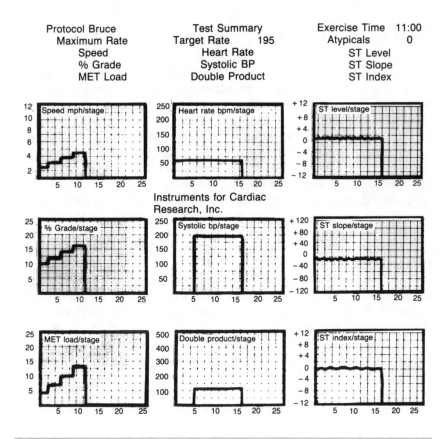

Figure 4.2. Computerized summary reports of exercise test.

belts, caliper brakes, and wheel rollers. Many of the bikes made today can be used for training, rehabilitation, and exercise research. Program directors should consider available space as well as purchase and maintenance costs of various ergometers before purchasing them. Many programs buy a dozen or more bikes and rent them on a monthly basis to the cardiac rehabilitation patients to help recover the purchase costs. Common maintenance of bicycle ergometers includes calibration, belt or caliper replacement, and chain and seat repair. Bicycle ergometer costs range from approximately $250 to $1,500.

Whether the equipment being purchased is major testing and/or rehabilitation or accessory equipment (paper, electrodes, cables, pens, etc.), directors need to assess the program needs and then closely match these needs with the options offered by the pieces of equipment. Shopping around for equipment can possibly save the program hundreds of dollars in purchase costs as well as later maintenance costs.

Cost Effectiveness

As one would expect, technological advancements in cardiac rehabilitation equipment and the current economic conditions have greatly increased manufacturing costs. From 1970 to 1983, the average cost of a motorized treadmill has more than quadrupled. The cost of a standard single channel ECG machine has, on the average, doubled in the last 10 years. Because the equipment cost is distributed to the hospital or clinic and in turn, passed on to the patient, it is a major consideration in the establishment of a cardiac rehabilitation program (Wilson et al., 1979). Rehabilitation program directors must discriminate among numerous factors to determine which equipment to purchase. One of the most important factors is the cost-effectiveness of the equipment. In other words, is the equipment capable of meeting the needs of the program and will the expenditure be recovered?

Cost-effectiveness of cardiac rehabilitation equipment can be projected for new rehabilitation programs as well as determined for current programs (Pyter & Doare, 1973). A problem that arises in projecting cost-effectiveness of equipment lies in the estimation of certain values. This problem will be addressed later. Figure 4.3 shows the steps involved in determining the cost-effectiveness of either single pieces of equipment or a total cardiac rehabilitation program.

The first step in the process is to determine equipment acquisition costs. This should include the actual equipment cost, and shipment and installa-

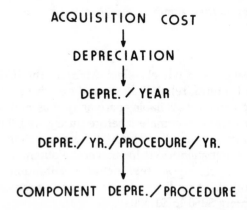

Figure 4.3. Steps involved in determining cost effectiveness.

tion fees. Maintenance contracts are often purchased by hospitals and clinics for equipment care, and this cost is included as part of the acquisition cost. Next, the depreciation value per year of the equipment must be determined. Most large equipment such as treadmills and ECG units has a 5-year depreciation value. Dividing the total acquisition cost of the equipment by five or the number of depreciation years will establish the depreciation value per year. To determine the actual expenditure recovery of the equipment, the component depreciation value per procedure is needed. This value is the component depreciation value per year by procedure per year as shown in the equation:

Component Depreciation Value/Year/Procedure/Year.

The years cancel out leaving the component depreciation value per procedure.

At this point the procedure cost has to be determined. The following expenses incurred by the program must be included in the procedure cost.

- Equipment
- Supplies
- Personnel (plus benefits)
- Rental
- Utilities
- Telephone
- Furnishings
- Marketing
- Miscellaneous

If the program costs are being projected, the number of tests performed monthly will be an estimate, whereas for programs already in existence, an actual number of tests is available. When the total monthly procedure cost is divided by the number of tests performed during a month, the cost per procedure is obtained. Once the cost per procedure is determined, the program director can easily look at the component value relative to the procedure cost and determine whether or not the procedural income is paying for the equipment.

Many program directors believe that cardiac rehabilitation and graded exercise testing equipment is very cost-effective if the program is properly organized. In a small survey (Hutchinson, 1983) of 18 cardiac rehabilitation programs in the South, program directors reported that equipment costs were generally recovered within a 2-year period (depending on the size of the program). Sixty-one percent (11 of 18) of the directors felt that when equipment companies offer options in the equipment, it is best to take as few options as possible to meet the program demands and keep the equipment costs down.

Summary

Program directors generally believe that properly organized and administered cardiac rehabilitation programs, offered in an area and at a time of need, recover all equipment costs and become self-supportive. Current and long-range program goals should be assessed relative to the options provided by the equipment before purchase. Procedure costs need to be adjusted to cover the expense of the program (including equipment) based on the patient volume. If possible the procedure costs should be great enough to cover all expenses incurred by the program and leave the program self-supportive. And finally, evaluations need to be made two to three times a year to assess the cost-effectiveness of the program and the equipment.

References

Harrison, T.R. (1944). Abuse of rest as a therapeutic measure for patients with cardiovascular disease. *Journal of the American Medical Association,* **125**, 1075.

Hutchinson, P.L. (1983). *Cardiac rehabilitation programs of Atlanta and surrounding areas.* Unpublished manuscript, Doctors Memorial Hospital, Atlanta, GA.

Pyfer, H.R., & Doane, B.L. (1973). Aspects of community exercise programs: Economic aspects of cardiac rehabilitation programs. In J.P. Naughton, H.K. Hellerstein, & I.C. Mohler (Eds.), *Exercise testing and exercise training in coronary heart disease.* New York: Academic Press.

Seitz, N. (1976). *Financial analysis: A programmed approach.* Reston, VA: Reston.

Wenger, N.K. (1979). Research related to rehabilitation. *Circulation,* **60**, 1636.

Wilson, P.K., Edgett, J.W., & Porter, G.H. (1979). Rehabilitation of the cardiac patient: Program organization. In M.L. Pollock & D.H. Schmidt (Eds.), *Heart disease and rehabilitation.* Boston: Houghton-Mifflin.

Part II

Cardiac Rehabilitation and Exercise Prescription Concerns

Chapter 5

Recognizing and Preventing Medical Problems Associated With Early Cardiac Rehabilitation

Wendy Dion

The concept of early monitored exercise, surveillance, and preventative cardiology provided the catalyst for the development of structured cardiac rehabilitation programs in the early 1970s (Carn, Frasher, & Stiverman, 1961; Ehsani, Martin, Heath, & Coyle, 1982; Franklin & Rubenfire, 1980; Haskell, 1979; Hellerstein, 1968; Hellerstein & Ford, 1957). These programs have increased substantially in number and level of sophistication. Cardiac rehabilitation can be executed at the bedside, on the ward, in inpatient and outpatient centers, or in community settings. This chapter discusses recognition and prevention of medical problems associated with early cardiac rehabilitation, and summarizes medical problems associated with the inpatient and outpatient cardiac rehabilitation programs at Mount Sinai Medical Center. General guidelines are presented, followed by discussion of specific concerns for an inpatient or outpatient program.

Patient Safety

Regardless of the environment, patient safety should be of paramount concern to those working with and supervising cardiac patients. The rate of cardiovascular complications during medically supervised exercise training of cardiac patients varies substantially, but generally lower rates have been recorded since 1970 (Wenger & Hellerstein, 1984). Haskell's (1978) review of 30 cardiac rehabilitation programs in the United States and

Canada found that the average cardiovascular complication rate (cardiac arrest, myocardial infarction [MI], and cardiopulmonary events) was one nonfatal and one fatal event every 34,673 and 116,402 participant-hr, respectively. Such a low rate of complications is attributed to improved training of personnel, including widespread cardiopulmonary resuscitation training and the development of state-of-the-art resuscitation equipment. The evolution of standards and guidelines for exercise tests and training through the American Heart Association and American College of Sports Medicine has also had a positive influence on the rate of complications.

There are several points to consider in regard to patient safety and the prevention of medical problems. First, a major consideration for any cardiac rehabilitation program is the selection of staff employed to work with patients. Knowledge of exercise response and training principles is important, but familiarity with specific disease states and treatment is also necessary for safe patient management. This is best accomplished through a multidisciplinary team approach. A second important consideration is the staff's ability to evaluate situations. Knowing when to intervene can prevent a problem from occurring and will help maintain a reassuring environment for the participants. Third, it is important for team members to share information with each other. Weekly rounds should be held so that all staff members have the opportunity to discuss the patients as well as potential problems. Rounds may also be used as an educational time for prepared or spontaneous discussions. Finally, maintaining a low patient-to-staff ratio allows for closer supervision of patients, thereby preventing problems associated with the program.

Patient safety during exercise training can be enhanced by preliminary screening and patient selection. Obtaining a complete medical history of each participant via data retrieval or interview is crucial. All pertinent test results should be acquired as well as hospital discharge summaries if possible. It is often beneficial to include a "significant other" in the initial interview or to make arrangements to do so as soon as possible after program entry. Being aware of any ongoing, secondary medical/psychiatric diagnoses or symptoms is a must for total patient management, as this can significantly affect a participant's progress in the program.

Devising a list of contraindications (relative and absolute) to exercise and a list of conditions that require special consideration, such as conduction disturbances or marked obesity, serves as useful guidelines for the staff (see Table 5.1). *How* the contraindications are interpreted is equally important. Not every client with one of these special problems will be excluded from exercise; thus it is vital to use good judgment and/or to consult with the medical director to clarify individual situations.

Table 5.1 Contraindications to Inpatient Exercise

I. Absolute Contraindications

1. Patients on bedrest

2. Prolonged or unstable angina

3. Recent acute M.I. and unstable

4. Resting diastolic blood pressure over 120 mmHg or resting systolic blood pressure over 200 mmHg.

5. Inappropriate blood pressure response: orthostatic or exercise-induced and patient symptomatic.

6. Severe atrial or ventricular dysrhythmias

7. Second or third degree heart block

8. Recent embolism, either systemic or pulmonary

9. Thrombophlebitis

10. Dissecting aneurysm

11. Fever greater than 100 °F or acute illness

12. Excessive sternal movement—contraindication for upper extremity and trunk R.O.M. exercises

13. Uncompensated heart failure

14. Active pericarditis (primary) or myocarditis

15. Acute systemic illness

II. Relative Contraindications

1. Resting diastolic blood pressure over 110 mmHg or resting systolic blood pressure over 200 mmHg

2. Inappropriate increase in blood pressure with exercise and patient symptomatic.

3. Hypotension (refer to policy)

4. Moderate aortic stenosis (25 mm–50 mmHg gradient)

5. Compensated heart failure

6. Significant emotional stress

7. Pericarditis associated with myocardial revascularization surgery

8. Resting ST depression (> 3 mm)

9. Uncontrolled diabetes

10. Neuromuscular, musculoskeletal, or arthritic disorders which would prevent activity

11. Excessive incisional drainage

(Cont.)

Table 5.1 (Cont.)

12. Sinus tachycardia greater than 120 at rest
13. New ECG changes post-operative or post-MI indicative or suggestive of fresh infarct
14. Ventricular aneurysm
15. Symptomatic anemia (Hematocrit < 30%)

III. Conditions Requiring Special Consideration and/or Precautions

1. Conduction disturbances
2. Controlled dysrhythmias
3. Fixed rate pacemaker
4. Mitral valve
5. Angina pectoris and other manifestations of coronary insufficiency
6. Electrolyte disturbance
7. Cyanotic heart disease
8. Marked obesity (20% above optimal body weight)
9. Diabetes
10. Pulmonary disease
11. Intermittent claudication
12. Automatic implantable cardioverter defibrillator
13. Sternal movement in the post-operative client—contraindication for upper extremity and trunk R.O.M. exercises
14. Active pericarditis (primary) or myocarditis
15. Sinus tachycardia greater than 120 at rest

Staff members working with clients should be very familiar with individual medical regimens, including medications and diet, as well as with the current treatment plan. Prescribing an aggressive exercise program for a client who is waiting to have a surgical procedure may not be advisable or safe. The staff should also know each client's symptoms and what usually precipitates them. Participants with ongoing ischemia and angina should be routinely queried to document any change in anginal pattern or in the frequency/intensity of symptoms. This type of information must also be communicated, either verbally or by making notations in the client's chart, to part-time staff who may not be familiar with each participant.

Continuous electrocardiographic (EEG) monitoring during exercise is a major service of most inpatient and outpatient cardiac rehabilitation programs and may increase patient safety by identifying abnormal changes that indicate high risk (Haskell, 1978). In addition, knowing what dysrhythmias and signs and symptoms typically occur in a Phase I or Phase II program gives the added advantage of knowing what to expect and when to intervene. Serious ventricular dysrhythmias seem to occur more frequently (54% of coronary patients) in the initial 1–2 months of exercise (Fardy, Doll, Taylor, & Williams, 1982).

Inpatient Medical Problems

In a study of 521 hospitalized post-coronary artery bypass surgery patients (CABGS) (Dion et al., 1981), the most notable medical problems were incisional pain, lightheadedness, and dysrhythmias. Angina pectoris, claudication, ST-segment changes, and hypotension were also observed but less frequently. Ventricular dysrhythmias were found in 44% of patients, and 17% exhibited supraventricular dysrhythmias during monitored exercise. The rehabilitation program was responsible for detecting 22% of all the signs/symptoms reported in the study, which further validates the need for this type of early surveillance.

Outpatient Medical Problems

A study of 365 medical and surgical clients in an outpatient hospital-based cardiac rehabilitation program at the same institution was conducted to document the occurrence of medical problems in this type of setting (Sennett et al., 1984). Angina pectoris, dysrhythmias, and dyspnea were significant in both CABGS and myocardial infarction (MI) patients. Lightheadedness and supraventricular dysrhythmias were more frequent in the CABGS group, whereas ST-segment changes occurred more frequently in the MI patients. Ventricular dysrhythmias were noted in 32% of both groups. Interestingly, the CABGS group exhibited a significantly higher percentage of ventricular tachycardia than the MI group (12% vs. 4%). The higher incidence of ventricular tachycardia in the surgical group was an unexpected finding and may reflect the need for monitored exercise in this type of individual, despite claims to the contrary. It is important, however, that the cardiac rehabilitation staff members remember not to rely solely on monitoring equipment to tell them how a participant is tolerating the exercise. This serves as only one parameter and must be viewed in context.

Some adverse subjective responses to exercise may include shortness of breath, dizziness, palpitations, chest or arm discomfort, and fatigue. Although it is easy to discount fatigue as an endpoint for exercise, often it is a reliable parameter and correlates well with objective measurements of the patient's exercise capacity (Underhill, 1982). This is especially true for individuals with cardiomyopathy or severely impaired left ventricular function. Patients with cardiomyopathy should avoid static exercise due to an increase in diastolic blood pressure that can be twice over the resting value and a marked decrease in stroke work index. Training individuals with low ejection fractions can be done provided certain precautions and guidelines are followed. Dr. Williams at Duke University has found that ejection fraction in itself is a poor indicator of acute work capacity. The ability to increase cardiac output, as well as heart rate and systolic blood pressure, is a better predictor of work performance with this type of patient. He suggests the following guidelines for patient selection in this group:

1. No active congestive heart failure.
2. No sustained exercise-induced hypotension.
3. Must be able to walk 50 yards without hemodynamic compromise.

A useful tool that can be used along with subjective symptoms is the Rating of Perceived Exertion (RPE) Scale developed by Borg (1962, 1978). This scale rates perceived exertion from 6 to 20, with a subjective verbal anchor at every odd number. When appropriately used, the perception score correlates well with physiological variables. The RPE scale is effective due to its high relationship to factors indicative of fatigue. Although the scale is not perfect and should be used in concert with common sense and other clinical psychological and physiological parameters, its use in exercise prescription does complement heart rate measurements. Clearly, the incorporation of perceived exertion to monitor training intensity can help prevent pushing clients beyond their tolerance.

Patients at high risk for cardiac arrest or MI are identified from graded exercise test data. Conditions that increase risk include the following: angina pectoris, significant ST-segment depression or elevation from resting values (particularly if ST-segment changes persist into recovery), inappropriate blood pressure response to exercise, significant dysrhythmia, and poor effort tolerance (<3 METs) (Granath, Sodermark, Winge, Volpe, & Zetterquist, 1977; Theroux, Waters, Halphen, Debaisieux, & Mizgala, 1979; Dillahurst & Miller, 1979; Davidson & DeBusk, 1980; Starling, Crawford, Kennedy, & O'Rourke, 1980). Moreover, the combination of poor left ventricular function and significant dysrhythmia increases the risk of sudden death (McNeer et al., 1978; Epstein, 1982). Individuals who exhibit these factors should be identified at the onset of participation in a structured cardiac rehabilitation program and monitored closely. The necessity of keeping this subset of cardiac patients training at their prescribed target heart rate (60–85% of maximum heart rate reserve) cannot be overemphasized. Exceeding the recommended target heart rate during training, along with the previously mentioned abnormal graded exercise test results, is associated with a higher risk of major cardiovascular events

(Hossack & Hartwig, 1982). As the exercise intensity approaches maximal effort, the relative risk of cardiovascular complications increases, as does the risk of orthopedic injury. An exercise program should therefore be designed to provide the greatest benefit with the least risk and does not have to be exhaustive to be beneficial.

Several guidelines should be reviewed with participants when they enter the program to help prevent exercise-related events (Wenger & Hellerstein, 1984):

1. Avoid tobacco and alcohol before and after exercise.
2. Avoid hot showers, steam rooms, saunas, and whirlpools before and immediately after exercise.
3. Avoid playing catch-up when a day of exercise is missed.
4. Avoid exercise during a febrile illness.
5. Avoid exercise for 1 to 2 hr after heavy meals. Also avoid beverages containing caffeine for 2 hr prior to exercise.
6. Avoid static exercise and activities producing the Valsalva maneuver.
7. Dress appropriately for exercise—avoid heavy clothes or rubber sweat suits.
8. Reduce the intensity of exercise in hot, humid weather or during ozone alerts.

Studies have not shown that hypertension during exercise is either hazardous at the time or indicates a poor prognosis for developing complications in the future (Hanson & Neede, 1970). The following guidelines have been developed to assess blood pressure response to exercise:

1. A small, initial decrease in blood pressure may be insignificant, provided the pressure stabilizes and a subsequent increase occurs with continued exercise.
2. A decrease in blood pressure associated with symptoms of decreased blood flow should always prompt termination of an exercise session.
3. A decrease in blood pressure that becomes more pronounced with persistent exercise should be regarded as evidence of cardiovascular decompensation.

Watching for subtle changes in the blood pressure either at rest, with exercise, or postexercise can indicate potential or impending problems. For example, postexercise hypotension may indicate a need for medication manipulation or closer monitoring of fluid intake.

It is appropriate at this point to mention the importance of the warm-up and cool-down in relation to exercise. Preparing the cardiovascular and musculoskeletal systems for activity is very important for injury prevention, as well as for the prevention of electrical instability or strain on the heart. It has been shown that lack of an adequate warm-up or cooldown may be the most common cause of exercise-related cardiovascular complications (Barnard, Gardner, Diaco, MacAlpin, & Kattus, 1973; Barnard, MacAlpin, Kattus, & Buckberg, 1973).

Inpatient Program

Day-to-day execution of the Inpatient Program at Mount Sinai Medical Center involves daily rounds to discuss clients in the program and, more specifically, to review individual exercise prescriptions and tolerance. All patients are evaluated by a physical therapist before they begin sessions in the Inpatient Exercise Center. Clients must be able to complete 10–15 repetitions of the range of motion (ROM) exercises and walk approximately 424 ft before they are allowed to use the exercise center. Readiness to begin this phase of exercise is best determined by the cardiac rehabilitation staff. Most patients view this step as progress in their recovery and are greatly disappointed if they are returned to their room because of inability to perform the exercise. Instituting this guideline has improved our assessment of the patient's readiness to begin treadmill ambulation or stationary cycling.

Prior to any patient treatment, the chart, graphic sheet, and nurse's notes are reviewed. The cardiac rehabilitation staff also discusses treatment time early in the morning with the primary nurse so as to organize and pace the client's day. Meal times are taken into consideration when scheduling group exercise classes, and clients are advised not to shower 2 hr before or after exercise to avoid problems with hypotension. Generally, the following conditions preclude exercise: resting heart rate > 120 beats/min, oral temperature > 100°, resting systolic blood pressure < 90 mm Hg.

Several years ago we developed policies for the inpatient program to help prevent the occurrence of medical problems. It is our feeling that these guidelines have helped detect problems early and helped prevent major setbacks in the client's recovery, especially with regard to hypotension:

INPATIENT CARDIAC REHABILITATION (ICR) POLICIES

I. Concurrent testing and coming to the Inpatient Exercise Center (IEC):

A. Patients may come to the IEC the day of cardiac catheterization for ROM/strengthening exercises and stair climbing only.

B. Patients undergoing an exercise test (predischarge-graded exercise test or nuclear dynamics) may attend classes in the IEC for ROM/strengthening exercises only on the day of the test.

C. To prevent undue fatigue, the patient will be advised to keep ambulation to a minimum on the day of the exercise test.

II. First day procedure for new patients (the following procedure is used to check for orthostatic and exercise-induced hypotension on the ward or in the IEC):

A. All patients will have orthostatic blood pressure measurements prior to beginning exercise. After obtaining a blood pressure on the patient in the sitting position, a second reading will be taken after the patient has been in a standing position for 30 s. Patients should be reminded to stand slowly from a sitting position to avoid lightheadedness. The systolic blood pressure should be at least 90 mm Hg prior to exercise. Typically systolic blood pressure and heart rate rise with exercise. However, patients may be anxious especially when first attending the IEC, and resting blood pressure and heart rate may be higher than usual. During exercise, systolic blood pressure and heart rate may not increase over resting levels in such cases.

1. Patients with symptomatic hypotension will not be exercised.

2. If the standing blood pressure is below 90 mm Hg (without symptoms), the attending physician will be notified and the patient will not be allowed to exercise until the nurse consults with the medical director.

3. If the patient exhibits a 10-20 mm Hg orthostatic drop in the systolic blood pressure (without symptoms), the medical director will be consulted prior to exercising the patient.

4. If the patient exhibits more than a 20 mm Hg orthostatic drop in the systolic blood pressure (without symptoms), the attending physician will be notified. If the attending physician wishes his/her patient to continue, the medical director will be consulted prior to beginning the exercise session.

5. Before consulting the medical director or the attending physician regarding hypotension, blood pressure measurements will be taken in both arms by two staff members.

B. Stair climbing procedure: Patients will climb stairs at a slow comfortable pace as tolerated. When taking exercise blood pressure reading post-stair climbing, the patient should alternately shift weight from one leg to the other (step in place) to help prevent venous pooling and hypotension.

1. *Medical patients*: Medical patients will climb stairs as outlined in the protocol (see Table 5.2). Blood pressure readings will be taken before and after stair climbing.

2. *Surgical patients*: Surgical patients may attempt stair climbing during their second visit to the IEC as outlined in the protocol (see Table 5.3). A blood pressure reading will be taken before and immediately after climbing six stairs. If there is less than a 10-20 mm Hg drop in the systolic blood pressure (without symptoms), the patient may climb six additional stairs and a final blood pressure reading should be taken. If the systolic blood pressure drops more than 20 mm Hg (without symptoms), no further stair climbing will be done that day and the attending physician will be notified.

3. *Surgical patients following MI protocol for ambulation*: Surgical patients following the MI protocol will climb stairs as outlined in the protocol. Blood pressure readings will be taken before and after stair climbing.

4. *Patients not coming to the IEC*: Stair climbing will be executed according to one of the previously mentioned protocols for patients being treated on the ward only.

C. Patients with new subclavicular permanent pacemaker implantation:

1. No upper extremity movement with affected arm for 24-48 hr.

2. After 48 hr, upper extremity exercise is limited to that associated with normal daily activity. No additional ROM will be executed for approximately the first 2 weeks to prevent pacemaker wire from dislodging. After this time, upper extremity ROM and strengthening exercises may commence.

Table 5.2 Post MI Inpatient Rehabilitation Program Guidelines; Heart Rates, Blood Pressures, and Comments are Recorded on Inpatient Data Record or Exercise Log

Step/Date	Cardiac Rehab/Physical Therapy	*Ward Activity	Patient Education
1 1.5 METs __/__/__	WARD TX: Passive ROM to major joints, active ankle exercises, 5 Reps, deep breathing (supine) BID.	1. Bedrest. 2. May feed self.	Orient to CCU. Orientation to exercise component of rehabilitation program. Answer patient and family questions regarding progress, procedures, reason for activity limitation. Explain perceived exertion (RPE).
2 1.5 METs __/__/__	WARD TX: Active-assistance ROM to major muscle groups, active ankle exercises, 5 Reps; deep breathing (supine/sitting) BID.	1. Feeding self. 2. Partial AM care (washing hands and face, brushing teeth in bed). 3. Bedside commode.	
3 1.5 METs __/__/__	WARD TX: Active ROM to major muscle groups, active ankle exercises, 5 Reps; deep breathing (sitting) BID.	1. Begin sitting in chair for short periods as tolerated 2×/day 2. Bathing self. 3. Bedside commode.	
4 1.5 METs __/__/__	WARD TX: Active exercises: shoulder: flexion, abduction; elbow flexion; hip flexion; knee extension; toe raises; ankle exercises; 5 Reps; deep breathing (standing) BID.	1. Bathroom privileges. 2. Sitting in chair 3×/day. 3. Up in chair for meals. 4. Bathing self, dressing, combing hair (sitting).	

(Cont.)

5 1.5-2 METs	WARD TX: Active exercises: shoulder: flexion, abduction, circumduction; elbow flexion; trunk lateral flexion; hip: flexion, abduction; knee extension; toe raises; ankle exercises; 5 Reps (standing); BID. Monitored ambulation of 100–200 ft., BID with physician approval	1. Bathroom privileges. 2. Up as tolerated in room. 3. Stand at sink to shave and comb hair. 4. Bathe self and dress. 5. Up in chair as tolerated.	Answer patient and family questions. Orient to ICCU phase of recovery. Present discharge booklet and other printed material (AHA). Encourage patient and family to attend group classes or do 1:1 sessions.
6 1.5-2 METs	WARD TX: STANDING: Exercises outlined in Step 5, 5-10 Reps; once daily. Monitored ambulation for 5 min (440 ft.) EXERCISE CENTER: Transport to Inpatient Exercise Center (IEC) for monitored ROM/strengthening exercises from Step 5, 5-10 Reps; leg stretching (posterior thigh muscles, gastrocnemius), 10 Reps; treadmill and/or bicycle	1. Continue ward activity from Step 5 2. Increase ambulation up to 1** Lap (440 ft.) with assistance if appropriate, 2 ×/day. 3. Walk short distance in hall (room and quad areas) as tolerated.	Instruction in pulse-taking and rationale. Explain value of exercise. Present T-shirt and activity log.

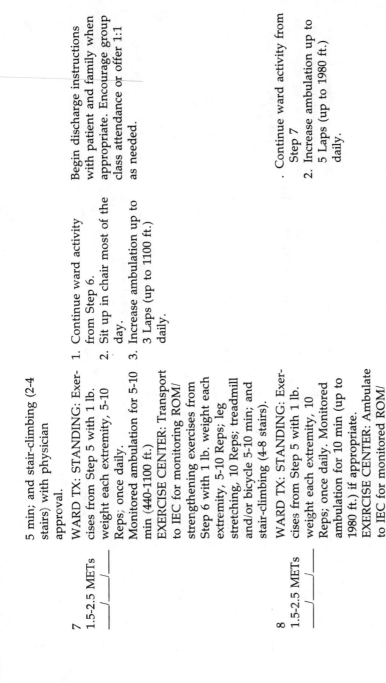

5 min; and stair-climbing (2-4 stairs) with physician approval.

7
1.5-2.5 METs

WARD TX: STANDING: Exercises from Step 5 with 1 lb. weight each extremity, 5-10 Reps; once daily. Monitored ambulation for 5-10 min (440-1100 ft.) EXERCISE CENTER: Transport to IEC for monitoring ROM/strengthening exercises from Step 6 with 1 lb. weight each extremity, 5-10 Reps; leg stretching, 10 Reps; treadmill and/or bicycle 5-10 min; and stair-climbing (4-8 stairs).

1. Continue ward activity from Step 6.
2. Sit up in chair most of the day.
3. Increase ambulation up to 3 Laps (up to 1100 ft.) daily.

Begin discharge instructions with patient and family when appropriate. Encourage group class attendance or offer 1:1 as needed.

8
1.5-2.5 METs

WARD TX: STANDING: Exercises from Step 5 with 1 lb. weight each extremity, 10 Reps; once daily. Monitored ambulation for 10 min (up to 1980 ft.) if appropriate. EXERCISE CENTER: Ambulate to IEC for monitored ROM/strengthening exercises from Step 6 with 1 lb. weight each

. Continue ward activity from Step 7
2. Increase ambulation up to 5 Laps (up to 1980 ft.) daily.

(Cont.)

extremity, 10 Reps; leg stretching, 10 Reps; treadmill and/or bicycle 10-20 min; and stair-climbing (10-12 stairs).

| 9 1.5-2.5 METs ___/___ | WARD TX: STANDING: Exercises from Step 5 with 2 lb. weight each extremity, 10 Reps; once daily. Monitored ambulation if appropriate. EXERCISE CENTER: Ambulate to IEC for monitored ROM/strengthening exercises from Step 6 with 2 lb. weight each extremity, 10 Reps; leg stretching, 10 Reps; treadmill and/or bicycle 20-25 min; and stair-climbing (12-14 stairs). | 1. Up as tolerated in room and quad area. 2. Increase ambulation up to 6 laps (up to 2640 ft.) daily. | Begin instruction in home exercise program. Initiate referral to Phase 2 if appropriate. Explain pre-discharge graded exercise test (PDGXT) and upper limit heart rate. |
| 10 1.5-3 METs ___/___ | WARD TX: Exercises from Step 5 with 2 lb. weight each extremity, 10 Reps; once daily. Monitored ambulation if appropriate. | 1. Up as tolerated in room and quad area. 2. Increase ambulation up to 8 Laps (up to 3300 ft.) daily. | Complete discharge instructions. Complete referral to Phase 2. |

| 11 | EXERCISE CENTER: Ambulate to IEC for monitored ROM/strengthening exercises from Step 6 with 2 lb. weight each extremity, 10 Reps; leg stretching, 10 Reps; treadmill and/or bicycle 25-30 min, and stair-climbing (14-16 stairs). | A pre-discharge graded exercise test is recommended at this time. | Continue previous ward activity. |

*Ward Activity = Activities performed alone, with family, or with primary nurse.
**Lap = Distance of approximately 424 feet or once around the square.

Table 5.3 Post Open Heart Surgery Inpatient Rehabilitation Program Guidelines; Heart Rates, Blood Pressures, and Comments Are Recorded on Inpatient Data Record or Exercise Log

Step/Date	Cardiac Rehab/Physical Therapy	*Ward Activity	Patient Education
1 1.5 METs __/__	AM WARD TX: SITTING: with feet supported: active-assistive to active ROM to major muscle groups, active ankle exercises, active scapular elevation/depression, retraction/protraction, 3-5 Reps, deep breathing. Monitored ambulation of 100 ft. as tolerated. PM WARD TX: SITTING: with feet supported: Active ROM to major muscle groups, 5 Reps; deep breathing. Monitored ambulation 100-200 ft. with assistance as tolerated.	1. Begin sitting in chair (when stable) several times/day for 10-30 min. 2. May ambulate 100-200 ft. with assistance, 1-2× daily.	Orient to CVICU. Reinforce purpose of physical therapy and deep breathing exercises. Orient to exercise component of rehabilitation program. Answer patient and family questions regarding progress.
2 1.5 METs __/__	WARD TX: SITTING: repeat exercises from Step 1 and increase repetitions to 5-10; deep breathing BID. Monitored ambulation of 200 ft. with assistance as tolerated (stress correct posture) BID.	Continue activities from Step 1.	Continue above.

3 1.5-2 METs	WARD TX: STANDING: Begin active upper extremity and trunk exercises bilaterally without resistance (shoulder: flexion, abduction, internal/external rotation), knee extension (if appropriate); ankle exercises; 5-10 Reps; BID. Monitored ambulation of 300 ft. BID.	Increase ambulation to 300 ft. or approximately 3 corridor lengths at slow pace with assistance, BID.	Begin pulse-taking instruction when appropriate and explain RPE scale. Answer questions of patient and family. Reorient patient and family to ICCU. Encourage family attendance at group classes.
4 1.5-2 METs	WARD TX: STANDING: Active exercises from Step 3, 10-15 Reps; BID. Monitored ambulation of 424 ft. BID.	Increase ambulation to 1 Lap** (424 ft. or once around square) at slow pace with assistance BID.	
5 1.5-2.5 METs	WARD TX: STANDING: Active exercises from Step 3, 15, Reps; once daily. Monitored ambulation for 5-10 min (424-848 ft.) as tolerated. EXERCISE CENTER: Walk to Inpatient Exercise Center (IEC) for monitored ROM/strengthening exercises from Step 3, 15 Reps; leg stretching (posterior thigh muscles, gastrocnemius), 10 Reps; treadmill and/or bicycle 5-10 min (refer to treadmill/bicycle protocol) with physician approval.	1. Increase ambulation up to 3 Laps (up to 1320 ft.) daily as tolerated. 2. Begin participating in daily ADL and personal care as tolerated. 3. Encourage chair sitting with legs elevated.	Orient to IEC. Continue instruction in pulse-taking and use of RPE scale. Explain value of exercise. Present T-shirt and activity log.

(Cont.)

| 6
1.5-2.5 METs | WARD TX: STANDING: Active exercises from Step 3 with 1 lb. weight each upper extremity, 15 Reps; once daily. Monitored ambulation for 10-15 min (up to 1980 ft.) if appropriate.
EXERCISE CENTER: Walk to IEC for monitored ROM/ strengthening exercises from Step 5 with 1 lb. weight each upper extremity, 15 Reps; leg stretching, 10 Reps; treadmill and/or bicycle 15-20 min; and stair-climbing (6-12 stairs) with assistance. | 1. Increase ambulation up to 5 Laps (up to 1980 ft.) daily.
2. Encourage independence in ADL.
3. Encourage chair sitting with legs elevated. | Give discharge booklet and general discharge instructions to patient and family. Encourage group class attendance. Individual instruction by physical therapist, nutritionist, pharmacist. |
| 7
2-3 METs | WARD TX: STANDING: Active exercises from Step 3 with 1 lb. weight each upper extremity, 15 Reps; once daily. Monitored ambulation for 15-20 min (up to 3300 ft.) if appropriate. | 1. Continue activities from Step 6.
2. Increase ambulation up to 8 Laps (up to 3300 ft.) daily. | Discuss referral to Phase 2 program if appropriate. |

| 8 2-3 METs ___/___ | EXERCISE CENTER: Walk to IEC for monitored ROM/ strengthening exercises from Step 5 with 1 lb. weight each upper extremity, 15 Reps; leg stretching, 10 Reps; treadmill and/or bicycle 20-30 min; and stair-climbing (up to 14 stairs) with assistance. WARD TX: STANDING: Exercises from Step 3 with 2 lb. weight each upper extremity, 15 Reps; once daily. Monitored ambulation if appropriate. | 1. Continue activities from Step 7 2. Increase ambulation up to 9 Laps (up to 3746 ft.) daily. | Reinforce prior teaching. Explain pre-discharge graded exercise test (PDGXT) and upper limit heart rate. Continue with possible referral to Phase 2. |
| 9 2-3 METs ___/___ | EXERCISE CENTER: Walk to IEC for monitored ROM/ strengthening exercises from Step 5 with 2 lb. weight each upper extremity, 15 Reps; leg stretching; 10 Reps; treadmill and/or bicycle 20-30 min; and stair-climbing (up to 16 stairs). WARD TX: STANDING: Exercises from Step 3 with 2 lb. weight each upper extremity, 15 Reps; once daily. Monitored ambulation if appropriate. | 1. Continue activities from Step 8. 2. Increase ambulation up to 12 Laps (up to 5060 ft.) daily. | Finalize discharge instructions. Complete referral to Phase 2. |

(Cont.)

EXERCISE CENTER: Walk to IEC for monitored ROM/strengthening exercises from Step 5 with 2 lb. weight each upper extremity, 15 Reps; leg stretching, 10 Reps; treadmill and/or bicycle 20-30 min; and stair-climbing (up to 18 stairs).

10
2-3 METs
____/____

WARD TX: STANDING: Exercises from Step 3 with 3 lb. weight each upper extremity, 15 Reps; once daily. Monitored ambulation if appropriate. EXERCISE CENTER: Walk to IEC for monitored ROM/strengthening exercises from Step 5 with 3 lb. weight each upper extremity, 15 Reps; leg stretching, 10 Reps; treadmill and/or bicycle 20-30 min; and stair-climbing (up to 24 stairs).

A pre-discharge graded exercise test (PDGXT) is recommended at this time.

1. Continue activities from Step 9.
2. Increase ambulation up to 14 Laps (up to 5940 ft.) daily.

*Ward Activity = Activities performed alone, with family, or with primary nurse.
**Lap = Distance of approximately 424 feet or once around square.

D. Patients with new abdominal permanent pacemaker implantation: No hamstring or gastrocnemius stretching for two weeks.

III. The upper limit exercise heart rate for both medical and surgical patients is 20 beats/min above the standing resting heart rate unless otherwise specified by the medical director.

Outpatient Program

As in our inpatient program, the outpatient staff meets routinely to discuss participants in the program and how they are adapting to exercise. The nurses and exercise leaders meet once a week to change individual exercise prescriptions and to assess home exercise. Upon entry into the program, each client is given basic information regarding appropriate exercise attire, the composition of the cardiac rehabilitation staff (physician, nurses, exercise physiologists, exercise leaders, physical therapist, nutritionist, and psychologist), emergency equipment, and signs and symptoms reportable to the physician/staff. All clients are asked weekly about changes in medication and are encouraged to report these as they occur.

During the final week of the outpatient program, clients are not monitored by telemetry, thus allowing the staff to evaluate the patient's proficiency in measuring self-pulse. This also enables the staff to view the client's perception of proper exercise intensity. Graduating participants are encouraged to return in 1 month for reevaluation and adjustment of the exercise prescription.

Emergency Protocol

A plan for emergency situations must be designed for each specific exercise area and posted where staff has access to it. Included in this plan should be a definition of roles in the event of a life-threatening emergency as well as individual responsibilities. It is advisable to review this plan periodically with staff due to the infrequent occurrence of life-threatening situations in cardiac rehabilitation programs. Following any type of emergency, involved staff should meet and discuss how it was handled and perhaps offer suggestions to enhance efficiency. A frank discussion of feelings about the situation is also helpful. All emergency equipment should be checked regularly and kept readily accessible. It goes without saying that all cardiac rehabilitation staff should be certified in basic life support. Dependent on hospital protocol, certification of at least one staff member in advanced cardiac life support may be desirable.

SUMMARY

This chapter discusses the recognition and prevention of medical problems associated with early cardiac rehabilitation. An important concept that cannot be overemphasized is the use of good judgment in any dangerous or potentially life-threatening situation. Providing a safe environment for cardiac rehabilitation participants is the responsibility of every staff member who comes in contact with participants. Having procedures readily available to staff as well as specific guidelines for common medical problems can help prevent confusion and will enhance efficiency. A review of the emergency protocol on a regular basis helps staff members maintain familiarity with individual roles and responsibilities. The reputation and safety of cardiac rehabilitation programs depend on maintaining these standards of care.

References

Barnard, R.J., Gardner, G.W., Diaco, N.V., MacAlpin, R.N., & Kattus, A.A. (1973). Cardiovascular response to sudden strenuous exercise— heart rate, blood pressure, and ECG. *Journal of Applied Physiology, 34*, 833-834.

Barnard, R.J., MacAlpin, R.N., Kattus, A.A., & Buckberg, G.D. (1973). Ischemic responses to sudden strenuous exercise in healthy men. *Circulation, 48*, 936-942.

Borg, G. (1962). *Physical performance and perceived exertion*. Lund, Sweden: Gleerup.

Borg, G. (1978). Subjective effort in relation to physical performance and working capacity. In *Psychology: From research to practice* (pp. 333-361). New York: Plenum.

Carn, H.D., Frasher, W.G., & Stiverman, R. (1961). Graded activity program for safe return to self care after myocardial infarction. *Journal of the American Medical Association, 177*, 111-115.

Davidson, D.M., & DeBusk, R.F. (1980). Prognostic value of a single exercise test 3 weeks after uncomplicated myocardial infarction. *Circulation, 61*, 236-242.

Dillahurst, P.H., & Miller, A.B. (1979). Early treadmill testing after myocardial infarction. *Chest, 76*, 150-155.

Dion, W.F., Grevenow, P., Pollock, M.L., Squires, R.W., Foster, C., Johnson, W.D., & Schmidt, D.H. (1982). Medical problems and physiologic responses during supervised inpatient cardiac rehabilitation: The patient after coronary artery bypass grafting. *Heart and Lung, 11*, 248-255.

Ehsani, A.A., Martin, W.H., Heath, G.W., & Coyle, E.F. (1982). Cardiac effects of prolonged and intense exercise training in patients with coronary artery disease. *American Journal of Cardiology*, **50**, 246-254.

Epstein, S.E. (1982). Implications of probability analysis on the strategy used for noninvasive detection of coronary artery disease. *American Journal of Cardiology*, **46**, 491-499.

Fardy, P.S., Doll, N., Taylor, J., & Williams, M. (1982). Monitoring cardiac patients: How much is enough? *The Physician and Sportsmedicine*, **10**, 146-152.

Franklin, B.A., & Rubenfire, M. (1980). Exercise training in coronary heart disease: Mechanisms of improvement. *Practical Cardiology*, **6**, 84-89.

Granath, A., Sodermark, T., Winge, T., Volpe, U., & Zetterquist, S. (1977). Early work load tests for evaluation of long-term prognosis of acute myocardial infarction. *British Heart Journal*, **39**, 758-763.

Hanson, J.S., & Neede, W.H. (1970). Preliminary observations on physical training for hypertensive males. *Circulation Research*, **27**(Suppl. 1), 149.

Haskell, W.L. (1978). Cardiovascular complications during exercise training of cardiac patients. *Circulation*, **57**, 920-924.

Haskell, W.L. (1979). Mechanisms by which physical activity may enhance the clinical status of cardiac patients. In M.L. Pollock & D.H. Schmidt (Eds.), *Heart disease and rehabilitation* (pp. 276-296). Boston: Houghton-Mifflin.

Hellerstein, H.K., & Ford, A.B. (1957). Rehabilitation of the cardiac patient. *Journal of the American Medical Association*, **164**, 225-231.

Hellerstein, H.K. (1968). Exercise therapy in coronary disease. *Bulletin of the New York Academy of Medicine*, **44**, 1028-1047.

Hossack, K.F., & Hartwig, R. (1982). Cardiac arrest associated with supervised cardiac rehabilitation. *Journal of Cardiac Rehabilitation*, **2**, 402-408.

McNeer, J.F., Margolis, J.R., Lee, K.L., Kisslo, J.A., Peter, R.H., Kong, Y., Behar, V.S., Wallace, A.G., McCants, C.B., & Rosati, R.A. (1978). The role of the exercise test in the evaluation of patients for ischemic heart disease. *Circulation*, **57**, 64-70.

Sennett, S.M., Pollock, M.L., Pels, A.E., Foster, C., Dolatowski, R., & Patel, S. (1984). Medical problems of cardiac patients in an outpatient cardiac rehabilitation program. *Medicine and Science in Sports and Exercise*, **16**(2), 149.

Starling, M.R., Crawford, M.H., Kennedy, G.T., & O'Rourke, R.A. (1980). Exercise testing early after myocardial infarction: Predictive value for subsequent unstable angina and death. *American Journal of Cardiology*, **46**, 909-914.

Theroux, P., Waters, D.D., Halphen, C., Debaisieux, J.D., & Mizgala, H.F. (1979). Prognostic value of exercise testing soon after myocardial infarction. *New England Journal of Medicine*, **301**, 341-345.

Underhill, S.L., & Woods, S.L. (1982). *Cardiac nursing*. Philadelphia: J.B. Lippincott.

Wenger, N.K., & Hellerstein, H.K. (1984). *Rehabilitation of the coronary patient*. New York: John Wiley and Sons.

Chapter 6

Exercise Prescription for the Well-Conditioned Cardiac Patient

Janet A. Lunn

Rehabilitation has been defined as the process by which an individual is restored to an optimal physical, social, emotional, psychological, and vocational status. This process must incorporate methods to reverse or retard the underlying disease (Hellerstein & Ford, 1957; Frommer, 1976). Hundreds of cardiac rehabilitation programs exist in the United States. Most are designed according to this basic philosophy, incorporating guidelines established by the American College of Sports Medicine (ACSM) (1980), and the American Heart Association (AHA) (1979). These guidelines represent the current standard of care for safe and effective rehabilitation programs.

At the end of 6 to 12 months of the cardiac rehabilitation process, most cardiac patients reach a satisfactory level of cardiorespiratory fitness (ACSM, 1980; Pollock, Ward, & Foster, 1979). At this point many individuals are no longer interested in increasing the conditioning load, and thus a new phase begins which is called the maintenance phase. However, many others seek to further their exercise tolerance and programs in terms of variety, duration, frequency, and intensity.

With the recognition of the tremendous potential of cardiac patients to make extraordinary improvements in physical work capacity (Kavanaugh, Shepard, & Pandit, 1974; Kavanaugh, Shepard, & Kennedy, 1977), there exists a need for guidelines not only to establish minimum training thresholds for physical improvements but also to exceed these thresholds if the patient desires. The well-conditioned cardiac patient may request guidelines for such activities as 10-km and marathon running events, triathlons, and various sports such as racquetball, tennis, and weight lifting.

Indeed, the popular and scientific literature has reported cases of post-myocardial infarction (MI) and coronary artery bypass (CABG) surgery patients attempting and safely completing 26-mi marathon runs (Kavanaugh et al., 1974; Kavanaugh et al., 1977; Dressendorfer, Scaff, Wagner, & Gallup, 1977).

This chapter attempts to define the well-conditioned cardiac patient and then to provide guidelines for a safe exercise prescription that reaches beyond the traditional recommendations. Guidelines will be confined to cardiorespiratory fitness.

Physiological Justification

Two investigators have reported the results of cardiac rehabilitation patients performing 26-mi marathons (Kavanaugh et al., 1974; Dressendorfer et al., 1977). It was concluded that the subjects in these groups made appropriate physiological adjustments to the stresses of marathon training and running and that myocardial function was unimpaired. The two groups showed similar changes in $\dot{V}O_2$max and body composition. The mean peak in $\dot{V}O_2$max was 38.4 and 43.5 ml.kg-1.min-1 for the Hawaii (Dressendorfer et al., 1977) and Toronto (Kavanaugh et al., 1974) groups, respectively. This value is comparable to that for active, healthy men of similar age (Dehn & Bruce, 1972) but considerably higher than values for coronary heart disease (CHD) patients following physical conditioning (Ferguson, Petitclerc, 1974).

The percentage of $\dot{V}O_2$max during running is estimated from average velocity (Margaria, Cerretelli, & Aghemo, 1963), and thus indicates overall metabolic demand. It has been estimated that national-class, long-distance runners utilize an average of 75% of VO_2max (range: 68–82%) during marathon running (Costill & Fox, 1969). Values of 67–79% VO_2max and an average of 81% were noted for the Hawaii and Toronto groups, respectively. Thus, relative VO_2, as well as oxygen transport and utilization during marathon running in trained CHD patients, appears similar to healthy, competitive runners.

Measurements of heart rate taken on the Hawaii group (Dressendorfer et al., 1977) indicate an elevation of 6 bpm-1 in the last stage of the marathon, compared to the first two stages. Increased heart rate is a common finding during prolonged steady-state work and generally accompanies an increase in body temperature (Costill, 1970). (Possible slide off of s.v.) In addition, participants experienced an average weight loss of 3.1%. It was estimated that without fluid replacement weight loss from the marathon run would have averaged 5.1%. The observed loss of fluids had no appreciable affect on serum electrolyte balance. Researchers noted a lower respiratory exchange ratio after the race, which is consistent with findings that indicate a metabolic shift to fatty acids as glycogen storage is reduced, and a lower lactate accumulation compared to a brief running bout (Costill, 1969).

All of the subjects except one showed decreased running speed in the final stage of the race. Muscular exhaustion was clearly evident in three of five subjects. The investigators concluded that because blood lactate levels were low, serum glucose was normal, dehydration was minimal, serum electrolytes were mostly unchanged, and body temperatures were well regulated, muscular exhaustion resulted from depletion of muscle glycogen stores. Furthermore, electrocardiograph (ECG) and (STI) measurements were not significantly altered by the marathon race. The investigators concluded that left ventricular performance was adequate.

Both the Dressendorfer et al. (1977) and the Kavanagh et al. (1974) studies concluded that many well-trained post-myocardial infarction patients will respond favorably to the heavy physiological demands of marathon running. They cautioned, however, that this task should be undertaken only under close medical supervision and coaching.

This paper is not intended to represent marathon running as the mode of activity appropriate or desirable for the well-conditioned cardiac patient. Running is, however, one type of activity that may be desired by some rehabilitation participants; the favorable results of the two rehabilitation groups indicate that, for some individuals at least, such a task can be accomplished in a safe manner. The physiological data indicate that physical activity of lesser stress than marathon running but more extensive than the traditional exercise prescription may be appropriate and safe for many individuals with CHD.

The Advanced Exercise Prescription

An absolute list of those patients who would qualify for an advanced exercise prescription does not exist. The following criteria are based on my personal experience as a rehabilitation program director, communication with other program directors, and the scientific literature identifying elements of safe exercise execution.

A patient should be considered for an advanced exercise prescription only after one year has passed since his or her myocardial infarction or CABG surgery. The individual should be stable in a supervised rehabilitation program for a minimum of 12 months. The expected increase in $\dot{V}O_2$max to 20% above the untrained level (Ferguson et al., 1974) should be achieved, and angina pectoris should be absent during exercise both at the appropriate training heart rate and at an intensity in excess of this, providing adequate warm-up has taken place. (Some individuals may elicit myocardial ischemia and develop symptoms of angina pectoris when they do not warm up properly; however, with adequate warm-up they may be able to sustain a physiologic training intensity free of myocardial ischemia and angina pectoris).

Myocardial ischemia should be absent at the target heart rate and within a 12-beat reserve above the training level. Malignant arrhythmias (e.g., paired or runs of premature ventricular contractions; multifocal, premature ventricular contractions; premature ventricular contractions that occur at a rate of 10 per minute or greater; tachyarrhythmias; and atrial-ventricular or ventricular conduction disturbances) should be absent on graded exercise test (GXT) and Holter monitoring. A normal inotropic and chronotropic response should be present. In addition, rehabilitation participants should have the desire to extend their exercise programs; it should not be a program or rehabilitation staff goal. A summary of these characteristics is presented in Table 6.1.

Table 6.1   Candidates for an Advanced Exercise Prescription

Minimum 12 months post-myocardial infarction/CABG surgery

Minimum 12 months in supervised cardiac rehabilitation program

Attainment of 20% improvement in VO_2max over untrained state

Angina pectoris absent

Myocardial ischemia absent to within a 12-beat reserve above target heart rate

Malignant arrhythmias absent

Normal inotropic response on GXT

Normal chronotropic response on GXT

Fundamentals of the Advanced Exercise Prescription

The following recommendations are based on the clinical experience of numerous cardiac rehabilitation program directors and the established guidelines for safe and effective exercise training programs (ACSM, 1980). Because cardiac rehabilitation deals with individuals in which coronary blood flow and impaired ventricular wall mechanics increase the variability of physiologic responses to acute and chronic exercise, a combination of objective and subjective factors should be considered when the individual progresses in an exercise program. Rehabilitation patients desiring to increase their exercise routine should attempt to do so in the following manner:

1. Increase frequency of exercise initially. Maintain the usual duration but add additional exercise days at no greater than one new bout per week, every other week. Five to six days per week should be the maximum frequency (five is the frequency of choice). A daily exercise program at conditioning intensity is usually undesirable.
2. Increase the duration of exercise by no greater than 10% every other week.
3. Alternate days of greater and lesser workouts. Less fatigue seems to result if the increase in duration is not repeated with each workout.
4. Maintain the existing target heart rate. At this point in the training regimen, the $\dot{V}O_2$max will undergo little if any change (Pollock et al., 1979). Because the target heart rate is a function of safe physical work capacity (ACSM, 1980), an increase in frequency and duration of the exercise regimen will not warrant an increase in target heart rate. The inclusion of anaerobic or speed workouts to improve performance times is probably contraindicated.

It is extremely important that individuals extending their exercise routines develop an unfailing sensitivity to such factors as fatigue and a change in perceived exertion. Individuals under all training circumstances should feel rested and not fatigued 1 hr following exercise (ACSM, 1980). The signs and symptoms of overexertion include:

- Insomnia
- Weakness
- Fatigue
- Muscular cramping
- Skeletal muscle pain
- Gastrointestinal disturbances
- Nausea
- Vomiting
- Light-headedness
- Arrythmias
- Continued high heart rate

The patient should be familiar with these symptoms and should immediately decrease the frequency, duration, and/or intensity of the exercise program.

Elements of the traditional exercise prescription such as adequate cardiovascular warm-up and cool-down, and consistency with the exercise routine cannot be overemphasized. As for all individuals with and without cardiovascular disease, the intensity, duration, and frequency of exercise should be decreased during extreme environmental conditions (Rowell,

1974; Wyndham, 1973; Drinkwater, Ravin, Horvath, 1974; Horvath, Ravin, & Dahms, 1975; Folinsbee, Silverman, & Shephard, 1975) and avoided during illness (ACSM, 1980). The incidence of these untoward symptoms will be minimized if patients maintain an exercise program free of competition with themselves (for an improvement in performance times) or others.

Continuing Evaluation

To assess their continued safety, patients should have an annual medical evaluation to include a GXT and a review of their exercise program by the physician or exercise specialist. In addition, the staff member should attach a Holter monitor to the patient during a routine exercise workout or have the patient undertake an ECG/blood pressure-monitored, simulated training session.

Comprehensive Rehabilitation Strategy

Success in the exercise aspect of the rehabilitation protocol does not preclude the necessity of continued adherence to modification of other coronary risk factors. The role of exercise in the prevention or retardation of atherosclerosis is unclear, although recent epidemiological and animal studies indicate a probable role (Paffenbarger, Wing, & Hyde, 1978; Saloren, Puska, & Tuomilehto, 1982; Kramsch, Aspen, & Abramowitz, 1981). The primary influences on the incidence and rate of atherosclerosis continue to be elevated cholesterol/HDL ratio, increased blood pressure, and cigarette smoking (Stamler, 1979). Whereas continuation of an appropriate exercise program is highly desirable, adherence to a lifestyle that optimizes the coronary risk factor profile is essential.

The clinical status of CHD patients can be greatly enhanced by a chronic cardiorespiratory exercise program due to a variety of physiological phenomena (Haskell, 1979). There is, however, no evidence to indicate the reversibility of the atherosclerotic process by exercise. One report (Selvester, Camp, & Sanmarcos, 1977) notes a relationship between exercise and rate of atherosclerosis but these results have been critically reviewed by Haskell (1979).

Because of the tremendous improvements in the clinical status of CHD patients, it is often easy to lose sight of the fact that the disease process not only continues to exist but may be progressing. Both rehabilitation staff and CHD patients need to be continually reminded of this fact to minimize heroic physical feats. As yet, no data indicate that an exercise program of high duration, frequency, and intensity is more beneficial physiologically or psychologically.

Conclusion

The participation of cardiac patients in modes of exercise that reach beyond the traditional exercise prescription is controversial, and its value often contested (Hellerstein, 1977). Although it seems reasonable to state that marathon running is an unrealistic and unnecessary goal for most cardiac patients, many of today's popular activities are well within the safe grasp of many of these individuals. Like individuals free of coronary heart disease, CHD patients want to feel physically competent and to enjoy social events that require an energy expenditure over and above that of the traditional rehabilitation program design. Given proper guidance for safe execution of such exercise programs, cardiac patients may experience the benefits and rewards granted those free of coronary disease.

References

American College of Sports Medicine. (1980). *Guidelines for graded exercise testing and exercise prescription* (2nd ed.). Philadelphia: Lea and Febiger.

American Heart Association. (1979). *The exercise standards book*. Dallas, TX: Author.

Costill, D.L. (1970). Metabolic responses during distance running. *Journal of Applied Physiology, 28*, 251-255.

Costill, D.L., & Fox, E.L. (1969). Energetics of marathon running. *Medicine and Science in Sports and Exercise, 1*, 81-86.

Dehn, M., & Bruce, R.A. (1972). Longitudinal variations in maximum oxygen intake with age and activity. *Journal of Applied Physiology, 33*, 805-807.

Dressendorfer, R.H., Scaff, J.H., Wagner, J.O., & Gallup, J.D. (1977). Metabolic adjustments to marathon running in coronary patients. *Annals of the New York Academy of Sciences, 301*, 465-483.

Drinkwater, B.L., Ravin, P.B., & Horvath, S.M. (1974). Air pollution, exercise, and heat stress. *Archives of Environmental Health, 28*, 177-182.

Fardy, P. In: Heart Disease and Rehabilitation.

Ferguson, R.J., & Petitclerc, G. (1974). Effect of physical training on treadmill exercise capacity, collateral circulation, and progression of coronary disease. *American Journal of Cardiology, 34*, 764-768.

Folinsbee, L.J., Silverman, F., & Shephard, R.J. (1975). Exercise responses following ozone exposure. *Journal of Applied Physiology, 38*, 996-1001.

Frommer, P.L. (1976). *Needs and opportunities for rehabilitating the coronary heart disease patient* (Report No. 76-750). Washington, DC: Department of Health, Education and Welfare.

Haskell, W.L. (1979). Mechanisms by which physical activity may enhance the clinical status of cardiac patients. In M.L. Pollock & D.H. Schmidt (Eds.), *Heart disease and rehabilitation* (pp. 276-296). Boston: Houghton-Mifflin.

Hellerstein, H. (1977). Limitations of marathon running in coronary patients: Anatomic and physiologic determinants. *Annals of the New York Academy of Sciences*, **301**, 484-494.

Hellerstein, H.K., & Ford, A.B. (1957). Rehabilitation of cardiac patients. *Journal of the American Medical Association*, **164**, 225-231.

Horvath, S.M., Ravin, P.B., & Dahms, T.E. (1975). Maximal aerobic capacity at different levels of carboxyhemoglobin. *Journal of Applied Physiology*, **38**, 300-303.

Kavanagh, T., Shephard, R.H., & Kennedy, J. (1977). Characteristics of postcoronary marathon runners. *Annals of the New York Academy of Sciences*, **301**, 455-465.

Kavanagh, T., Shepard, R.H., & Pandit, V. (1974). Marathon running after myocardial infarction. *Journal of the American Medical Association*, **229**, 1602-1605.

Kramsch, D.M., Aspen, A.J., & Abramowitz, B.M. (1981). Reduction of coronary atherosclerosis by moderate conditioning exercise in monkeys on an atherogenic diet. *New England Journal of Medicine*, **305**, 1483-1489.

Margaria, R., Cerretelli, P., & Aghemo (1963). Energy cost of running. *Journal of Applied Physiology*, **18**, 367-370.

Paffenbarger, R.S., Wing, A.L., & Hyde, R.T. (1978). Physical activity as an index of heart attack risk in college alumni. *American Journal of Epidemiology*, **108**, 161-175.

Pollock, M.L., Ward, A., & Foster, C. (1979). Exercise prescription for rehabilitation of the cardiac patient. In M.L. Pollock & D.H. Schmidt (Eds.), *Heart disease and rehabilitation* (pp. 413-445). Boston: Houghton-Mifflin.

Rowell, L.B. (1974). Human cardiovascular adjustments to exercise and thermal stress. *Physiological Review*, **54**, 75-159.

Salonen, J.T., Puska, P., & Tuomilehto, J. (1982). Physical activity and risk of myocardial infarction, cerebral stroke and death: A longitudinal study in eastern Finland. *American Journal of Epidemiology*, **115**, 526-537.

Selvester, R., Camp, J., & Sanmarcos, M. (1977). Effects of exercise training on progression of documented coronary atherosclerosis in men. *Annals of the New York Academy of Sciences*, **301**, 495-508.

Stamler, J. (1979). Research related to risk factors. *Circulation*, **60**, 1575-1587.

Wyndham, C.H. (1973). The physiology of exercise under heat stress. *Annual Review of Physiology*, **35**, 193-200.

Chapter 7

Upper Extremity Exercise in the Phase II Setting

Ruth M. Anderson

The comprehensive multiphasic approach to cardiac rehabilitation implicitly encourages a lifetime commitment to proper health habits as a means to achieving and maintaining cardiovascular health. During the initial stages of an organized program the main objective is to return the heart and general body functions to their optimum performance levels. This is accomplished by focusing educational and therapeutic modalities on the improvement of the psychologic, social, physiologic, and vocational status of the patient. Although the rehabilitation team is responsible for facilitating this process, it is the participant's acceptance of the goals and motivation for accomplishing them that determine the final outcome.

Medically supervised clinic- or hospital-based outpatient programs designed to achieve these objectives during the 2-4 months following hospital dismissal for myocardial infarction and coronary artery bypass surgery are commonly referred to as Phase II. This chapter will focus on the use of upper extremity exercise modalities in the Phase II setting.

The safe and effective supervision of the activities of cardiac patients during the rehabilitative Phase II process requires an awareness of the individual's cardiac capacity and the assignment of work loads that will assure that the patient maintains an adequate cardiac reserve. Although certain limitations must be established and observed during the convalescent stages, it is important to recognize that activities that will maximize the recovery and restoration of the patient for return to vocational activity must be implemented as early as possible.

Safety is achieved in the Phase II setting by offering continuous electrocardiograph (ECG) monitoring and periodic blood pressure measurements during activity. In the initial stages of the supervised Phase II program, the participant is gradually introduced to calisthenic and dynamic activities that will increase heart rate up to 60% of maximal capacity. Over the subsequent weeks the intensity and duration of these activities are increased as cardiovascular adaptation occurs. All too often in the past, Phase II programs have focused their attention on lower extremity training to the exclusion of upper extremity muscle strengthening and flexibility exercises (Hellerstein & Franklin, 1978). Walking, jogging, bicycling, and swimming are most often used in organized cardiac rehabilitation programs (Meyer, 1984; Wilson, 1975). Of these, only swimming demands use of both arm and leg muscles. During the early stages of rehabilitation, swimming is not commonly prescribed due to lack of available facilities and the higher interindividual variability in energy cost between patients of varying skill levels (Haskell, 1978; Hellerstein & Franklin, 1978). Walking, jogging, and bicycling are activities that do not require a great deal of skill to maintain a prescribed exercise intensity and are beneficial in developing cardiovascular endurance. However, most recreational and job-related tasks require a predominant amount of upper extremity activity and minimal sustained lower extremity exercise (Ford & Hellerstein, 1958; Ford, Hellerstein, & Turell, 1959). Further, there is no transfer of cardiovascular training effect to the arms when leg exercises are performed exclusively (Clausen, Trap-Jensen, & Lassen, 1970). Exercise training is muscle specific; therefore all muscle groups must be stressed if general body conditioning is to occur in preparation for return to occupational tasks and leisure-time pursuits.

It is important to recognize that the circulatory and metabolic demands of upper extremity work loads are augmented in comparison with lower extremity work. Generally, systolic blood pressure and heart rate response will be greater at a given MET level for arm work; as a result, ischemic responses will occur at lower work loads (Astrand & Rodahl, 1977; Schwade, Blomqvist, & Shapiro, 1977). Additionally, there may be significant interindividual variability in the hemodynamic responses to arm exercise.

If indeed we are interested in returning the cardiac patient to a functional capacity that will allow for safe return to activities of daily living and to gainful employment, it becomes imperative to institute upper extremity strengthening exercises in the supervised Phase II program where deleterious responses may be disclosed and appropriate recommendations made (Haskell, 1978). This is particularly significant when dealing with an industrial-based or manual labor populations in which the vocational demands for upper extremity strength and flexibility may be more prevalent and the socioeconomic burdens are powerful enough to encourage a return to work (Ford & Hellerstein, 1958; Ford et al., 1959; Hellerstein & Franklin, 1978).

Hellerstein and Friedman (1970) have reported evidence that patients who did not experience symptoms were far more likely to return to work and sexual activity after myocardial infarction. Work evaluation units have been established to examine the issues pertinent to cardiac patients returning to work, and to problems that may prevent them from returning to work (Levenson, 1969).

If the work environment and physical tasks involved can be simulated during the outpatient therapy sessions, patients who experience symptom-free success in completing exercise utilizing the upper extremity may be more confident about returning to their jobs requiring arm movement. If the patient is unable to accomplish job-related tasks involving the upper extremity without injury or symptomatic episodes, it is the responsibility of the rehabilitative team to communicate alternative recommendations via the physician so that the patient is protected.

Functional Evaluation

Because hemodynamic response to exercise can vary in cardiac patients, primarily relative to myocardial status, clinical interest should be focused on the assessment of functional capacity. Initially a good medical history and cardiovascular examination should be obtained. Exercise response will vary according to age, sex, pharmacological intervention, and myocardial function. Also, the history should elicit a response to the basic question of what the patient's exercise desires are and the completion of an occupational activity profile (see Figure 7.1).

The purpose of the graded exercise test is to detect exertional dangers ahead of time. Continuous ECG monitoring and interval measurement of blood pressure should be done in order to assess heart rate and blood pressure response and changes that might be related to therapy and prognosis, such as ST-segment changes, frequent arrhythmias, or excessive exertional hypotension.

Secondary to detecting dangers of physical exertion, the purpose of the exercise test is to individually assess functional capacity in METs, which can then be correlated to the approximate level and amount of exercise the patient may engage in on his or her own. The ability to hemodynamically adapt well to measured work loads during clinical testing enables the physician to prescribe a safe yet adequate level of exercise for the Phase II participant wishing to pursue sport or work activities. Periodic reevaluations are used to update the exercise prescription and assess the value of the rehabilitative process.

OCCUPATIONAL ACTIVITY

WHAT IS YOUR JOB TITLE?_____

HAS YOUR JOB TITLE CHANGED IN THE LAST YEAR?_____

IF YOU ARE RETIRED OR UNEMPLOYED, DO YOU HAVE A SOURCE OF INCOME? _____

DESCRIBE WHAT PHYSICAL ACTIVITY YOU DO DURING A TYPICAL WORKING DAY _____

_____

WHAT IS THE DISTANCE FROM YOUR HOME TO YOUR PLACE OF EMPLOYMENT?_____ mile

HOW LONG DOES IT TAKE TO GET TO WORK ONE WAY? _____ minute

HOW MANY HOURS A DAY DO YOU USUALLY WORK? _____ hour

HOW MANY TIMES PER MONTH DO YOU WORK OVERTIME? _____ times per month

HOW MANY HOURS DO YOU USUALLY WORK OVERTIME ON EACH OCCASION?_____ hour

HOW MANY REST PERIODS DO YOU HAVE DURING THE DAY INCLUDING LUNCH? _____ rest period

DOES YOUR JOB INVOLVE THE OPERATION OF MACHINERY? ___ YES ___ NO   DESCRIBE_

_____

ARE YOU RESPONSIBLE FOR THE SAFETY OF OTHERS? ___ YES ___ NO   DESCRIBE ___

_____

_____

ARE YOU OR ANYONE AROUND YOU IN DANGER SHOULD YOU FAINT? ___ YES ___ NO

DESCRIBE _____

_____

ARE YOU UNDER ANY EMOTIONAL STRESS AT WORK? ___ YES ___ NO   DESCRIBE_____

_____

_____

DURING A TYPICAL WORKING DAY LIST THE NUMBER OF HOURS YOU SPEND DOING THESE THREE ACTIVITIES. SITTING _____ HOURS STANDING _____ HOURS WALKING _____ HOURS. DOES YOUR WORK INVOLVE ANY OF THE FOLLOWING? CHECK THE FOLLOWING AND DESCRIBE THE ACTIVITY, HOW MUCH AND HOW OFTEN IT IS DONE. GIVE APPROXIMATE OR EXACT WEIGHTS IF KNOWN

___ PUSHING _____

___ PULLING_____

___ CARRYING_____

___ LIFTING _____

___ ARMS ABOVE HEAD _____

___ CRAMPED POSITION_____

___ STAIR CLIMBING_____

___ CRAWLING _____

___ OTHER _____

___ NONE OF THESE _____

ARE YOU EXPOSED TO ANY OF THESE ENVIRONMENTAL CONDITIONS? CHECK AND DESCRIBE.

___ COLD _____

___ HEAT _____

___ HUMIDITY _____

___ ALTITUDE _____

___ FUMES _____

___ OTHER _____

___ NONE OF THESE _____

Figure 7.1.   Occupational activity profile.

Exercise Tests for Upper and Lower Extremities

Because habitual daily activities and vocational tasks require both dynamic (isotonic) and static (isometric) muscular contractions, involving both the upper and lower extremities, the effects of these on heart rate and blood pressure must be equally evaluated. Hemodynamic responses differ between dynamic and static exercise as well as between arm and leg work (Hellerstein & Franklin, 1978; Painter & Hanson, 1984). Common isometric activities are characterized by an effort in which tension develops within the muscle group but no muscle shortening or joint movement occurs. When an effort involves the development of tension with muscle shortening and movement, it is an isotonic activity.

Isometric contractions demand a greater increase in systolic and diastolic blood pressure when compared with isotonic contractions. This increased blood pressure is met by an increase in cardiac output. The magnitude of the hemodynamic responses to isometric contractions augment as the percentage of maximal voluntary contraction increases beyond 20%. These responses will differ in cardiac patients with varying degrees of myocardial left ventricular dysfunction, systemic vascular resistance, and pharmacological intervention. Those with poor left ventricular function will not have the expected increase in cardiac output to meet the demands of isometric contractions. They can be expected to have lower ejection fractions as a result of an increased end-systolic volume (Painter & Hanson, 1984). In addition, significant rhythm and ST-T changes can occur as myocardial oxygen demand increases (Hellerstein & Franklin, 1978).

Standard treadmill or bicycle exercise tests should be used to assess tolerance for isotonic activities. It will then be possible to proceed with testing such moderate isometric exercise as will keep the rate pressure product (RPP) within the RPP tolerated on the treadmill or bike. The specific isometric task or arm exercise the patient may desire or need to engage in to accomplish recreational and vocational tasks may be tested (Schwade et al., 1977). For example, a patient may be asked to lift a specific weight or object such as a concrete block if bricklaying is the goal or carry golf clubs while walking on the treadmill if playing golf is the goal. It is unlikely that the exercise test will precisely simulate all of the actual physical and emotional demands of the occupational or recreational environment. Ford and Hellerstein (1958) and Ford et al. (1959) have studied industrial settings and concluded that the cardiovascular responses to exercise testing fluctuate from actual on-the-job responses. The exercise test will, however, reveal useful information about the patient's myocardial aerobic capacity and hemodynamic response to equal energy expenditures. Relative energy costs for many occupational, recreational, and daily life activities have been established (Astrand & Rodahl, 1977; Fox, Naughton, & Gorman, 1972).

Numerous arm ergometer devices and test protocols are now available, which can be used to accurately assess tolerance for arm exercise utilizing a variety of muscle groups and skills (Hellerstein & Franklin, 1978). These devices can then serve as a training modality during the monitored Phase II program.

For isotonic activities a percentage of the peak heart rate or MET value attained during testing can be prescribed. The patient's heart rate and rhythm are then monitored at the prescribed level during the Phase II exercise sessions. Moderate isometric activities can be prescribed in a similar manner; however, a 20-25% further cutback on heart rate or MET level should be calculated in order to allow for the higher blood pressure response elicited by this type of effort.

For activities of daily living and occupational tasks, the patient can be given a MET chart (Fox et al., 1972) listing various leisure-time and work activities and instructed to match the prescribed MET level with desirable activities on the list. Approximate allowances must be made for variations in environmental temperature, surface area on which the activity is performed, and speed at which the activity is accomplished. For an unsupervised home-based exercise program the work loads should be conservatively prescribed to minimize the risk of adverse responses due to overexertion.

Phase II Therapy Sessions

The purpose of the Phase II exercise therapy sessions is to progressively improve the patient's functional capacity while monitoring for any adverse signs or symptoms of intolerance. The exercise prescription should outline guidelines for safely achieving a conditioning effect of the upper and lower extremities. Cardiovascular conditioning improves with exercise engaged in three times per week for 20-40 min in duration and of an intensity that is 60-80% of functional capacity as assessed by the graded exercise test (Hellerstein & Franklin, 1978). This can be accomplished with continuous endurance activity, interval work, or a combination of both. Generally, interval work can be accomplished at a higher heart rate or MET work load than endurance work because it is not sustained for longer than 5-min intervals and allows for a recovery period between work phases. Lactate accumulation is thus minimized and the patient is able to perform greater total work before muscle fatigue limits continuation. Circuit-interval training, alternating upper and lower extremity modalities, is advantageous in reducing the degree of fatigue of specific muscle groups while assuring that conditioning effects will occur in both the arm and leg muscles (Meyer, 1984). Intermittent work loads of high-intensity effort followed by 3-4 min recovery periods correlate better with actual occupational demands (Blomqvist, 1978). The nature of each patient's job requirements in terms of peak work loads and overall average work load must be considered when prescribing the modalities and intensity during Phase II.

During the initial Phase II sessions the focus should be on gradually introducing the patient to the exercise routine and encouraging the formation of a trusting relationship with the program staff. This will enhance communication among the patient, program staff, and physician, thereby facilitating the rehabilitative process (Task Force on Cardiovascular Rehabilitation of the National Heart and Lung Institute, 1974).

EXERCISE RECORD

NAME _____   PHYSICIAN _____

DIAGNOSIS _____   TARGET HEART RATE _____

WEEK _____ DATE _____ DATE _____ DATE _____

RESTING PULSE RATE: _____   _____   _____

WARM-UP TIME (PR): _____ (   ) _____ (   ) _____ (   )

(FLEXIBILITY)

ENDURANCE EXERCISE	ENDURANCE EXERCISE	ENDURANCE EXERCISE
TDM TIME _____	TDM TIME _____	TDM TIME _____
MPH _____ GRADE _____	MPH _____ GRADE _____	MPH _____ GRADE _____
BIKE TIME _____	BIKE TIME _____	BIKE TIME _____
WORK LOAD _____	WORK LOAD _____	WORK LOAD _____
PEAK PULSE RATE: _____	PEAK PULSE RATE: _____	PEAK PULSE RATE: _____

INTERVAL EXERCISE (3–5 min)	INTERVAL EXERCISE (3–5 min)	INTERVAL EXERCISE (3–5 min)
AIR-DYNE _____	AIR-DYNE _____	AIR-DYNE _____
ROWING _____	ROWING _____	ROWING _____
ARM ERGOMETER _____	ARM ERGOMETER _____	ARM ERGOMETER _____
SHOULDER WHEEL _____	SHOULDER WHEEL _____	SHOULDER WHEEL _____
WALL PULLEY _____	WALL PULLEY _____	WALL PULLEY _____
PEAK PULSE RATE: _____	PEAK PULSE RATE: _____	PEAK PULSE RATE: _____

STRENGTH TRAINING	WT	SETS/REPS	WT	SETS/REPS	WT	SETS/REPS
SIT- OR CURL-UPS	___	___ / ___	___	___ / ___	___	___ / ___
BENCH PRESS	___	___ / ___	___	___ / ___	___	___ / ___
ARM CURLS	___	___ / ___	___	___ / ___	___	___ / ___
ARM RAISE	___	___ / ___	___	___ / ___	___	___ / ___
WRIST CURLS	___	___ / ___	___	___ / ___	___	___ / ___
HAMSTRING CURLS	___	___ / ___	___	___ / ___	___	___ / ___
FRENCH PRESS	___	___ / ___	___	___ / ___	___	___ / ___
FLIES	___	___ / ___	___	___ / ___	___	___ / ___
OTHERS	___	___ / ___	___	___ / ___	___	___ / ___
COOL-DOWN TIME (PR)	( )		( )		( )	

COMMENTS: _____   COMMENTS: _____   COMMENTS: _____

Figure 7.2. Record for monitoring exercise.

The exercise routine should consist of a warm-up period involving over-all body stretching and bending exercises for improving flexibility, a training period utilizing various arm and leg modalities for cardiovascular conditioning and muscular strengthening, and a cool-down period where the stretching and bending exercises are repeated in reverse order.

Aquatic exercise, if pool facilities are available in the Phase II setting, can be very useful in improving both strength and flexibility of upper extremity muscle groups. Activities isolating specific groups may be performed in shallow water requiring minimal skill execution and maximal safety. The buoyancy of the water and its added resistance will encourage strength development while minimizing orthopedic concerns.

Muscle groups that are particularly weak or are needed for performing specific occupational tasks should be identified. Specific strengthening exercises can then be introduced progressively under monitored conditions (see Figure 7.2). Modalities that can be used include the rowing machine, arm ergometer, shoulder wheel, free weights, Schwinn Air-Dyne, and wall pulley (see Figures 7.3-7.8).

In advanced phases of the rehabilitative process, enjoyable recreational activities that focus on upper torso movements such as volleyball, basketball, racquetball, and badminton can be introduced to maintain upper extremity training and encourage program adherence. These activities should be modified to discourage competition while enhancing the participant's fun and achievement.

Special attention should be focused on muscle groups affecting the lower back and proper body mechanics for bending and lifting in patients with a history of low back pain. In particular, these individuals should be discouraged from hyperextending the back during the pull-back phase of the rowing machine movement. These participants should be prescribed abdominal strengthening exercises as well.

The shoulder wheel is a particularly useful device for patients recovering from coronary bypass surgery who tend to restrict movement of the chest musculature. The wheel encourages a full range of movement of the shoulder girdle for improved flexibility, and resistance can be set to progressively increase strength development of these same muscles.

Weight training with free weights can effectively develop upper extremity strength. Patients should be supervised closely during weight training to assure that they are not performing a Valsalva maneuver, which can result in significant deleterious changes in hemodynamic responses and ST-T wave changes (Hellerstein & Franklin, 1978). They should be initially encouraged to use low resistance with increased repetitions and should be closely monitored with rhythm checks and interval blood pressure measurements. The response of blood pressure to weight lifting is linear to the percentage of maximal voluntary contraction

(Donald, Lind, & McNicol, 1967). As the patient achieves an increase in upper extremity strength through free resistive weight training he or she should be able to perform occupational tasks that require lifting, pushing, pulling, or carrying objects with a lower percentage of maximal voluntary contraction and therefore a lower blood pressure response (Hellerstein & Franklin, 1978). This would also be transferable to recreational activities such as golfing in which the improved muscular strength and efficiency of upper extremity muscle groups should result in a better golf score as well as lower blood pressure response to swinging or carrying golf clubs. To simulate the actual response to such activities, encourage the patient to bring his or her golf clubs into the Phase II environment and perform a typical swing while being monitored.

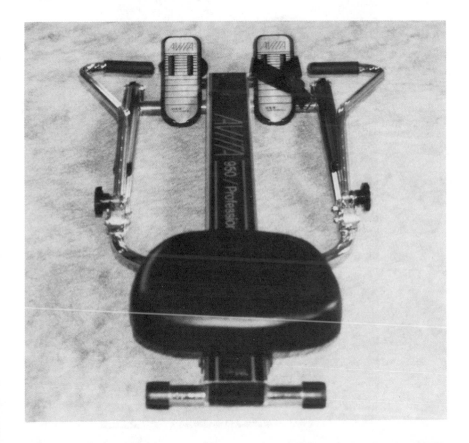

Figure 7.3. Rowing machine. Utilized to strengthen muscle groups of the back, stomach, arms, shoulders, and legs. Resistance is regulated by moving the position of the oars on the tension device.

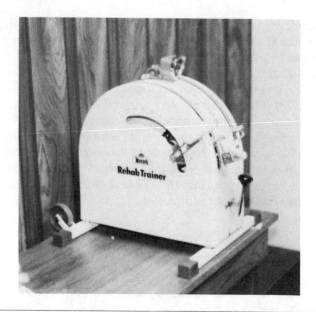

Figure 7.4. Arm ergometer. This machine uses muscles of the back, shoulder, arms, and chest and can be adjusted to increase or decrease work loads.

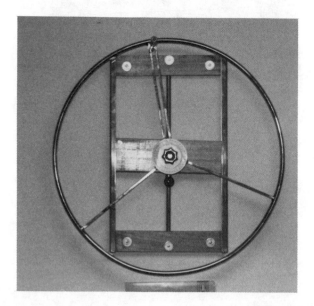

Figure 7.5. Shoulder wheel. Excellent for achieving range of motion of the shoulder, upper back, and chest muscles, which is especially helpful for postsurgical patients. The wheel, which is attached to a wall, can be adjusted to various heights and tensions to vary the work load.

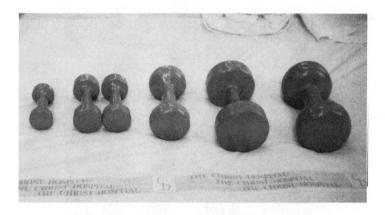

Figure 7.6. Free weights. Dumbbells in 1, 2, 3, 5, 6.6, 10, 12, and 15 lb are used while performing various upper body exercises. The number of repetitions and amount of weight are adjusted to gradually increase muscular strength and endurance of isolated muscle groups. Similar arm exercises, once learned in the monitored setting, may be done at home with household items such as canned goods or milk jugs filled with sand serving as the weights.

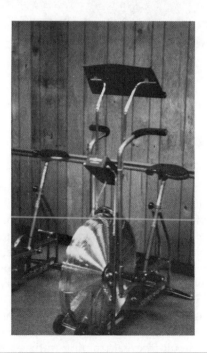

Figure 7.7. Schwinn Air-Dyne. This versatile bike is used for leg or arm work, or a combination of the two. The work load is determined by the exerciser's pedaling faster or slower as tolerated.

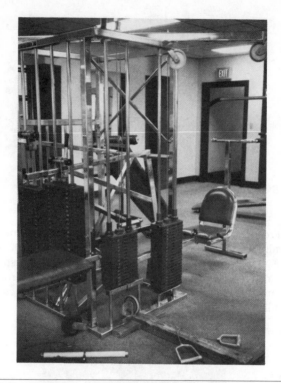

Figure 7.8. Wall pulley. These weights are attached to the wall. A rope and pulley system attached to the weights can be moved in various ways to exercise different muscle groups with varying resistance added as tolerated.

Summary

If Phase II cardiac rehabilitation programs are to achieve their goal of restoring patients to their optimal functional capacity for safely accomplishing activities of daily living and employment, they must incorporate a blend of exercises to improve cardiovascular endurance and muscular strength and flexibility of the upper and lower extremities. The training effect should result in a lowering of heart rate and blood pressure response and, therefore, lower demand on the cardiac reserve for a given submaximal work load. Because exercise training is specific to the muscle groups utilized, it is important to train both arms and legs if the desired hemodynamic adaptations are to occur for performing tasks that will use these extremities. Circuit-interval training initiated during the Phase II outpatient program will allow the participant to perform higher work intensities with a lower level of lactic acid and therefore an ameliorated sense of fatigue with each work load (Meyer, 1984).

References

Åstrand, P.O., & Rodahl, K. (1977). *Textbook of work physiology*. New York: McGraw-Hill.

Blomqvist, C.G. (1978). Clinical exercise physiology. In N.K. Wenger & H.K. Hellerstein (Eds.), *Rehabilitation of the coronary patient* (pp. 133-148). New York: John Wiley.

Clausen, J.P., Trap-Jensen, J., & Lassen, N.A. (1970). The effects of training on the heart rate during arm and leg exercise. *Scandinavian Journal of Clinical Laboratory Investigations, 26*, 295.

Donald, K.W., Lind, A.R., & McNicol, G.W. (1967). Cardiovascular responses to sustained (static) contractions. *Circulation Research, 20-21*, 1-15.

Ford, A.B., & Hellerstein, H.K. (1958). Work and heart disease: I. A physiologic study in the factory. *Circulation, 18*, 823.

Ford, A.B., Hellerstein, H.K., & Turell, D.J. (1959). Work and heart disease: II. A physiologic study in a steel mill. *Circulation, 20*, 537.

Fox, S.M., Naughton, J.P., & Gorman, P.A. (1972). Physical activity and cardiovascular health: III. The exercise prescription: Frequency and type of activity. *Modern Concepts of Cardiovascular Disease, 41*, 25.

Haskell, W.L. (1978). Design and implementation of cardiac conditioning programs. In N.K. Wenger & H.K. Hellerstein (Eds.), *Rehabilitation of the coronary patient* (pp. 203-241). New York: John Wiley.

Hellerstein, H.K., & Franklin, B.A. (1978). Exercise testing and prescription. In N.K. Wenger & H.K. Hellerstein (Eds.), *Rehabilitation of the coronary patient* (pp. 149-202). New York: John Wiley.

Hellerstein, H.K., & Friedman, E.H. (1970). Sexual activity and the post-coronary patient. *Archives of Internal Medicine, 125*, 987.

Levenson, R.M. (1969). Work evaluation units as a resource in exercise programs. *Journal of the South Carolina Medical Association, 65*(12), 69.

Meyer, G.C. (1984). The role of circuit interval and continuous conditioning in cardiac rehabilitation. In L.K. Hall (Ed.), *Cardiac rehabilitation: Exercise testing and prescription* (pp. 193-204). Spectrum.

Painter, P.L., & Hanson, P. (1984). Isometric exercise: Implications for cardiac rehabilitation. In L.K. Hall (Ed.), *Cardiac rehabilitation: Exercise testing and prescription* (pp. 223-242). Spectrum.

Schwade, J., Blomqvist, C.G., & Shapiro, W. (1977). A comparison of the response to arm and leg work in patients with ischemic heart disease. *American Heart Journal, 94,* 203.

Task Force on Cardiovascular Rehabilitation of the National Heart and Lung Institute. (1974). *Needs and opportunities for rehabilitating the coronary heart disease patient.* Washington, DC: Department of Health, Education, and Welfare.

Wilson, P.K. (Ed.). (1975). Adult fitness and cardiac rehabilitation. Baltimore: University Park Press.

Chapter 8

The Role of Computers in Cardiac Rehabilitation

Daniel R. Timmons

Computer information management systems have been accepted as an integral part of the modern health care facility including both hospital and clinical settings. However, individual departmental computerization in most facilities has not met the challenge of this technological marvel.

Most hospitals and clinics have adopted the computer to perform typical duties such as billing, inventory, word processing, and other administrative data management tasks. Another accepted function of medical computing is in the highly developed area of medical instrumentation. The newest and probably the most underdeveloped medical computer application is in the area of patient management.

This chapter will be devoted to the application of computers in a cardiac rehabilitation setting. Many applications will be presented ranging from administrative tasks to patient education. To date no integrated software packages have been developed specifically for cardiac rehabilitation centers. Therefore, a basic understanding of computers and specifically selected generic software application is required to implement a program. These skills can be either self-acquired or provided by a trained programmer. In either case, this chapter will be most valuable in giving cardiac therapists innovative ideas to integrate into their specific situations.

Cardiac rehabilitation programs currently exist at hospital outpatient departments, clinics, and free-standing centers. These preexisting facilities may already have computer systems that can be integrated into the cardiac rehabilitation program. This would drastically reduce the start-up cost by eliminating the need for hardware. However, there may be a need for an additional terminal, a printer, and memory devices.

This chapter considers primarily the tasks that a computer can perform in a cardiac rehabilitation center. It does not deal with specific hardware and software, beyond giving general recommendations, because, as this document is in print, new and innovative hardware and software will be developed to make it obsolete.

Computers have a place as partners in health care and will undoubtedly become more integrated with the cardiac rehabilitation program and with the total health care network in the future. Computers will serve as filing cabinets, word processors, statisticians, organizers, and schedule books to enable more efficient use of time.

Does Your Cardiac Rehabilitation Program Really Need a Computer?

Before deciding whether to computerize your cardiac rehabilitation center, you must first decide whether it would be cost-effective in this specific setting. Cost is not the only factor to consider when deciding to utilize a computer. Other benefits that are equally as important are presented in the section on the "Benefits of Computerizing a Cardiac Rehabilitation Program." There is no special formula to determine cost impact, but general guidelines will be presented to offer some objective information.

Center Evaluation

A center evaluation cannot be performed until it is decided what specific tasks the computer will perform in the cardiac rehabilitation setting and what tasks the current staff are performing. The section in this chapter titled "Specific Tasks That a Computer Can Perform in a Cardiac Rehabilitation Setting" offers a variety of ideas, which can easily be implemented into a rehabilitation setting. These fall under the four main application categories of data base management, word processing, administration, and education.

First, evaluate the current duties performed by the rehabilitation staff. This should reflect a period of time to include special as well as everyday duties. Each staff member should record all the various duties he or she performs and the estimated time spent for each duty, both daily and monthly. Compile the lists of the staff members; the end result should reflect the percentage of monthly time that is spent doing various tasks in the rehabilitation center. For instance, if the secretary spends an average of 70% of the time filing, typing standard reports, and billing, then it may be possible to accomplish these tasks more efficiently with a computer and have the secretary work only part-time in the center. If the center does not have secretarial support, and a large percentage of the medical staff's time is spent doing such things as billing, filing, and filling out reports and forms then a computer would probably be cost-effective. The other benefits of a computer should be analyzed along with the pure cost analysis (e.g., time, organization, and quality of patient care).

After analyzing the current tasks that the staff is performing, decide which of these tasks can be performed by a computer. Someone knowledgeable in computers and computer software should be consulted at this point. Probably the best source is a computer programmer, program consultant, or program analyst, who is associated with one of the reputable, local computer stores or services. This person should be able to demonstrate both hardware and software that meet your specifications. It will most likely take several trips to a variety of computer stores before you become comfortable with one store and one programmer or sales representative. For more information on selecting a computer see the section in this chapter on "Selecting the Right Computer for a Cardiac Rehabilitation Program."

Determine the approximate cost of the computer that will meet the cardiac rehabilitation center's needs. Include all the hardware, software packages, supplies, and ongoing service charges in this cost. You should be able to recoup this cost in a reasonable time period by saving staff time, managing the center more efficiently, and providing better patient care and follow-up. Also, additional services may be possible with the use of the computer and special software packages (see "Specific Tasks That the Computer can Perform in a Cardiac Rehabilitation Setting").

By evaluating your center's needs according to these criteria, you can identify the specific tasks which will be performed by the computer on a daily basis. In other words, you will learn how a computer can be used to its full capacity based on the specific functioning of your cardiac rehabilitation center.

The answer to the question of whether your cardiac rehabilitation program really needs a computer will depend on many factors. But, the cost-to-benefit relationship should be carefully analyzed. Let's now look at some of the other benefits to help answer the question.

The Benefits of Computerizing a Cardiac Rehabilitation Program

Cost-effectiveness or cost impact is not the only benefit that can be derived from computerizing the cardiac rehabilitation program. Two other major areas include administrative support and medical decision-making assistance.

Cost Impact

In the late seventies, the cost of computerized medical information systems was cost-prohibitive in all but experimental hospital or clinical facilities. Now, as hardware is becoming less expensive and more reliable and software is becoming more sophisticated, the cost-effective applications are emerging. Original investigation into the cost impact of the older systems did not indicate clearly a beneficial cost impact. Unfortunately, the newer, more economical systems, which may have a beneficial cost impact, have not been thoroughly evaluated.

The market for hospital information systems in 1977 was $419 million and grew to nearly $1 billion in 1982 (U.S. General Accounting Office [USGAO], 1980). Most of the growth has been centered on financial and administrative aspects. A report to Congress (Office of Technology Assessment, 1977) summarized the cost of computerized information systems as follows:

> Medical information systems are an expensive technology. Operating costs for a hospital-based system range from $4 to $9 per patient per day. For systems based on ambulatory care sites, costs range from $0.50 to $14 per patient visit. Costs of implementation are high. Costs are, however, likely to decrease in the future, because of lower prices for computer hardware and higher volume. Moreover, a majority of both hospitals and ambulatory care facilities now using medical information systems report overall savings in institutional costs due to their computer systems. At least one study has documented cost savings. In particular, savings are experienced in labor expenses.

This 1977 report reflects the higher cost of new technology.

An analysis of the methods for evaluating the cost of automated systems is beyond the scope of this chapter (for an excellent summary, see Drazen & Metzger, 1981; they concluded that improvements in information flow provided the major motivation to implement a computerized information system). A study at El Camino Hospital (Gall et al., 1977) demonstrated that interhospital labor trends over time were reduced when compared with the costs of other similar hospitals. However, they failed to demonstrate savings based on before-after studies.

Less objective analysis has been done in the evaluation of ambulatory care facilities, which more closely simulate the cardiac rehabilitation setting. Kuhn et al. (1984) states:

> There continues to be a lack of economic data to evaluate benefits derived from the Ambulatory Automated Medical Records System (AAMRS). Where cost savings are realized, they are most often realized from the administrative services provided by the system. While

most system developers believe that the medical benefits of an AAMRS are the primary justification for the system, there is some evidence that the administrative services may be a primary justification to those who purchase and install the systems. For some of the modular systems, the administrative services are the first to be implemented, and in some cases, they are the only ones that are implemented.

A realization of cost impact will be seen most likely in the administrative aspects of the system and will be directly related to a reduction of clerical and financial personnel. The system assumes the tasks of immediate billing and rapid claims processing, minimizes the cost of health care mistakes, and provides complete resource utilization through proper management. Health care may be improved through more accurate and accessible medical records, prompting the provider to follow up on patient care and monitoring appointments for preventive care, which would enhance overall patient care and stimulate patient satisfaction with the service provided.

No study has analyzed the cost impact of computerization of a cardiac rehabilitation program. Therefore, it is necessary to apply the information regarding the hospital and ambulatory systems to cardiac rehabilitation settings. If the need for a computer system can be justified economically, the reduction in manpower requirements and the meeting of increased data management needs should make the system an important component of cardiac rehabilitation programs.

Administrative Support

Patient care in the rehabilitation center involves many administrative tasks. These range from tasks involving patient interaction (appointments and schedules) to clerical tasks (charting, typing, filing reports, etc.). A computer system can provide benefits by performing the same functions both more efficiently and more effectively than existing administrative personnel.

The process of administering health care has been called *information intensive* (Blum, 1984). Jydstrup and Gross found that about one-fourth of all activity in the hospitals they studied was devoted to information processing, which was defined as any action involving the recording, reading, or transmitting of information. Although much of this information processing cannot be handled by the computer information system, it can be effective in

- modifying work flow,
- improving timeliness,
- reducing errors, and
- providing access to new functions.

Let's now look at each of these four areas and apply them to the cardiac rehabilitation setting.

Modifying Work Flow.   The computer system can reduce redundancy of information processing. For example, it is not uncommon in the cardiac rehabilitation setting to fill out insurance forms, billing forms, progress report forms, referral forms, and so forth. Each of these forms, although unique, contain many of the same questions and are generated from a common data base, the patient's medical records. These include patient name, address, age, sex, date of birth, social security number, diagnosis, date of current incident, referring physician, and type of insurance. All of this information can be stored in a computer information system and programmed to print on various generic forms. All common forms would need to be standardized and the computer would do the work upon request for any particular patient.

The Joint Commission for Accreditation of Hospitals (JCAH) requires that the following basic requirements be met for all outpatient rehabilitation services:

1. Establishment of goals
2. Development of a plan of treatment
3. Regular and frequent assessment
4. Maintenance of treatment and progress records
5. Periodic assessment of the quality and appropriateness of care provided

Each of these five areas could be easily generated on a computerized system by the cardiac therapist and health care team for each patient. All of these combined would only take a matter of minutes to complete, thus reducing medical staff and secretarial time and improving the care plan of each patient.

The JCAH also requires that records for each patient referred to the rehabilitation program service shall include at least the following data:

1. The diagnosis and problem list pertinent to the rehabilitation process
2. Precautions necessitated by the patient's general medical condition or other factors
3. The short- and long-term goals of the treatment program as appropriate
4. A statement regarding the frequency of review, when it is desired more often than monthly, of the patient's progress

Thus, to meet the requirements of the JCAH, specific processing of information is necessary. The ability of the computer to organize, centralize, assist in the generation of, update, and extract information provides the potential for the reorganization of work flow to decrease time and provide better patient care with a more complete care plan. The computer also allows the reassignment of some clerical tasks that were normally performed by health care professionals.

One study (Coffey, 1980) at El Camino Hospital demonstrated that a computerized information system improved the efficiency of nursing care by freeing nurses up to care for a greater number of patients. It also demonstrated a reduction of nursing cost per patient by 5%. This cost reduction could also be accomplished in the cardiac rehabilitation setting with the help of a computer.

Improving Timeliness. Computerized information systems improve timeliness by generating and transferring reports and forms moments after they have been entered into the system. For instance, in many facilities you literally have to wait days or weeks for a testing physician to interpret and sign a patient's exercise tolerance test results or exercise prescription after transcription has prepared the document. This often delays the process of beginning cardiac rehabilitation. It is possible to computer-generate any form simultaneously during the exercise tolerance test and to generate an exercise prescription and complete the entire procedure before the physician leaves the testing laboratory.

Another common experience is when a physician wishes to see a progress report on an individual participant who will be seen in just a few minutes or hours. A computer-generated report could be prepared in seconds that details the average training heart rate, blood pressure, rate pressure product, current signs or symptoms, and update on risk factor reduction. This would take at least one-half hour to generate by hand for the requesting physician. As stated earlier, these reports are required monthly by the JCAH.

Reducing Errors. Many tasks in the cardiac rehabilitation setting require the cardiac therapist to work with numbers or formulas, for instance:

Target training heart rate = (max heart rate) − (resting heart rate) × .70 + (resting heart rate) ± 5 bpm

K/cal per min expenditure during walking on flat surface =

$$\frac{[(26.82 \times \text{mph}) \times .1] \times [(\text{body weight in kg}) + 3.5] \times 5}{1000}$$

Functional aerobic inpatient =

$$\frac{(\text{predicted MET level} - \text{attained MET level})}{\text{predicted MET level}} \times 100$$

It would take several minutes to determine the results of these equations with an accuracy level with which you would be comfortable. The computer can correctly solve these equations in a fraction of the time it takes to do them manually.

In addition to performing mathematical problems, the computer has the ability to examine and reflect data that are inconsistent with pre-established criteria. Thus, if a heart rate of over 200 (or any predetermined number) is entered into a system as an exercising heart rate, then a cue or input prompt would occur to make sure the input was correct. One study (Simborg, 1973) comparing an automated to unautomated physician order system demonstrated that the automated system consistently received less errors in transcription, communication, uninterpreted information, and failure to carry out exactly the order than the unautomated system.

Provides Access to New Information.   Yearly or even quarterly reports in a cardiac rehabilitation program should examine the following statistics:

1. The referring physician base
    - cardiologists
    - internists
    - family physicians
2. The insurance base
    - Medicare
    - BC/CS
    - other private companies
3. The patient base
    - number of patients
    - age
    - sex
    - MI, CABG, or angina
    - patient improvement
4. Compliance
    - percent of patient base
    - length of program
5. Follow-up
6. Patient flow
    - summer
    - winter

This type of information can be very helpful in determining the success or weakness of the cardiac rehabilitation program. It can identify trends in insurance coverage, physician referral, and patient demographics. A yearly evaluation of the program with program goals should be based on this type of information. The computer can very easily keep an on-going record of these entities.

Medical Decision-Making Assistance

The previous two sections on cost impact and administrative support have indicated how a computer information system could benefit cardiac rehabilitation program management. This section will deal with the benefits of the system to the actual provider or cardiac therapist.

Displaying Clinical Information. When clinical data are stored and displayed in an organized manner on a computerized information system the result is a more complete and accurate data base. For instance, when a cardiac therapist is seeing 20–30 patients three times per week it becomes difficult to recall detailed information on each patient. With a computer information system, this information is always readily available both to the cardiac therapist and to the other staff members in the primary cardiac therapist's absence. The referring physician can also access this information at any time.

Automatic Surveillance. The computer information system provides quick access to all patient's clinical data. This allows the computer to

- identify patients who are not progressing,
- identify patients who are not compliant,
- identify patients who are not losing weight, and
- identify any other patients who need to be analyzed more closely.

A list of any of these classifications of patients can be produced, and those identified are then available for special treatment or a revised care plan.

Surveillance of signs, symptoms, and angina threshold ST-segment depression can also be watched more closely during exercise tolerance testing and/or training. The computer can pick up particular changes that the cardiac therapist and/or physician have overlooked.

Automatic Reminders. The computer information system can generate a list or surveillance report to either the provider or the patient. A surveillance list can be generated on participants who have missed two cardiac rehabilitation sessions in a row; this list would include phone numbers for reminder calls. This step would be beneficial to improve patient compliance with the cardiac rehabilitation program.

Reminders may also be generated to all participants concerning a special educational offering that will be sponsored by the facility. Another approach may be to send reminders to patients for yearly exercise tolerance tests or a monthly Phase II cardiac rehabilitation program. In these and other ways, reminders and surveillance can enhance the cardiac rehabilitation program.

Decision-Making Support. By displaying clinical information, providing surveillance, and issuing reminders, the computer system indirectly supports the decision-making process. In more direct application, the system can help determine, with the application of Bayes' Theorem, the likelihood of an event based on certain pre- and post-test events. With this statistical information at the physician's fingertips it may be possible to make a more accurate treatment decision. One such system, the Duke Prognostogram (Rosati, McNeer, Stamler et al., 1975), can be used to predict the outcome of either surgical or medical treatment for patients with angina. It has been reported that this system has been significantly successful in reducing unnecessary surgery.

Many benefits exist in favor of the computerized information system. Therefore, it is likely that the development of the system's application will continue to extend into health care including cardiac rehabilitation programs as the technology of computers continues to advance and their benefits are realized by the medical community.

Selecting the Right Computer for a Cardiac Rehabilitation Program

Computers and computer systems have improved tremendously in the last few years and will continue to do the same in the future. Specific computers and software will not be mentioned in this section because this information would be outdated by the time this work is published. Instead, general guidelines are provided, which should continue to be applicable in the years to come.

Probably the two most important points that need to be emphasized about computers are compatibility and expandability. The computer must be compatible with a large variety of software packages both now and in the near future. The computer must also be expandable to handle upgraded hardware. It is also best to look for a computer that is supplied by a reputable company that will still be in business 5–10 years from now.

Brickman, Ashton, and Balsam (1984) present a complete list of vital questions to ask when purchasing a computer for medical needs.

1. Will the computer company provide names of current users? (If not, forget about them. Be sure to check out the referrals; they will tell you a lot more than the salesman can about the product.)
2. How easy-to-use is the system?
3. Will the computer company thoroughly train your office staff, and is this training included in the cost of the system?
4. How many systems are currently in the field?
5. How long has the company been in business?
6. How much training is required before the system can be operated by your staff?
7. Can you understand what the salesperson is showing you? (If not, the office staff will probably have even more trouble.)
8. Can you enter your own data into the system and see the reports, or are you seeing only a prearranged demonstration?
9. Will the computer company provide on-site maintenance? What is the cost?
10. How are software updates handled? (Every system needs periodic updates.)
11. Does the computer company offer one-stop service or will you have to deal with two, three, or more vendors to maintain the computer? (With more than one vendor, it is possible that no one will accept responsibility for the problem.)
12. How thorough and well written is the user's manual?
13. What enhancements are in the works?
14. What reports does the computer supply?
15. How are you protected in case of power failure or system malfunction?
16. Are hard copy printouts readily available for all transactions and other valuable information?
17. Who makes the hardware, and how reliable is it?
18. How many patients can the system handle?
19. How many doctors can the system handle?
20. How many daily transactions can the system handle?
21. How many patients can be maintained for a year?
22. Does the system maintain a permanent record of all patients, or are they removed periodically?
23. Does the system support the CP/M operating system? (There is more software available for this operating system than for any other.)
24. Is it a hard disk or floppy system? A floppy system is definitely not recommended except for exceptionally small centers.
25. Can the system be easily and cost-effectively expanded and/or upgraded?

The hardware for a cardiac rehabilitation program should include at least a versatile and expandable central processing unit, a hard disk drive system for storage, a quality printer (either word processing or dot matrix, depending on tasks), and at least one monitor and input device. The initial software packages should include a large, programmable, data base management system; a word processing package; and an accounting type or billing program. These three pieces of software enable the user to perform a majority of the daily tasks of a cardiac rehabilitation center. In most cases the software will have to be customized to your setting by a professional programmer.

Specific Tasks That a Computer Can Perform in a Cardiac Rehabilitation Setting

This section will be devoted to the variety of tasks that the computer can perform in a cardiac rehabilitation setting. The computer can function as an integral part of the cardiac rehabilitation program by acting as an integrated patient data base and information system being involved in almost every day-to-day function. In addition, it can be used to support the current organization.

An Integrated Patient Data Base

The most complex system is the integrated patient data base. Theoretically, this system stores all pertinent patient information until it is needed for further processing, review, updates, reports, or billing. The most difficult task in this system is deciding what information to store on the data base. Data should be collected not because they are available but only if their use in a decision-making process can be identified. For example, in a cardiac rehabilitation program it would not be necessary to store information regarding a patient's appendectomy of 10 years ago; however, it would be important to know the referring physician's name and his or her diagnosis. This information can be used directly in filing for reimbursement. Once this information is entered into the data base it should never have to be entered again unless it is changed. The following list of items should be considered as data entry into the integrated data base because of their frequency of use in a cardiac rehabilitation program.

- Participant demographic file
- Medical history file
- Current medications file
- Exercise tolerance test file

- Exercise prescription file
- Exercise therapy file
- Insurance information and billing
- Risk factor lifestyle changes
- Education file

Each of the items listed may have 10–20 variables of its own. The computer organizes all the information and stores it until the user requests the information presented in a specific manner. Several tasks can be performed with this type of integrated patient data base.

Form Completion. With the appropriate input, various types of forms (e.g., progress report forms) could be generated during a cardiac patient's rehabilitation program. This requires no additional time by the cardiac therapist if data are entered as they are collected during the exercise session.

Reports. Exercise-tolerance-test flow sheets and reports can be completed at the time of the exercise test, eliminating the delay of results to referring physicians.

Billing and Insurance. Bills can be submitted to insurance carriers on a daily basis through processed forms or even telecommunication with some insurance carriers.

Surveillance. The computer can generate lists of poor compliance, follow-up appointments, patients with hypertension, or any variable that is entered.

Reminders. Reminders of Phase III, follow-up visits, yearly exercise tolerance tests, or follow-up visits with the physician can be issued. Also, referring physician lists can be easily generated to enhance referrals.

Program Analysis. The system may be programmed to provide a yearly report of referral pathways, patient demographic data, insurance mix, and other information that is important to yearly evaluation of a cardiac rehabilitation program.

Non-Data Base Tasks

There are many other tasks the computer can perform besides utilizing the integrated patient data base. These can be done independently of the data base or integrated into the entire system to store information.

Patient Education. Patient education will probably be one of the most exciting advancements that computers will bring to medical education.

Currently patient interaction programs are available in which the patient participates in the learning process by performing tasks and answering questions asked by the computer. If the task is performed incorrectly the computer may assist in the answer until the correct response is given. Then the program continues on to the next question or task. A lot of work is currently being done with videodiscs and with the integration of video with computer programs. These types of applications would revolutionize education.

Telecommunication. With a modem the computer can communicate with any other compatible computer system. The most common medical application is with a medical data base to medical literature. The American Medical Association (AMA) has a data base that includes medication and diagnostic information, courses for CME credit, and schedules of professional meetings.

Statistics. Statistics are a vital part of clinical medicine. A computer package in statistics allows the clinical practitioner to perform group comparisons and easily determine significant differences among them.

Summary

This chapter has described computer application to the medical field of cardiac rehabilitation. Much of the information has been taken from studies of hospital and ambulatory care facilities using computerized systems. Currently, cardiac rehabilitation programs across the United States are not actively using the computer. The benefits of using a computer for this purpose have been described. Also several applications have been suggested to those interested in computerizing a cardiac rehabilitation center. I hope that this chapter will stimulate more use of computers in cardiac rehabilitation.

References

Blum, B. (1984). *Information systems for patient care.* New York: Springer-Verlag.

Brickman, D., Ashton, J., & Balsam, J. (1984). Medical computing: Realities for the private practitioner. In B. Blum (Ed.), *Information systems for patient care.* New York: Springer-Verlag.

Coffey, R. (1980). *How a medical information system affects care: The El Camino Hospital experience.* (Research Summary Series, DHEW Publication No. PHS 80-3265). National Center for Health Service Research.

Drazen, E., & Metzger, J. (1981). *Methods for evaluating costs of automated hospital information systems*. (Research Summary Series, DHHS Publication No. PHS 81-3283). National Center for Health Service Research.

Gall. (1977). *Demonstration and evaluation of a total hospital information system*. (Research Digest Series No. 77-3188). National Center for Health Service Research.

Kuhn, I. (1984). Automated ambulatory medical record systems in the U.S. In B. Blum (Ed.), *Information systems for patient care* (pp. 199-217). New York: Springer-Verlag.

Office of Technology Assessment. (1977). *Policy implications of medical information systems*.

Rosati, R., McNeer, F., & Stamler, F. (1975). A new information system for medical practice. *Archives of Internal Medicine, 135*.

Simborg, D. (1973). The development of a word information management system. *Methods of Information in Medicine, 12*(1), 17-26.

U.S. General Accounting Office. (1980). Computerized hospital medical information systems need further evaluation to ensure benefits from huge investments. *AFMD, 81*, 3.

Chapter 9

Assessment of the Energy Costs of Various Occupations

Daniel R. Timmons

In the prescription of occupational activities for cardiac patients, each patient's clinical status must be quantitatively assessed in relation to the physical, emotional and environmental stress of a particular occupation. The patient's physical status should be ascertained from a current medical profile and a symptom-limited, maximum exercise tolerance test (ETT) with continuous electrocardiography (EKG) and blood pressure (BP) monitoring performed. The physiological data obtained should be tested against the total and myocardial energy demands of the patient's occupational activities.

The typical exercise tolerance test or total energy cost assessment of a particular occupation is limited in its ability to evaluate such factors as the psychological stress of emotion, environmental factors, or the utilization of muscle groups in a manner not used during the ETT or work assessment. With these limitations in mind, this chapter will present the total energy cost of various simple and complex activities in terms of kilocalorie (kcal) expenditure or oxygen (O_2) consumption. A comparison will be made between cardiac and noncardiac groups when possible. Various factors effecting the use of energy cost will also be presented.

The myocardial energy cost in relation to energy demand will be discussed in a separate section. This factor plays the most important role in the assessment of an occupation for the cardiovascularly impaired individual. I hope that, as a result of the information in this chapter, the medical practice of modestly restricting occupational and recreational activity of noncomplicated cardiac patients will be totally eliminated.

Expressions of Energy

Energy cost is a very ambiguous term. The term may be interpreted as an expression of either the work output or work input. These two expressions are unique measurements, but comparisons can be made by representing them as identical units. The relationship between these units of energy are presented in Table 9.1. With the use of Table 9.1, work in watts, foot-pounds, and kilopound-meters can be represented as energy in kilocalories. This conversion becomes quite useful in the evaluation of various energy-requiring tasks and occupations.

Table 9.1   Relationship and Conversion Table for Various Expressions of Energy

Power	Work and energy
1 watt = 0.001 kilowatt	1 kilocalorie = 4.186 × 10^{10} ergs
1 watt = 0.73756 ft-lb s^{-1}	1 kilocalorie = 4,186 joules
1 watt = 1 × 10^7 ergs s^{-1}	1 kilocalorie = 3.9680 British Thermal Units
1 watt = 0.056884 British Thermal Units 1 min = 3.41304 BTU-hr	1 kilocalorie = 3087.4 ft-lb
1 watt = 0.01433 kilocalories min^1	1 kilocalorie = 426.85 kpm
1 watt = 1.341 × 10^{-3} hp (horsepower)	1 kilocalorie = 1.5593 × 10^{-3} hp-hr
1 watt = 1 J s^{-1}	1 erg = 2.3889 × 10^{-11} kcal
1 watt = 6.12 kpm min^{-1}	1 erg = 1 × 10^{-7} joule
1 kilocalorie per minute = 69.767 watts	1 erg = 9.4805 × 10^{-14} British Thermal Units
1 kilocalorie per minute = 51.457 ft-lb s^{-1}	1 erg = 7.3756 × 10^{-8} ft-lb
1 kilocalorie per minute = 6.9770 × 10^8 ergs • s^{-1}	1 erg = 1.0197 × 10^{-8} kpm
	1 erg = 3.7251 × 10^{-14} hp-hr
1 kilocalorie per minute = 3.9685 British Thermal Units min^{-1}	1 joule = 2.3889 × 10^{-4} kcal
1 kilocalorie per minute = 0.093557 hp	1 joule = 1 × 10^7 ergs
1 horsepower = 745.7 watts	1 joule = 9.4805 × 10^{-4} British Thermal Units
1 horsepower = 550 ft-lb s^{-1}	1 joule = 0.73756 ft-lb
1 horsepower = 7.457 × 10^9 ergs s^{-1}	1 joule = 0.10197 kpm
1 horsepower = 42.4176 British Thermal Units min^{-1}	1 joule = 3.7251 × 10^{-7} hp-hr
1 horsepower = 10.688 kcal min^{-1}	1 BTU = 0.25198 kcal

(Cont.)

1 horsepower = 745.7 joules s^{-1}

1 horsepower = 75 kpm s^{-1}

1 BTU = 1.0548×10^{10} ergs

1 BTU = 1054.8 joules

1 BTU = 777.98 ft-lb

1 BTU = 107.56 kpm

1 BTU = 3.9292×10^{-4} hp-hr

1 foot-pound = 3.2389×10^{-4} kcal

1 foot-pound = 1.35582×10^{7} ergs

1 foot-pound = 1.3558 joules

1 foot-pound = 1.2854×10^{-3} British Thermal Units

1 foot-pound = 0.13825 kpm

1 foot-pound = 5.0505×10^{-7} hp-hr

1 kilogram-meter = 2.3427×10^{-3} kcal

1 kilogram-meter = 9.8066×10^{7} ergs

1 kilogram-meter =9.8066 joules

1 kilogram-meter = 9.2967×10^{3} British Thermal Units

1 kilogram-meter = 7.2330 ft-lb

1 kilogram-meter = 3.6529×10^{-6} hp-hr

1 watt = 6.12 kpm min^{-1} (approx. = 6 kpm min^{-1})

50 watts = approx. 300 kpm min^{-1}

1 kpm min^{-1} = 0.1635 watt

1 kp = 9.80665 newtons

1 kpm = 9.80665 joules

Note. From *Textbook of Work Physiology* (p. 657) by P. Åstrand and K. Rodahl, 1977, New York: McGraw Hill. Copyright 1977 by McGraw Hill. Reprinted by permission.

Energy Output

In physics, the term *energy* is defined as the capacity to perform work and overcome resistance. This resistance may be the naturally occurring gravitational force of the earth, a person's body weight, the fly wheel of a bicycle ergometer, or any external object carried, pushed, or moved in any way by an individual.

In the physical sense, *work* is objectively defined as force acting through a distance, where force is mass times acceleration. Another expression commonly used for work is power. Power is simply work per unit of time. By definition, units of work can be quantified as:

Energy—the capacity of performing work
Work—force × distance
Force—mass × acceleration
Power—work per unit of time (work/time)

If external work or work output can be measured it can be converted into kcal equivalents. For example, on the bicycle ergometer with a fly wheel of 6 m and a pedaling resistance of 50 RPM, (300 m total distance) with 1 kg resistance, 300 kg of work are performed (300 m × 1 kg). According to Table 9.1 this can be converted into .7 kcal of work output [(2.3427 × 10⁻³ kcal) × 300].

Energy Input

Energy in another sense, energy input or energy cost for work, refers to the energy utilized to produce the work output. At first glance, you might assume that the work input should be equal to the work output. This would represent 100% efficiency. This is not the case. A percentage of the energy input is dissipated in metabolic or mechanical energy transformations. The conventional formula to represent this discrepancy termed *mechanical efficiency* (ME) is (Taylor, 1960)

$$ME\% = \frac{(\text{kcal external work produced})}{(\text{kcal net energy used})} \times 100$$

Based on the previous example on the bicycle on an individual with a measured net O_2 consumption of .6 l or 2.88 kcal (1 l of O_2 = 4.8 kcal) (Lust, 1928), the following ME can be calculated.

$$ME\% = \frac{(.7)}{2.88} \times 100$$

$$ME\% = 24.3\%$$

The result of this measured work output in relation to work input is a 24.3% mechanical efficiency, which can also be expressed as a 75.7% energy loss. It can easily be seen that if an activity were more efficient it would require less energy to perform a known work output. Thus, the efficiency of a particular occupation or activity will directly effect the energy cost in work with identical work outputs.

Evaluation of Total Energy Cost

Several methods are available to measure and categorize energy cost. The method chosen depends on a variety of factors including the accuracy, mobility, time, and cost considerations of the particular technique utilized. The energy cost (energy input) not the energy output is the term that will be used when dealing with the cost of various occupations and activities.

Direct Measurement of Energy Cost

Heat exchange calorimeters have been utilized as a direct measurement of energy cost. However, these methods require expensive and extensive instrumentation. For these reasons indirect methods to evaluate the energy cost of man have been developed.

Indirect Measurement of Energy Cost

The indirect methods, as their name implies, do not measure the energy of an activity directly. They are based on the fact that all energy metabolism in the body ultimately depends on the utilization of oxygen. Therefore, oxygen consumption is measured, and an energy equivalent is determined. The methodology of various oxygen consumption techniques is described extensively in the literature (Åstrand & Rodahl, 1977; Consolazio, Johnson, & Pecora, 1963; Mellerowicz & Smodlaka, 1981). The early studies by Carpenter (1939) showed that the energy equivalent for 1 l of oxygen based on the respiratory exchange ratio (RER) (an indicator of intensity) ranged from 4.686 kcal per l of O_2 at rest (RER .70) to 5.047 kcal per l of O_2 during near maximal effort (RER 1.0). At a work load of 50% maximum capacity, a respiratory exchange ratio in the range of .81 to .84 or approximately 4.8 kcal min (Pruett, cited in Åstrand & Rodahl, 1977) would be common. This constant of 4.8 kcal per l of O_2 will be used throughout this chapter when transformations are made.

Automated Systems.   The most common technique to measure oxygen consumption today is with an automated or semiautomated system that provides relatively instantaneous values of O_2 consumption after measurements of the volume of air inspired as well as oxygen and carbon dioxide fractions are recorded. These automated systems (see Figure 9.1) are not portable and do not lend themselves to evaluations outside the laboratory setting (e.g., occupational, sports, or recreational evaluations). However, the most reliable physiological data on energy cost are obtained from the controlled laboratory setting by measuring oxygen consumption and its interaction with work.

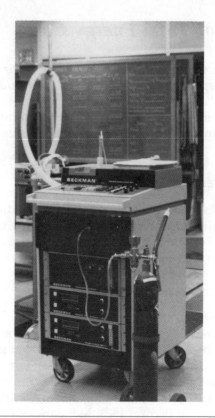

Figure 9.1. An automated gas analysis system.

Portable Spirometers. In the working environment, portable spirometers have been used (see Figure 9.2). Their reliability and validation as an alternative technique for the measurement of oxygen cost during daily functional activities have been reported (Harrison, Brown, & Belyavin, 1982; Van Baak & Binkhorst, 1981).

The most accurate values of the energy cost of occupations would be attained with the use of a portable spirometer. However, its use in the clinical setting to evaluate the energy cost of various occupations does not seem practical. Besides, physiological studies have been performed on groups of individuals at various worksites evaluating numerous occupations. These data can provide a framework for the energy cost of various individual occupations. However, they do not use large populations or take into account the individual variations of mechanical efficiency or intensity of the type of work performed in the referenced activity. When predicting a person's energy cost of an occupation, which can be considered a complex activity, there is a much greater variation than in predicting the energy cost of simple repetitive activities such as bicycle ergometry or walking. Therefore these two categories of complex and simple activities need to be looked at independently. The analysis of simple activities will provide the groundwork for analyzing complex activities.

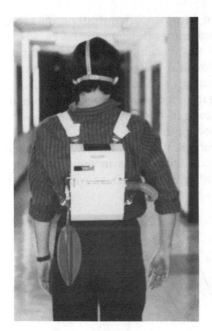 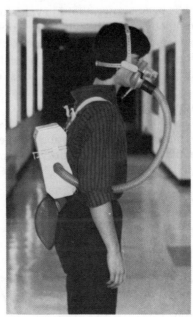

Figure 9.2. A portable spirometer used during activity to measure O_2 consumption.

Predicted Energy Costs (O_2 Consumption)

Activities can be grouped into two general categories: simple and complex. Simple activities refer to activities that are repetitive in nature, continue for a specified continuous time at the same intensity, use an isolated muscle group, and have a precise measurable work output. Complex activities are defined as activities that are not repetitive in nature, are intermittent, change considerably from one activity and intensity to another, do not use isolated muscle groups, and have a work output that is difficult to measure and complicated in nature. Most occupations are classified as complex activities. Work performed on the bicycle ergometer or treadmill is classified as simple activity. When predicting energy cost the accuracy depends on the nature of the activity, either simple or complex.

A greater error is attained when predicting the energy cost of complex activities as opposed to simple activities.

Simple Activities

It has been shown that in evaluating known work output on the bicycle ergometer and arm ergometer, a positive linear relationship exists between oxygen consumption and work output (in kcal/min or O_2 consumption). Figure 9.3 demonstrates this relationship with data compiled from 10 authors in different publications and presented by Boffert (1960).

An evaluation of various investigators using a variety of methods has found slightly different values of oxygen consumption during performance on the bicycle ergometer (see Figure 9.4).

These variations are probably due to the varying efficiency of muscular, circulatory, and respiratory mechanisms involved in the work output (Mellerowicz & Smodlaka, 1981). Other factors such as weight, stature,

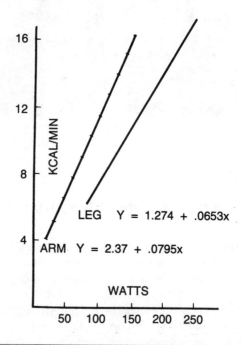

Figure 9.3. The linear relationship between work in watts and energy cost in kcal per min in arm and leg ergometry. *Note.* From ''Physiological Comparison of Three Types of Ergometry'' by A. Bobbert, 1960, *Journal of Applied Physiology*, **15**(6), p. 1007. Copyright 1960 by *Journal of Applied Physiology*. Adapted by permission.

age, physical capacity, different subject populations, different mechanical properties of ergometers used, different physiological ranges of variation in the O_2 consumption at equal performances, and errors in calibration and measurement may also effect the work input of performing the work (Åstrand & Rodahl, 1977; Mellerowicz & Smodlaka, 1981).

Oxygen consumption at a given submaximal rate of work on a bicycle ergometer has been shown to be very constant even if the work is performed under different conditions (Åstrand & Rodahl, 1977); therefore it can be predicted quite accurately. This has been shown under conditions of high altitude (Klausen, 1966; Pugh, 1964) (see Figure 9.5) and various temperatures (Rowell, 1974) (see Figure 9.6). This does not hold true for cardiovascular or hemodynamic indexes such as heart rate (HR) and blood pressure (BP) as will be shown in the following section.

Ambulatory activities such as walking and many occupational tasks, when compared to stationary activities such as the bicycle ergometer, are considered weight bearing. In all weight-bearing activities there is a positive linear correlation between body weight and absolute oxygen consumption or absolute kcal (see Figure 9.7). This is simply due to the fact that the body weight adds to the work output. For example, an individual who weighs 75 kg expends approximately 955 ml of O_2 per min when walking at 3.5 mph. A 100-kg man walking the same 3.5 mph would consume approximately 1290 ml of O_2 per min. This can be converted to 4.6 and 6.2 kcal, respectively.

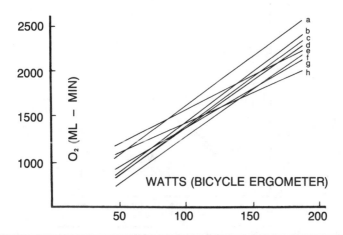

Figure 9.4. The linear relationship between work in watts and energy cost in ml per min in untrained individuals (a composite of eight authors). *Note.* From *Ergometry: Basics of Medical Exercise Testing* (p. 182) by H. Mellerowicz and V. Smodlaka, Baltimore: Urban and Schwarzenberg. Copyright 1981 by Urban and Schwarzenberg. Adapted by permission.

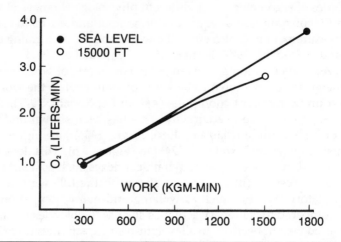

Figure 9.5. The linear relationship between workloads of 300 and 1,800 kgm on a bicycle ergometer and energy cost in liters of O_2 per min at sea level and at 15,000 ft. *Note.* From "Muscular Exercise at Great Altitudes" by L. Pugh, 1964, *Journal of Applied Physiology,* **19**, p. 431. Copyright 1964 by *Journal of Applied Physiology.* Adapted by permission.

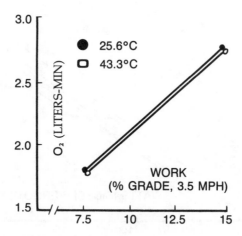

Figure 9.6. The linear relationship between work on a treadmill (walking 3.5 mph at a 7.5% to 15% grade) and energy cost in liters per minute at temperatures of 25.6 °C and 43.3 °C. *Note.* From "Human Cardiovascular Adjustments to Exercise and Thermal Stress" by L. Rowell, 1974, *Physiological Reviews,* **54**, p. 75. Adapted by permission.

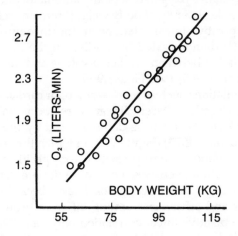

Figure 9.7. The linear relationship between body weight in kg and energy cost in liters per minute. *Note.* From *Exercise Physiology: Energy, Nutrition, and Human Performance* (p. 116) by W. McArdle, F. Katch, and V. Katch, 1981, Philadelphia: Lea and Febiger. Copyright 1981 by Lea and Febiger. Adapted by permission.

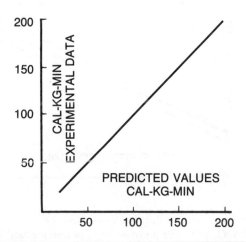

Figure 9.8. The linear relationship between predicted values of O_2 consumption (based on a composite of 9 authors) and experimental (measured) O_2 consumption. *Note.* From "Physiological Comparison of Three Types of Ergometry" by A. Bobbert, 1960, *Journal of Applied Physiology, 15*(6), 1015. Copyright 1960 by *Journal of Applied Physiology*. Adapted by permission.

Therefore the relative oxygen cost of any ambulatory activity (O_2 per kg of body weight or kcal per kg of body weight) remains relatively constant and presents a positive linear relationship for uncomplicated work outputs. This can be demonstrated by studies on the treadmill that show a positive correlation between predicted values and measured values as shown by Bobbert (1960) (see Figure 9.8).

When subpopulations such as men, women, or cardiac men are studied independently, slightly different linear correlations will exist between work load and $\dot{V}O_2$. This can be demonstrated by the work of Bruce, Kusumi, and Hosmer (1973) (Figure 9.9), in which three different regression lines and equations were presented for specific subgroups of individuals. This method decreases the error in the prediction of $\dot{V}O_2$ from work load. These slight differences probably exist because of varying functional capacities and efficiencies among different groups.

There is also a positive linear correlation between VO_2 and HR that is unique to each individual when performing a simple activity. However, the slope and y-intercept of this linear correlation will change as different

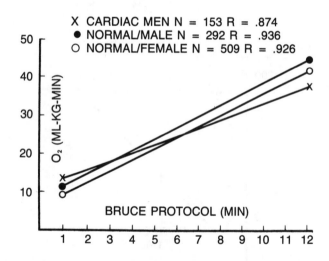

Figure 9.9. The linear relationship between work on the Bruce protocol and energy cost in ml of O_2 per kg of body weight per min for cardiac males, normal males, and normal females. *Note.* From "Maximal Oxygen Intake and Nomograhic Assessment of Functional Aerobic Impairment in Cardiovascular Disease" by R. Bruce, T. Kusumi, and D. Hosmer, 1973, *American Heart Journal*, **85**, p. 546. Copyright 1973 by *American Heart Journal*. Adapted by permission.

simple activities are performed (see Figure 9.10). It has also been shown to change between individuals who are trained and untrained, and also in individuals beginning a training program. The unique correlation that exists between each individual's HR and $\dot{V}O_2$ will fluctuate with variations in environmental and psychosocial situations and level of functional capacity. It appears, then, that this method of determining $\dot{V}O_2$ from HR could be used only in situations where simple activities were being performed in a controlled setting with a unique group of individuals that did not change its functional capacity. This is not applicable to the worksite at which complex activities are performed under a variety of environmental and psychosocial stresses by individuals with different functional capacities.

The activities discussed so far (bicycle ergometry and treadmill walking) are simple activities, and we can predict their energy cost within an acceptable range. There are greater individual variations in mechanical efficiency and oxygen consumption if an activity becomes complex. It also becomes increasingly difficult to perform complex activities at identical intensities to evaluate the oxygen consumption. This becomes apparent in evaluating the energy cost of occupations in light of the variety of individuals and individual working intensities and paces.

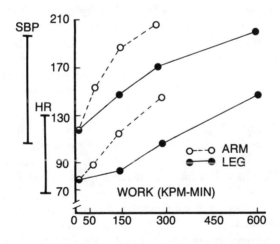

Figure 9.10. Comparison of heart rate (HR) and systolic blood pressure (SBP) responses at rest and during submaximal arm and leg ergometry in patients with ischemic heart disease. *Note.* From J. Schwade, 1977, *American Heart Journal*, **94**, p. 203. Copyright 1977 by *American Heart Journal*. Adapted by permission.

Complex Activities

The most complete review of human energy expenditure during work and leisure-time activities was presented by Passmore and Durnin (1955). A more recent compilation of the energy cost of various activities, which reviewed the work of several sources (Bannister & Brown, 1968; Howley & Glover, 1974; Passmore & Durnin, 1955), is presented by McArdle, Katch, and Katch (1981). It is necessary to understand several assumptions that have been implied in the construction of many energy cost tables before utilizing them.

Sample Size.   A review of the original studies revealed that the number of individuals tested was very small in many cases. This type of data collection does not provide an accurate representation of a particular activity and allows for a large deviation when assuming energy costs of activities. The assumptions that many tables make are that all individuals represent the small sample population, which is not true, and thus generalizations should not be made from small samples.

Energy Expressions.   Many tables often present their data in absolute units such as kcal per min or liters of O_2 per min. Use of these tables would assign the same energy cost of weight-bearing activities for individuals of all body weights. This would not be accurate because of the relation that body weight has to energy expenditure (see Figure 9.7). A relative expression such as ml/kg/min, METs, or kcal/kg/min would be much more accurate when considering individual variations in body weight. Several tables are presented in this manner (American College of Sports Medicine [ACSM], 1980; McArdle et al., 1981). The assumption that many tables make is that individuals performing activities have the same body weight, and thus the tables do not allow a greater absolute energy expenditure for individuals with increased weight.

Activity Variation.   Many tables do not take into account the variations in intensity or mechanical efficiency of the activities evaluated. Some tables are presented with mean energy expenditure and ranges (Åstrand & Rodahl, 1977), which is a more accurate approach that allows variation to account for work performed at different intensities. The assumption that many tables make is that all activities are performed at the same intensity and mechanical efficiencies. Therefore, when assessing the energy cost for any purpose, these assumptions have a direct effect on the accuracy of the energy assessment based on tables. They must be considered or at the minimum realized when assessing energy cost with tables.

All of the previously mentioned assessments of energy were performed on individuals without cardiovascular disease. But, can the assumption be made that individuals with cardiovascular disease will perform activities at the same energy cost as those without cardiovascular disease? Or will their work be less intense dictating a decrease in energy expenditure in this population?

Occupational Energy Cost of Individuals With Cardiovascular Disease

Only a small amount of literature has been presented in which oxygen consumption has been measured during occupational activities in a cardiac population. The following section will look at a variety of occupations ranging from relatively light factory work to work in a steel mill. The energy evaluation of business and professional fields will also be reviewed.

Factory Work.   A study on factory workers (Ford & Hellerstein, 1958), which included 30 types of work, revealed that the average rates of energy expenditure in kcal per min between the cardiac group and a matched noncardiac group (controls) were not significantly different (see Table 9.2). The average rate of energy expenditure of workers with heart disease was 1.97 kcal per min compared to 2.13 kcal per min in the matched controls. Figure 9.11 represents the results of this study by job classification. The intermittent nature of work is responsible for the lower energy cost of the entire shift when compared to the energy cost of actual work. The actual working energy costs were not significantly different between the two groups: 2.29 in the cardiac group and 2.51 in the control group ($p < .4$). The energy cost of the individual jobs increased as the work involved the use of progressively larger muscle groups. There was also no significant difference in the average peak kcal expended per min ($p < .2$). These values were 3.45 kcal/min in the control and 3.04 kcal/min in the cardiac group. Only one individual exceeded 5 kcal per min during the entire work evaluation; however, this was only for a short period of time.

Table 9.2   Average Rates of Energy Expenditure (calories per minute)

	Cardiacs (N = 36)		Controls (N = 26)	
	Average	S.D.	Average	S.D.
At rest	1.30	0.25	1.40	0.20
During shift	1.97	0.48	2.13	0.45
During actual work	2.29	0.64	2.51	0.68

The mean and standard deviation values for kcal of energy expenditure during factory work in cardiacs and controls. There is no significant difference between the two groups ($p < .4$). *Note.* From "Work and Heart Disease: I. A Physiologic Study in the Factory" by A. Ford and H. Hellerstein, 1958, *Circulation*, **18**, p. 825. Copyright 1958 by *Circulation*. Adapted by permission.

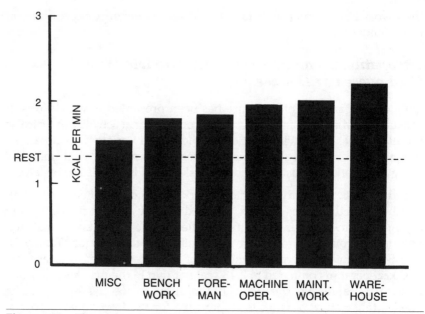

Figure 9.11.   The mean rate of energy expenditure during an 8-hr shift of 36 factory workers with heart disease. *Note*. From "Work and Heart Disease: I. A Physiologic Study in the Factory" by A. Ford and H. Hellerstein, 1958, *Circulation*, **18**, p. 823. Copyright 1958 by *Circulation*. Adapted by permission.

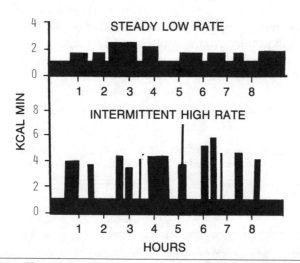

Figure 9.12.   The pattern of energy expenditure during a 3-hr shift for two types of jobs representing a steady low rate and an intermittent high rate of work. *Note*. From "Work and Disease: I. A Physiologic Study in the Factory" by A. Ford and H. Hellerstein, 1958, *Circulation*, **18**, p. 823. Copyright 1958 by *Circulation*. Adapted by permission.

Two patterns of work were observed in the work evaluations: (a) a low rate of energy expenditure maintained fairly steadily and (b) higher peaks of energy expenditure alternating with inactive periods (see Figure 9.12). The majority of jobs resembled the low, steady pattern.

Steel Mill. Another evaluation of the energy assessment of individuals with cardiovascular disease was performed on workers holding 34 different jobs in a steel mill (Ford, Hellerstein, & Turell, 1959). The jobs held by the workers with cardiovascular disease were matched with a group of workers without cardiovascular disease (controls) who held similar jobs. Two main types of stress were identified in the steel mill: (a) heat stress and (b) energy expenditure of the activity. However, temperature does not appear to alter the actual kcal expenditure of activity (see Figure 9.6). But, heat will alter both HR and BP responses at identical work loads. These cardiovascular alterations that will significantly effect myocardial oxygen consumption will be discussed in greater detail in the following section.

The energy expenditure, like that of the factory workers, was related to the muscular involvement of the job. The average energy expenditure of the most demanding job classification (furnaceman) was 3.03 kcal/min. The energy in kcal per min for each job classification is represented in Figure 9.13.

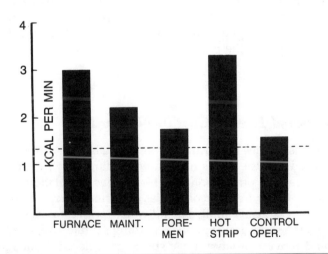

Figure 9.13.   The mean rate of energy expenditure during an 8-hr shift of five job categories of steel mill workers in individuals with and without heart disease. *Note.* From ''Work and Heart Disease: II. A Physiologic Study in a Steel Mill'' by A. Ford, H. Hellerstein, and D. Turrell, 1959, *Circulation,* **20,** p. 537. Copyright 1959 by *Circulation.* Adapted by permission.

The individual job with the highest energy expenditure was that of furnaceman-second helper. The average and highest single energy expenditure of this job was 4.50 and 8.3 kcal/min, respectively. However, no workers with cardiovascular disease held this position. It has been estimated that 5 kcal/min is the maximum tolerable limit of sustained energy expenditure for an 8-hr work shift in a healthy man (Passmore & Durnin, 1955).

The results of this study demonstrate that the average energy expenditure during the shift and during actual work, maximum energy expenditure, and the proportion of resting to working time showed no significant differences between the cardiovascular disease group and control group. The previous two studies support the fact that individuals with cardiovascular disease can maintain jobs in relatively low-energy cost (factory) and relatively high-energy cost (steel mill) jobs based on their energy expenditure alone. This can be attributed to the intermittent pattern of work.

Businessmen.   An investigation of businessmen (Hellerstein, 1978) with old myocardial infarctions represented one subsample of this larger study. The results showed that the energy cost averaged 1.97 kcal/min with an average peak value of 2.29 kcal/min. These values were much the same as the energy requirements of the factory workers. However, there was a difference in the peak energy expenditure values. As expected, the factory workers averaged higher peak energy expenditures (3.45 kcal/min) in comparison with the businessmen (2.29 kcal/min).

Occupational Energy Cost of Noncardiacs

The previous studies performed on individuals with cardiovascular disease showed that there was no significant difference in energy cost between the cardiac population and noncardiac population. Therefore it appears that the energy cost of studies performed on noncardiac populations can be reasonably applied to individuals with cardiovascular disease. However, the same assumptions regarding sample size, energy expressions, and activity variation must still be considered. It must always be recognized that these energy costs are only estimations and should be used in that manner, and that this type of energy cost evaluation does not take into account hemodynamic limitations that may exist in individuals with cardiovascular disease.

Sedentary Work.   The average energy costs for miscellaneous office work while sitting and standing have been estimated at 1.6 and 1.8 kcal/min, respectively (Passmore & Durnin, 1955). The energy expenditure of this so-called mental work, which includes office work, is not different from sitting or standing at leisure unless such occupations involve a greater amount of physical demand, such as walking, bending, or opening and closing drawers (Åstrand & Rodahl, 1977).

It has been shown that mental work requires only a minor rise in energy cost (Hellerstein, 1978; Bendict & Bendict, 1933); however, it has been shown that mental work can be associated with muscular tension as a result of emotional stress (Eiff & Gopfert, cited in Åstrand & Rodahl, 1977) and with increasing energy cost as much as 11%. This says nothing about the effect that stress has on myocardial energy cost.

Manual Labor.   Occupational activities such as coal mining (3.0–10.5 kcal/min), iron and steel work (5.5–16 kcal/min), and lumber work (5.5–20 kcal/min) have been reported as peak energy cost in European occupational evaluations. These types of intensities can only be maintained in an intermittent fashion but can require as much as 6,000 kcal per day. To perform at this energy cost a very high degree of muscular strength and functional capacity is required, and only a select few can work at this level.

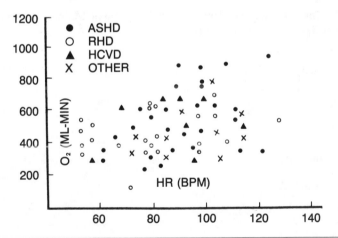

Figure 9.14.   The relationship between heart rate and energy cost of 36 factory workers with heart disease. *Note.* From "Work and Heart Disease: I. A Physiologic Study in the Factory" by A. Ford and H. Hellerstein, 1958, *Circulation, 18,* p. 823. Copyright 1958 by *Circulation.* Adapted by permission.

Attempts have been made to use the relationship that exists between HR and $\dot{V}O_2$ to determine the energy cost of an activity from the HR alone. As discussed earlier, this method must be used with caution because of the many factors that have been shown to alter this relationship (e.g., environmental factors, psychosocial factors, and individual functional capacity). Ford and Hellerstein (1958) verified that this method could not be used for the prediction of the energy cost of factory workers (see Figure 9.14). This method of predicting energy cost at kcal expenditures has been shown to be accurate in occupations that require greater than 5 kcal per min of energy (Lundgren, 1946).

The Energy Cost of an 8-Hr Work Shift

The effect that an activity has on an individual over an extended period of time and its relative effect on the cardiovascular load must be viewed in relation to the maximal working capacity. As an example, running a mile in 12 min would be extremely demanding for an individual with a maximal capacity of 35 ml/kg/min (approx. 87% of maximum). It would be quite easy for an individual with a maximal capacity of 60 ml/kg/min (approx. 50% of maximum) to perform this task. Similarly, in the work setting, individuals with higher work capacities can produce a greater amount of work for the same relative percent of energy expenditure or perform the same amount of work at a much lower percent of maximum.

Table 9.3   The Percent of O_2 Consumption That Can be Maintained for an 8-Hr Work Bout Based on Maximal Aerobic Capacity

Aerobic capacity (max $\dot{V}O^2$)	Relative % of $\dot{V}O_2$ (8 hr)
Superb physical condition 4.5 l O_2 (60 ml-kg-min)*	38.5
Average condition 3.0 l O_2 (40 ml-kg-min)*	25
Very poor condition 2.25 l O_2 (30 ml-kg-min)*	20

*Based on a 75-kg male
Note. From "Proceedings of the First Canadian Fitness Seminar" by B. Balke, 1968, in H. Falls (Ed.), *Exercise Physiology* (p. 301), New York: Academic Press. Copyright 1968 by Academic Press. Adapted by permission.

It has been reported that work loads approximating 50% of maximal capacity are the upper limit of the optimal work load for a 1-hr period, without disturbing the physiological equilibrium (Åstrand, Åstrand, & Rodahl, 1959). Different ranges of relative energy cost have been reported for the limits of an 8-hr work shift. Passmore and Durnin (1955) reported that an upper limit for healthy men was 5 kcal/min (approx. 14.7 ml/kg/min). This method however does not take into account the maximal capacity. Åstrand and Rodahl (1977) and others (Caldwell, 1863; Blomqvist, 1969) have reported relative values of 30–40% of maximal capacity as a reasonable average upper limit for physical work performed regularly over an 8-hr workday.

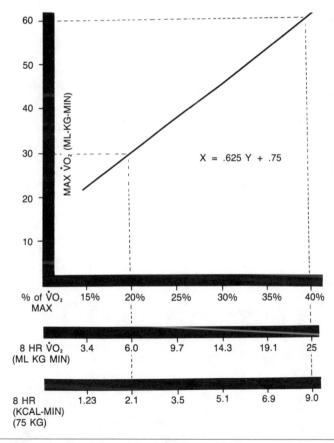

Figure 9.15. The linear regression equation and line to determine the percent of maximal capacity that can be maintained for an 8-hr work shift without undue fatigue. *Note.* From ''Proceedings of the First Canadian Fitness Seminar'' by B. Balke, 1968, in H. Falls (Ed.), *Exercise Physiology* (p. 301), New York: Academic Press. Copyright 1968 by Academic Press. Adapted by permission.

Table 9.4 Classification of Physical Work Recommended From the Work Capacity Test

Classification of work	HR/min	MR O₂ cc/min	MR cal/min	Ventilation vol. l/min	Ventilation rate/min	RQ	Lactic acid in multiples of rest. val.	Time of duration work can be sustained
I. Light								
1. Mild	< 100	< 750	< 4	< 20	< 14	.85	Normal	Indefinite
2. Moderate	< 120	< 1500	< 7.5	< 35	< 15	.85	Within normal limits	8 hr daily
II. Heavy								
3. Optimal	< 140	< 2000	< 10	< 50	< 16	.9	1.5 ×	8 hr daily for few weeks (seasonal work; military maneuvers, etc.)
4. Strenuous	< 160	< 2500	< 12.5	< 60	< 20	.95	2 ×	4 hr. two or three times a week for few weeks (special physical training)
III. Severe								
5. Maximal	< 180	< 3000	< 15	< 80	< 25	< 1.0	5-6 ×	1 to 2 hr occasionally (usually in competitive sports)
6. Exhausting	> 180	> 3000	> 15	< 120	< 30	> 1.0	> 6 ×	Few minutes, rarely

The classification of physical work recommended from the work capacity test based on heart rate (HR), metabolic rate (MR), ventilation, respiratory exchange ratio (RQ), and lactic acid. *Note.* From "Lactic Acid Accumulation During Work: A Suggested Standardization of Work Classification" by G. Wells, B. Balke, and D. Fossan, 1957, *Journal of Applied Physiology, 10*(1), p. 51. Copyright 1957 by *Journal of Applied Physiology.* Adapted by permission.

Balke, in Falls (1968), described the relationship between maximal capacity and ability to work at certain levels of energy expenditure. This study showed that noncardiac individuals with higher maximal capacities could work at higher intensities for an 8-hr work period. The results of this study are presented in Table 9.3 and displayed as a linear regression in Figure 9.15.

Another classification system (Wells, Balke, & Fossan, 1957) offers six classification categories of work (see Table 9.4). This study also took into account lactate accumulation, heart rate, metabolic rate, ventilation, and respiratory exchange ratio in their classification system. Energy costs from 4 to 7.5 kcal/min were suggested to be an energy cost that could be tolerated for 8 hr of daily work on a permanent basis. These values appear much higher than those of Balke (1968), and neither study took into account body weight.

It appears that as an individual increases in age the maximal capacity decreases; but, occupational work remains fairly constant throughout the working years (Muller, 1962). One explanation for this plateau in occupational energy cost is that older workers may be more highly skilled than younger workers and thus able to perform at a lower caloric expenditure. Another explanation may be that the pace of the work remains relatively constant for a particular occupation and is usually independent of individual capacities. In other words, workers tend to keep up with the pace set by their peers independent of their relative energy expenditure. The average maximal capacity for individuals with cardiovascular disease (Bruce, 1977) is 30–40 ml/kg/min. Therefore, work on a long-term basis should not tax greater than 20–25% of this maximal capacity. This would be approximately a 7–9 ml/kg/min level of work, or approximately 2.6–3.3 kcal per min for a 75-kg man.

This level would enable participation in factory work (Ford & Hellerstein, 1958), where the average caloric cost was 1.97 kcal/min with peak energy expenditures of 2.13 kcal per min, without causing an unusual metabolic stress. Many jobs in a steel mill (Ford et al., 1959) could also be tolerated where the average energy cost was 2.51 kcal per min with peak levels of 4.05 kcal per min.

Based on the classification presented by Balke, in Falls (1968) and the determination of an individual's maximal functional capacity, the following equation can be used to determine the approximate Kcal per min that can be tolerated during an 8-hr day for an extended period of time:

$$kcal/min = (max/kcal/min \times .625) + .75$$

where kcal/min is equal to the kilocalories that can be tolerated for an 8-hr day, and max/kcal/min is equal to the maximal capacity represented in kilocalories. Figure 9.15 represents this equation in graphic form. A common error exists when performing an occupational or recreational energy assessment when an activity exceeds that of the individual's recommended daily kcal per min prescription or exceeds the individual's functional capacity. First it should be recognized that the daily kcal per min prescription represents an average of intermittent work, some work performed above and some below the average. This can be demonstrated in Figure 9.12, which shows two common patterns of energy expenditure during an 8-hr shift of two types of factory jobs in individuals with cardiovascular disease (Ford & Hellerstein, 1958). It can be seen that an individual working at an intermittent high rate of work often exceeds 3.5 kcal per min and even reaches 6 kcal per min but only averages 2 kcal per min for the entire 8-hr shift.

An individual therefore should not be restricted from performing intermittent activities greater than the recommended daily kcal per minute if there are no other contraindications such as abnormal BP, rhythm, angina, or electrocardiographic (EKG) changes.

Another common problem exists when an individual exceeds the predicted maximal capacity derived from an exercise tolerance test (ETT). This also can occur during intermittent activities where activities of short duration and high intensity are performed. This will occur because during the ETT the individual performs a progressive continuous test and reaches maximal cardiovascular capacity and when performing the intermittent work the individual reaches local muscle fatigue but not total cardiovascular fatigue. Activities of short duration and relatively high intensity that appear to elicit a high energy cost may be performed by many individuals with or without cardiovascular disease if there are no other cardiovascular complications such as hypertension, aneurysm, left ventricular dysfunction, or severe coronary artery disease. The final decision should be based on signs or symptoms when stressing the myocardial O_2 consumption.

Subjective Assessment of Energy Cost

The *Dictionary of Occupational Titles* (U.S. Department of Labor [USDOL], 1981) lists and defines the characteristics of approximately 8,000 job titles. This type of information may assist in the energy assessment of a particular occupation. A more accurate subjective assessment would be obtained by interviewing the worker in a prospective situation or interviewing someone who was familiar with the intricacies of the particular job in a prospective situation. The system of analyzing a particular job presented in the directory provides valuable guidelines when conducting a job assessment interview.

Table 9.5 The Classification System to Evaluate the Physical Demands and Working Conditions

Physical demands

1. Strength (lift, carry, push, pull):

	Maximum lift	Frequent lift
S Sedentary	10 lb	
L Light	20 lb	up to 10 lb
M Medium	50 lb	up to 25 lb
H Heavy	100 lb	up to 50 lb
V Very heavy	over 100 lb	over 50 lb

2. Climb and balance

3. Stoop, kneel, crouch, crawl

4. Reach, handle, finger, feel

5. Talk, hear

6. See (acuity, depth perception, field of vision, accommodation)

Working conditions

1. I Inside (75% or more)

   O Outside (75% or more)

   B Both

2. Extremes of cold plus temperature changes

3. Extremes of heat plus temperature changes

4. Wet and humid

5. Noise and vibration

6. Hazards

7. Fumes, odors, toxic conditions, dust, poor ventilation

Note. From *Selected Characteristics of Occupations Defined in the Dictionary of Occupational Titles* (p. 479) by the U.S. Department of Labor, 1981, Washington, DC: U.S. Government Printing Office. Copyright 1981 by U.S. Government Printing Office. Reprinted by permission.

The physical demands (strength) of a particular occupation have been classified and expressed in terms of sedentary, light, medium, heavy, and very heavy activity. These strength categories are grouped according to specific pounds lifted, carried, pushed, or pulled (see Table 9.5). Other attributes such as balancing, crouching, handling, and using visual perception have also been included in the assessment. The strength classifications may be very helpful in assessing the requirements for an individual with hypertension, aneurysm, or left ventricular dysfunction who should not place a further pressure overload on the cardiovascular system. Lifting and pushing activities may also lead to complications encountered due to a Valsalva maneuver.

Working conditions are also categorized in the *Dictionary of Occupational Titles* (USDOL, 1981). The conditions identified include extremes in environmental conditions such as temperature, humidity, noise, or fumes.

Table 9.6   Energy Cost of Work Classifications

Work classification	Energy cost (kcal/min)
S (Sedentary)	2.5 and below
L (Light)	2.6 to 4.9
M (Medium)	5.0 to 7.5
H (Heavy)	7.6 and above
V (Very heavy)	7.6 and above

Note. Adapted from *Recreational and Occupational Recommendations for Use by Physicians Counseling Young Patients With Heart Disease* (AHA publication 71-008-A) by the American Heart Association, 1971. Copyright 1971 by the American Heart Association, Inc. Adapted by permission.

Table 9.7   Average and Peak Average Heart Rate and Blood Pressure Values Recorded on the Job of Several Occupations in Cardiac and Noncardiac Patients

Occupation	HR		BP	
	Avg	Peak	Avg	Peak
Factory	102	122	136/81	153/89
Steel mill	87	158		
Radio-Television	92	116	126/81	136/89
Businessmen	82	103		
Anesthetists	83	108	121/79	140/86
Firemen	89	140	116/80	156/108
Surgeons	104	118	132/84	147/92

Note. From "Prescription and Vocational Leisure Activities" by H. Hellerstein, 1978, *Advances in Cardiology,* **24,** p. 105. Copyright 1978 by *Advances in Cardiology.* Adapted by permission.

Attempts to correlate the physical demands, as listed in the *Dictionary of Occupational Titles*, with energy cost (see Table 9.6) have been performed (American Heart Association, 1971). However, these must be used only as estimations because the myocardial O_2 consumption will vary in individuals at the same MET levels.

Thus far I have discussed only one expression of energy—total energy cost or kcal per min. Another expression of energy cost, which is of prime consideration to the individual with cardiovascular disease, is myocardial energy cost ($M\dot{V}O_2$). Often the $M\dot{V}O_2$ is the limiting factor when individuals with cardiovascular disease are performing occupational and recreational activities.

Evaluation of Myocardial Energy Cost ($M\dot{V}O_2$)

The total energy cost or $\dot{V}O_2$ of an activity can be measured quite accurately and without much discomfort or risk to the individual. The total energy cost measures the metabolic load placed upon the entire system including skeletal and smooth muscle function and organ functions including the myocardial oxygen consumption. The ability to perform an activity depends in large part on the capacity of both the skeletal and myocardium to extract and utilize oxygen. The quantity of oxygen consumed depends on the load placed on the skeletal muscles and the myocardium, respectively. There is a direct linear relationship between total energy cost ($\dot{V}O_2$) and energy output (see Figure 9.3) and also between $M\dot{V}O_2$ and myocardial work (see Figure 9.16). However, there is a poor relationship between myocardial work and energy output because of various factors that may raise MVO_2 without an accompanying rise in $\dot{V}O_2$ such as a sympathetic rise in heart rate and blood pressure brought on by psychosocial factors and environmental conditions. An increase or decrease in any one of the major determinants of $M\dot{V}O_2$ (see Figure 9.17) would cause a disproportionate relationship to total energy consumption. For this reason both total energy cost and, more importantly, myocardial oxygen consumption of various occupations and activities should be considered in a cardiac population.

Myocardial oxygen consumption cannot be measured directly by noninvasive techniques. However, it can be estimated from its relationship to a combination of its major determinants: heart rate, intramyocardial tension, and myocardial contractility. In the clinical setting, $M\dot{V}O_2$ may be estimated from the relationship of the product of the HR and systolic blood pressure (SBP) termed *double product* (Kitamura, Jorgensen, Gobel, et al., 1970) or *triple product*, which is the product of HR, SBP, and left ventricular ejection time (LVET). Figure 9.18 represents the relationship between $M\dot{V}O_2$ and double product with a correlation coefficient of .90. This relationship has been shown to be consistent with and independent of variations in type, intensity, and duration of exercise (Robinson, 1967), as demonstrated in Figure 9.19 in a group of individuals with cardiovascular disease.

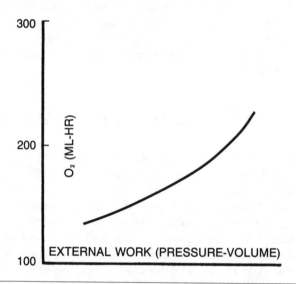

Figure 9.16. The relationship between external myocardial work (pressure volume) and O_2 consumption. *Note.* From *Physiology of the Heart* (p. 218) by A. Katz, 1977, New York: Raven Press. Copyright 1977 by Raven Press. Adapted by permission.

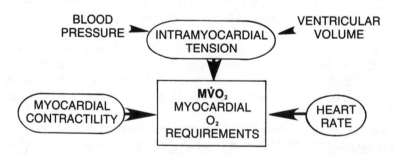

Figure 9.17. The major determinants of myocardial O_2 consumption. *Note.* From "Physiologic Approach to the Medical and Surgical Treatment of Angina Pectoris" by E. Amsterdam, J. Hughes, R. Miller, R. Massumi, R. Zelus, and D. Mason, in J. Naughton, H. Hellerstein, and I. Mohler (Eds.), *Exercise Testing and Exercise Training in Coronary Heart Disease* (p. 104), New York: Academic Press. Copyright 1973 by Academic Press. Reprinted by permission.

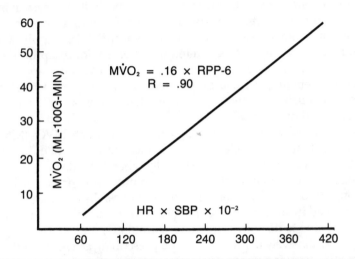

Figure 9.18. The relationship between myocardial O_2 consumption and double product (HR $\times$ SBP $\times$ 10^{-2}). *Note.* From R. Kitamura, 1972, *Journal of Applied Physiology, 32,* p. 516. Copyright 1972 by *Journal of Applied Physiology.* Adapted by permission.

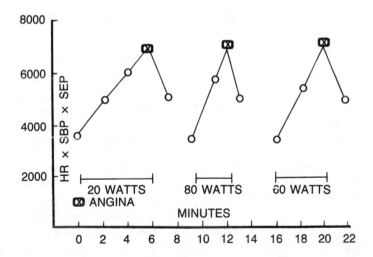

Figure 9.19. The relation of onset of angina to duration and intensity of exercise on the bicycle ergometer and the triple product (HR, SBP, SEP). Angina occurs at a constant triple product. *Note.* From "Relation of Heart Rate and Systolic Blood Pressure to the Onset of Pain in Angina Pectoris" by B. Robinson, 1967, *Circulation, 35,* p. 1073. Copyright 1967 by *Circulation.* Reprinted by permission.

Occupational and recreational activities may be limited in certain individuals with coronary artery obstruction by establishing a level that does not precipitate an imbalance between myocardial O_2 supply and O_2 demand. Activity may also be limited in patients with compromised left ventricular function where ejection fraction decreases due to a specific myocardial demand, cardiac output falls, and coronary perfusion decreases. Rate-related dysrhythmias are another complication that may also be precipitated at a set $M\dot{V}O_2$, which must be considered.

Heart rate can also be used as a single factor to estimate MVO_2 (Kitamura et al., 1970; Robinson, 1967). This single measurement of HR has limitations for use in assessing $M\dot{V}O_2$, especially when BP is disproportionately elevated. This may occur during upper extremity work or isometric work, or in conjunction with emotions. However, HR can be easily and accurately determined in almost any occupational or recreational activity. For this reason and due to its high correlation with $M\dot{V}O_2$, heart rates have been used quite extensively in proscribing and prescribing activity in individuals with cardiovascular disease during typical activities.

Hung, McKellop, & Savin (1982) found HR to track the onset of ischemic abnormalities as effectively as the product of HR and BP. This was limited to the clinical setting, however, and did not take into account disproportionate rises in BP.

Laboratory and Clinical Evaluation of Myocardial Energy Cost

Because the $M\dot{V}O_2$ can be noninvasively assessed by monitoring HR and BP during activity, this method has been applied in both the clinical and the work setting. In the clinical setting, HR and BP can be measured during an ETT. Likewise, HR and BP can be assessed during occupational tasks. From these evaluations, guidelines can be established regarding safe working levels for individuals with cardiovascular disease.

Laboratory Evaluation. Previous work in assessing a patient's response to a particular work setting emphasized laboratory simulation of the patient's work environment (Franklin & Hellerstein, 1982). These so-called realistic performance tests document the cardiovascular response taking into account the type and duration of skeletal muscle contraction and the specific cardiovascular stress, which may be either a volume or pressure overload performed during a particular vocational activity. These realistic performance tests can be very useful in specific instances (e.g., when a patient is returning to a job that requires excessive lifting, climbing, or heavy manual labor). Independent of the method of evaluation, the laboratory evaluation should be a symptom-limited dynamic test, which elicits a clinically maximal cardiovascular response. This symptom-limited maximal test is most likely to elicit clinically important myocardial ischemia and left ventricular dysfunction (Debusk & Dennis, 1982). These two entities, myocardial ischemia and left ventricular function, are major determinants of both prognosis and functional capacity.

Leg ergometry has been shown to be more effective than arm ergometry (Debusk, Convertina, Hung, et al., 1982) and equally effective as a combination static effort (Debusk, Pitts, Haskell, et al., 1979). It has also been shown that there are no differences in eliciting ischemic responses and angina pectoris when testing patients in a cold environment (Lassvik & Areskog) or in a postprandial state (Hung, McKellop, Savin, et al., 1982).

It appears that, when possible, a symptom-limited dynamic test using the lower extremities in the typical laboratory setting may be the most accurate, efficient, and cost-effective approach to take when evaluating work capacity. As always HR, BP, signs, and symptoms should be documented throughout the evaluation. From this information an individualized work prescription can be formulated and presented to the patient. The activities of work should not exceed the HR and/or BP limits established by the laboratory evaluation.

Occupational Evaluation.   The evaluation of an individual at work would provide the most accurate method of assessing $M\dot{V}O_2$ through HR and BP. Heart rate evaluation with the use of radio telemetry systems and more recently Holter monitoring systems have been used quite extensively for this purpose. These portable, lightweight units are valuable tools in identifying excessive HR responses and dysrhythmias, which may not have occurred during the clinical evaluation and may be directly related to occupational work. Recently, portable blood pressure units have also been used to assist in the detection of inappropriate BP response of occupational and other daily tasks. If a particular occupation or task elicits an abnormal HR and/or BP response that is associated with angina, ventricular dysfunction, arrhythmias, or an ischemic response, then the particular task or occupation should be discontinued.

HR and BP responses have been evaluated during various occupations in cardiac populations. But, as previously discussed and displayed in Figure 9.14, HR can not be predicted accurately from work load.

In studies evaluating HR and BP responses during steel mill work (Ford & Hellerstein, 1958), BP was shown to rise an average of 6mm Hg systolic and 3mm Hg diastolic for 33 noncardiac subjects. These changes were no greater for men with arteriosclerotic heart disease. The men with heart disease did show a significantly higher average heart rate during low-energy-related tasks than noncardiacs. This difference persisted from before work (rest) to the end of the shift. Average and peak HR and BP statistics are presented in Table 9.7, which represents seven studies of various occupations on both cardiac and noncardiac subjects. These data indicate that neither mean HRs or BPs appear to be excessive in any of the listed occupations. These values did have wide ranges and should not be used in occupational work prescription because of individual variation. However, most individuals with noncomplicated myocardial infarction and post-coronoary artery bypass surgery should be able to tolerate these relatively small increases in HR and BP. One study with a cardiac population of post-myocardial infarction and post-coronary artery bypass patients in an outpatient rehabilitation program summarized mean training HRs to be 131-142 bpm (Pollock, Ward, & Foster, 1979).

Table 9.7 Average and Peak Average Heart Rate and Blood Pressure Values Recorded on the Job of Several Occupations in Cardiac and Noncardiac Patients

Occupation	HR		BP	
	Avg	Peak	Avg	Peak
Factory	102	122	136/81	153/89
Steel mill	87	158		
Radio-Television	92	116	126/81	136/89
Businessmen	82	103		
Anesthetists	83	108	121/79	140/86
Firemen	89	140	116/80	156/108
Surgeons	104	118	132/84	147/92

Note. From "Prescription and Vocational Leisure Activities" by H. Hellerstein, 1978, *Advances in Cardiology*, **24**, p. 105. Copyright 1978 by *Advances in Cardiology*. Adapted by permission.

Summary and Application

When assessing the energy cost of various occupations both total energy cost and myocardial energy cost should be considered. The total energy cost can provide information concerning occupations that can be tolerated without undue fatigue for an 8-hr work shift. The myocardial oxygen consumption provides information concerning the individual's ability to perform an occupation at levels that do not cause an imbalance between O_2

supply and O_2 demand. The following summary is offered to assist in the assessment of various occupations and activities.

1. The average total energy cost of most occupations is approximately:

    2-3 kcal min
    5.3-8 ml-kg-min
    1.5-2.3 METs

   However, intensity is a significant factor.
2. The average myocardial energy cost of most occupations is also relatively low as represented by HR and BP:

    Average HR = 91
    Average BP = 126/81
    Average RPP $\times$ 10^{-2} = 115

   However, these values may be affected by environmental, psychosocial, and individual working differences.
3. An individual should not work at an occupation at an intensity that elicits abnormal physiological responses:

    Dangerous arrhythmias
    Ischemic EKG changes (HR $\times$ BP)
    Angina (HR $\times$ BP)
    Ventricular dysfunction
4. An individual should not work at an occupation at an intensity that elicits undue fatigue at the end of an 8-hr shift—usually 20-40% of maximum aerobic capacity.

References

American College of Sports Medicine. (1980). Guidelines for graded exercise testing and exercise prescription. Philadelphia: Lea and Febiger.

American Heart Association. (1971). *Recreational and occupational recommendations for use by physicians counseling young patients with heart disease* (AHA publication 71-008-A).

Åstrand, I., Åstrand, P., & Rodahl, P. (1959). *Journal of Applied Physiology*, **14**, 562.

Åstrand, P., & Rodahl, K. (1977). *Textbook of work physiology*. New York: McGraw Hill.

Bannister, R., & Brown, S. (1968). The relative energy requirements of physical activity. In H.B. Falls (Ed.), *Exercise physiology* (pp. 267-322), New York: Academic Press.

Bendict, F., & Bendict, C. (1933). *Mental effort in relation to gasious exchange, heart rate, and mechanics of respiration* (Report No. 446). Washington, DC: Carnegie Institute.

Blomqvist, G. (1969). Exercise and performance evaluation. *Journal of the South Carolina Medical Association,* (Suppl. December), 1-4.

Bobbert, A. (1968). Physiological comparison of three types of ergometry. *Journal of Applied Physiology,* **15**(6), 1007-1015.

Bruce, R. (1977). Methods of exercise testing: Steptest, bicycle, treadmill, isometrics. In E. Amsterdam, J. Wilmore, & A. DeMaria. *Exercise in cardiovascular health and disease* (pp. 149-160). New York: Yorke Medical.

Bruce, R., Kusumi, F., & Hosmer, D. (1973). Maximal oxygen intake and nomographic assessment of functional aerobic in cardiovascular disease. *American Heart Journal,* **85**, 546-562.

Caldwell, L. (1963). *Journal of English Psychology,* **2**, 155.

Carpenter, T. (1939). *Tables, factors and formulas for computing respiratory exchange and biological transformation of energy* (3rd ed.). Washington, DC: Carnegie Institute of Washington.

Consolazio, F., Johnson, R., & Pecora, L. (1963). *Physical measurement and metabolic function in man.* New York: McGraw Hill.

Debusk, R., Convertina, V., & Hung, J. (1982). Randomized trial of exercise training following bed rest in normal middle aged men: Relevance to patients recovering from myocardial infarction. *Clinical Research,* **30**, 6A.

Debusk, R., & Dennis, C. (1982). Occupational work evaluation of patients with cardiac disease: A guideline for physicians. *The Western Journal of Medicine,* **137**(6), 515-520.

Debusk, R., Pitts, W., & Haskell, W. (1979). A comparison of cardiovascular responses to combined static-dynamic and dynamic effort alone in patients with chronic ischemic heart disease. *Circulation,* **59**, 977-984.

Falls, H. (1968). *Exercise physiology.* New York: Academic Press.

Ford, A., & Hellerstein, H. (1958). Work and heart disease: I. A physiologic study in the factory. *Circulation,* **18**, 823-832.

Ford, A., Hellerstein, H., & Turell, D. (1959). Work and heart disease: II. A physiologic study in a steel mill. *Circulation,* **20**, 537-548.

Franklin, B., & Hellerstein, H. (1982). Realistic stress testing for activity prescription. *Journal of Cardiovascular Medicine,* 570-586.

Harrison, M., Brown, G., & Belyavin, A. (1982). The oxylog: An evaluation. *Ergonomics,* **25**(9), 809-820.

Hellerstein, H. (1978). Prescription of vocational and leisure activities. *Advances in Cardiology,* **24**, 104-115.

Howley, E., & Glover, M. (1974). The caloric cost of running and walking one mile for men and women. *Medicine and Science in Sports*, **6**, 235.

Hung, J., McKellop, J., & Savin, W. (1982). Comparison to cardiovascular response to combined static-dynamic effort, to postprandial dynamic effort and to dynamic effort alone in patients with chronic ischemic heart disease. *Circulation*, **65**, 1043-1048.

Kitamura, K., Jorgensen, C., & Gobel, O.F. (1970). Hemodynamic correlates of coronary blood flow and myocardial oxygen consumption during upright exercise. *American Journal of Cardiology*, **26**, 643.

Klausen, K. (1966). Cardiac output in man at rest and work during and after acclimatization to 3800 m. *Journal of Applied Physiology*, **21**, 609.

Lassvik, C., & Areskog, N. (1980). Angina pectoris during inhalation of cold air: Reactions to exercise. *British Heart Journal*, **43**, 661-667.

Lundgren, N. (1946). The physiological effect of time schedule work on lumber workers. *Acta Physiologica Scandinavica*, **13** (Suppl. 41), 1-157.

Lust, G. (1928). *Science of nutrition* (4th ed.). Philadelphia: W.B. Saunders.

McArdle, W., Katch, F., & Katch, V. (1981). *Exercise physiology: Energy, nutrition, and human performance.* Philadelphia: Lea and Febiger.

Mellerowicz, H., & Smodlaka, V. (1981). *Ergometry: Basics of medical exercise testing.* Baltimore: Urban & Schwarzenberg.

Muller, E. (1962). *Ergonomics*, **5**, 445.

Passmore, R., & Durnin, J. (1955). Human energy expenditure. *Physiological Reviews*, **35**, 801.

Pollock, M., Ward, A., & Foster, C. (1979). Exercise prescription for rehabilitation of the cardiac patient. In M. Pollock & D. Schmidt (Eds.), *Heart disease and rehabilitation* (pp. 413-415). New York: John Wiley.

Pugh, L. (1964). Muscular exercise at great altitudes. *Journal of Applied Physiology*, **19**, 431.

Robinson, B. (1967). Relation of heart rate and systolic blood pressure to the onset of pain in angina pectoris. *Circulation*, **35**, 1073-1083.

Rowell, L. (1974). Human cardiovascular adjustments to exercise and thermal stress. *Physiological Reviews*, **54**, 75.

Taylor, H. (1960). In W.R. Johnson (Ed.), *Science and medicine of exercise and sports* (p. 133). New York: Harper.

U.S. Department of Labor. (1981). *Selected characteristics of occupations defined in the Dictionary of Occupational Titles.* Washington, DC: U.S. Government Printing Office.

Van Baak, M., & Binkhorst, R. (1981). Oxygen consumption during outdoor recreational cycling. *Ergonomics*, **24**(9), 725-733.

Wells, G., Balke, B., & Fossan, D. (1957). Lactic acid accumulation during work: A suggested standardization of work classification. *Journal of Applied Physiology*, **10**(1), 51-55.

Chapter 10

Leisure Counseling and the Cardiac Patient

Janet Treftz
Thomas T. Gushiken

Since the late 1970s, changes have been made in the treatment of the myocardial infarction and bypass patient. The mortality rate for individuals admitted to hospitals with a myocardial infarction has decreased from 30 to 15%. Statistics show that 85% of those who suffer a myocardial infarction survive and return to normal lifestyles. Patients resume activities much sooner and are discharged much earlier from the hospital (Montiero, 1979). Several studies have demonstrated the effects of conservatively treated myocardial infarction patients (Wenger, 1971; Siegel, 1969). These studies have given the medical profession a basis for recommending early activity for the cardiac patient. Goldbarg (1973) showed that complete bed rest was psychologically harmful to the patients studied.

Patients who are considered medically stable are good candidates for early ambulation. These patients comprise one-half of all patients admitted to coronary care units. This phase of rehabilitation is generally considered to be Phase I or the inpatient phase of cardiac rehabilitation (Wenger & Hellerstein, 1978). In Phase I, activities are of very low intensity and typically will progress in intensity with each additional day of hospitalization. These activities generally include eating, learning self-care, using the commode, and performing active and passive exercises. Once the patient is removed from the coronary care unit, activities are designed to increase endurance so that the individual can perform household and other light activities without difficulty prior to returning home. The program may include occupational or recreational therapy as a regular part of the patient's daily routine. Patients perform light craft activities in their room, and this activity is considered a regular part of their progressive physical activity (Wenger & Hellerstein, 1978).

Once discharged, the patient may return to the hospital for exercise sessions two to three times a week. This phase of rehabilitation is called Phase II or outpatient cardiac rehabilitation. These sessions generally consist of regular exercise classes using the treadmill or stationary bicycle. The patients are monitored for electrocardiograph (EKG) responses while exercising, and a nurse, therapist, or exercise physiologist supervises each session. The patient remains in this phase anywhere from 4 to 12 weeks.

Cardiac patients who are unable to return to the hospital for outpatient exercise sessions are sent home with an exercise prescription that will often include either a walking program or a stationary bicycle program. Generally, periodic follow-up sessions are scheduled to check patient progress.

Impact of Increased Free Time

Wishnie (1971) studied the psychological hazards of the cardiac patient after returning home. Twenty-three patients reported that they felt frustrated with their inactivity at home. A few patients walked and others watched television during their free time. Three of the patients became involved in former hobbies. All the patients felt a lack of structure in their lives because they did not return to work. In all of the patients' families there was evidence of significant emotional conflict after the myocardial infarction. Seventy-five percent of the problems were the result of differences over medical instructions.

Patients who do not return to work are often depressed. Nagel and Gargola (1971) found that of the patients they studied who did not return to work, 55% were depressed. In more than half of the patients there was no clinical evidence of residual heart damage. They concluded that the emotional reactions were unrelated to the severity of the heart attack, but seemed to be associated with inadequate medical instructions about exercise and how to resume normal activities.

Finlayson and McEwen (1977) looked at the impact of a myocardial infarction on the patient's family and leisure activities. The men in the study reported a reduction in physical and social activities 4 years after the event. They spent less time gardening, were less involved in sports and clubs, went out less, and did less maintenance work around the house.

Totman (1979) studied those factors that promoted better adaptation to stressful life events. The results of the study indicated that the extent to which a person adjusted to a stressful life event could be determined by examining two factors before and after the event. The first factor was the overall extent of the patient involvement in leisure and work projects such as hobbies, yard work, carpentry, and others. The second factor was the patient's social improvements. If the individual's participation in projects and social activities increased or remained the same as before the event, it was inferred that the adjustment was good. A decline in socializing and activity involvement indicated that adjustment to a stressful life event such as a heart attack was poor or incomplete. Cardiac patients in the study were shown to have less goal-directed activities after their heart attack than control subjects. It was concluded that a reduction in activities and social contacts was potentially harmful to the health of the patient.

Role of Leisure Counseling in Cardiac Rehabilitation

When an individual is ill or handicapped, the need for meaningful leisure time activities is magnified. The ultimate goal of rehabilitation is to restore the functional capabilities of the patient so that he or she can return to the community as independently as possible. Vocational adjustment is very important, but for those patients who will not return to their same job or must modify their jobs, an excess of free time may be a problem (Hayes, 1977).

One way to individualize a program of physical activity and recreational involvement is through a process called leisure counseling. Leisure counseling is a process that uses all information gathered about a person to further explore interests and attitudes about leisure, recreation, and social relationships to enable the patient to identify, locate, and utilize community resources (O'Morrow, 1977). Leisure counseling can assist cardiac patients in returning to former hobbies and adapting to new restrictions by providing activities for leisure involvement (both active and passive).

Wenger and Hellerstein (1978) suggest that counseling may be a necessary component of cardiac rehabilitation programs. Hoeft (1979) conducted a study that examined the impact of leisure counseling in altering leisure attitudes, work self-concepts, work attitudes, leisure self-concepts, and leisure satisfaction of cardiac patients. The study concluded that leisure counseling significantly affected leisure self-concept and leisure satisfaction in the patients studied. A follow-up study was conducted to determine whether leisure counseling had sustained an increase in the participants' leisure satisfaction and leisure self-concept since the original leisure counseling sessions. It was concluded that those patients who participated in leisure counseling sustained a positive leisure self-concept after a period of 2 years (Hoeft, 1982).

The literature revealed several approaches to be used in the leisure counseling process (McDowell, 1977; Peterson, 1977). The approach or orientation that will be used with the client depends on the needs, strengths, and problems of the individual. Because people and their situations differ, the method or methods used to deal with these situations will also differ. The three orientations outlined by McDowell (1977) are leisure resource guidance, therapeutic-remedial-normalizing service, and lifestyle development education service.

A 7-Step Leisure Counseling Program

A leisure counseling program was developed for myocardial infarction and bypass patients (see Figure 10.1). From existing research in the area of leisure counseling a 7-step program was developed. The purpose of this model was to outline various approaches to leisure counseling that might be effective in improving the quality of leisure-time activities for cardiac patients, and to provide guidelines for cardiac rehabilitation personnel interested in establishing this type of program in their hospitals.

It is important to note that each step of the leisure counseling program can be independent of the others. The patient who has more problems participating in leisure activities may progress through all 7 steps. The patient's needs will dictate which steps are appropriate.

Step 1—Inpatient Occupational or Recreational Therapy

Step 1 is the 14-step program for Phase I of cardiac rehabilitation developed by Wenger and Hellerstein (1978) for the inpatient or a modified version of this. The 14-step program begins with range of motion exercises and activities of daily living and progresses the patient to ambulation on the hospital floor. The 14-step program also specifies that in certain steps patients read or perform light craft activities as part of their program. The general guideline is that the activity should not exceed 1–2 METs. A MET is a unit indicating intensity of activity. The therapist should refer to a MET chart to determine which activities are appropriate. Each step of the 14-step program is ordered or signed by the physician when he or she feels that the patient is capable of completing that step. Patients generally complete all 14 steps prior to discharge. In most hospitals the 14-step program will begin 1–2 days after admission for those patients who are not experiencing complications. The use of craft activities in the inpatient setting serves to increase each patient's functional capacity. In this setting, recreational activities are used to keep patients active during their hospital stay.

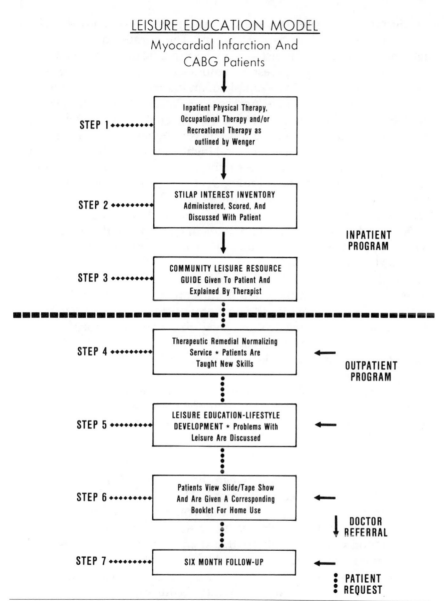

Figure 10.1. Leisure counseling program for myocardial infarction and bypass patients.

Step 2—Leisure Interest Inventory

Step 2 involves administering a leisure interest inventory to patients, evaluating the findings of the inventory, and discussing the findings of the inventory with patients while they are inpatients in the hospital following their heart attack or bypass surgery. The purpose of this step is to help the patient and therapist identify leisure-time interests and deficiencies. There are many interest inventories currently in use for leisure counseling purposes. One example of an interest inventory is the State Technical Institute's Leisure Assessment Process (STILAP), developed by Peterson and outlined by Navar (1977). This interest inventory has been field-tested and evaluated through continuous implementation over the past 4 years at the State Technical Institute and Rehabilitation Center in Plainwell, Michigan. The researcher chose this particular inventory because it has been in use at Lutheran Hospital in La Crosse, Wisconsin for several years as a part of the Recreational Therapy Department and because it is based on a normal or nondisabled population.

The STILAP was designed to provide the therapist with objective data, which enables both the client and staff to become involved in leisure decision making. It also provides the therapist with valuable information about the needs of the client. To accomplish this, the STILAP categorizes the types of activities that the client is currently involved in and identifies those in which the individual does not participate. These categories are referred to as competencies. By categorizing the inventory responses patients will become more aware of the leisure activities available and the types of leisure activities or competencies that are not currently incorporated into their lives.

Following the completion of the interest inventory and scoring by the therapist, the results should be discussed with the patient. The overall objectives of this step of the leisure counseling model include the following:

- To promote discussion between the patient and therapist.
- To identify skill areas or former hobbies of the patient.
- To relate interest areas to existing resources in the community.
- To provide any contacts necessary with community agencies.
- To identify skills or hobbies that the patient has an interest in, but has not participated in previously due to lack of skill or knowledge.
- To identify blocks or problems with leisure participation.
- To promote the use of community resources.

The interest inventory can be used to identify the needs and interests of the patient. The therapist should make a follow-up appointment with the patient and proceed with Step 3 (distribution of community resource guide) to provide the appropriate resources based on the results of the interest inventory.

Step 3—Distribution of Community Leisure Resource Guide

This step of the leisure counseling program is designed to match leisure interests with existing resources. Once the patient has progressed to this step, he or she should have an idea of some interests or activities in which he or she would like to become involved.

In order to provide the appropriate resources for patients' varied interests, it is necessary to develop a community resource guide, which can be designed based on the community resources in any city. The purpose of this guidebook is to supply patients with a variety of community resources that can be used for leisure-time activities. This guide not only lists the various clubs, agencies, and recreational opportunities, but also attempts to instruct patients as to the function of these organizations and how they could best be utilized.

The information contained in the guidebook can be entered into a computer. Each time an organization changes its address or the individual in charge, the listing can be updated on the computer. In this way an accurate record of each organization is available to make periodic revisions of the entire guide.

During the session, the therapist explains the various sections of the book and emphasizes that no activity should be done that exceeds the doctor's recommendation for the patient.

The general objectives of this step are the following:

1. To help the patients become aware of the resources available in the community.
2. To give the patient a permanent copy of the resource guidebook for home use.
3. To make the patient aware of various volunteer jobs and opportunities.
4. To explain the services of various agencies in the community and to inform the patient of how they might be utilized.
5. To determine whether further counseling is necessary.

In this step, the therapist attempts to match leisure interests and needs with existing resources in the community. The patient may wish to learn a new craft or skill that is not offered within the community. The therapist would then set up a follow-up appointment and proceed with Step 4.

Step 4—Therapeutic Remedial Normalizing Service

This approach or component of the leisure counseling program attempts to define problems that the patient may have with leisure involvement that relate to a lack of skill in that area. The therapist can be instrumental in teaching patients new skills or providing the resources necessary for new skill acquisition. The following objectives outline how the therapist might help patients in this step:

1. Plan appropriate teaching sessions for patient-expressed interests.
2. Utilize community resources for the teaching session (bring in outside personnel to assist).
3. Give the patient the opportunity to try out the new skill. If teaching a craft, let the patient create his or her own project with the guidance of the therapist.
4. Have appropriate materials available for use. For example, if the patient expresses an interest in ceramics, make ceramic materials available at the session.
5. Be available to help the patient if problems or questions arise with the new activity or skill.

The emphasis of the session should be centered on introducing the skill rather than attempting to teach the patient every aspect of that skill. The therapist should be prepared to discuss further resources such as books or classes in the community that the patient might utilize to develop the skill area. The session should be approximately 1 hr in length and, because of time and money limitations, be confined to one session.

Step 5—Leisure Education-Lifestyle Development

Patients sometimes do not engage in leisure activities because of obstacles or difficulties with participation. These obstacles or difficulties may be due to attitudes, physical limitations, or values. Counseling provides planned intervention into the patient's existing lifestyle to help him or her become involved in activities and experiences that are satisfying and appropriate.

As a means to facilitate discussion, the therapist should ask patients to list several activities or projects that they would like to do in the next 5 years. These activities could be done for recreational purposes (enjoyment), for the patient's family, for friends, or for community service. Patients should be encouraged to brainstorm ideas and to list activities that seem somewhat impossible at this time. A patient might list, for example, taking a cruise, learning to scuba dive, or going dancing more often as activities he or she would like to do. After the patient has listed the activities, the therapist then asks the individual what is preventing him or her from doing each activity. The therapist may suggest that the patient contact an agency or person familiar with that activity. For example, the patient interested in taking a cruise may see financial obstacles as the block to doing this activity. This patient could be referred to a travel agent to determine the actual cost of the trip. Lower priced cruises or special-priced package deals might be suggested by the travel agent to make this activity possible for the patient.

This process of identifying the reasons why patients are not participating in activities or projects they would like to do is an important step in helping them initiate a plan to accomplish their objectives. The therapist functions as a mediator in helping patients do those activities that they express an interest in. The following are the general objectives of Step 5:

1. To identify specific problems patients have with leisure involvement. One example of this is lack of finances to participate in the activity.
2. To explore with the patient possibilities for adapting activities of interest so that involvement is possible. For example, if the patient is unable to play an entire game of golf, the therapist suggests that the patient play less holes and ride in a cart.
3. To make the therapist available for questions the patient might have after the counseling session is completed (patient feels free to call).

This step of the leisure counseling model might involve more than one session if the patient requests more assistance. There are no specific forms for this step; however, therapists might develop their own forms based on the needs of their particular programs.

Step 6—Slide/Tape Show and Corresponding Booklet

Many patients are unable to attend Phase III programs in the community or are not interested in group exercise programs. For this reason a slide/tape program was developed to provide the information necessary for patients to exercise safely on their own. The slide/tape program was designed to be used in conjunction with a Phase II outpatient program. The following goals were formulated for Step 6. After viewing the program the patient should

1. understand how to choose safe activities based on his or her MET level prescription,
2. be aware of the appropriate frequency and duration of exercise that will promote the best conditioning effect,
3. be able to monitor activity intensity using the heart rate method,
4. be able to choose aerobic activities with a knowledge of the wide variety of exercise opportunities that are appropriate, and
5. understand the value of recreational and social activities.

A corresponding booklet was developed to clarify the ideas presented in the slide/tape program. The booklet includes the following:

1. A MET value chart with the MET costs of various recreational, occupational, and daily activities. In this way patients are able to choose appropriate activities.
2. A windchill chart for determining the safety of exercising outside in the winter.
3. A temperature-humidity index for determining the safety of exercising in the heat.
4. General precautions for certain types of activities including isometrics.
5. General activity guidelines.
6. Warning signs of a heart attack.
7. A detailed explanation of each of the exercise modes presented in the slide/tape program.
8. Information about angina and the use of nitroglycerin.

The booklet is passed out to the patient after viewing the slide/tape program.

Step 7—6-Month Follow-Up Appointment

Most cardiac patients do not experience problems with adjustment to their cardiac event until a few months after the cardiac event. This step of the leisure counseling program should include all patients for this reason. This step is included in the leisure counseling program to ensure that patients are receiving the necessary assistance with problems they may be having with leisure-time involvement. The following topic areas are suggested as a means to establish how well the patient is doing and to facilitate discussion:

Exercise Routine. Has the patient been participating in regular physical activity? If so, what has he or she been doing? Have there been any problems with participation such as physical symptoms? If the patient has not been participating, what was the reason? Is there a need to discuss this problem with the patient's physician?

Recreational Activities. In what recreational activities has the patient been participating? If the patient learned a new skill, has he or she had any problems or questions about it? Has the patient been doing any activities with family members? Does the patient feel limited in any way with activity involvement? Does the patient have any new interest areas about which he or she may need help finding classes or information?

Social Activities. Has the patient returned to normal social activities (church, card clubs, etc.) that he or she participated in prior to the cardiac event? If not, what problem has the patient had with returning to these activities? Has the patient been fearful of activity involvement because of physical limitations? Does the patient need to see the exercise physiologist to reinforce in which activities the patient should and should not participate?

References

Finlayson, A., & McEwen, J. (1977). *Coronary heart disease and patterns of living*. New York: Prodist Books.

Goldbarg, A.N. (1973). Rehabilitation of the coronary patient. *Medical Clinics of North America*, 57, 231-241.

Hayes, G. (1977). *Leisure education and recreation counseling*. Springfield, IL: Charles C Thomas.

Hoeft, T.M. (1979). The effect of leisure counseling upon selected attitudes of potential cardiac clients (Doctoral dissertation, Virginia Polytechnic Institutional and State, 1979). *Dissertation Abstracts International*, 40(5), 2481A. (Ann Arbor University Microfilms No. 7924110, 219)

Hoeft, T.M. (1982). The long term effect of leisure counseling upon selected attitudes of potential cardiac clients: A follow-up study. In *Applied leisure research: Therapeutic services and counseling for special populations*. Symposium presented at the meeting of the National Recreation and Parks Association, Louisville.

McDowell, C. (1977). *Leisure counseling*. Springfield, IL: Charles C Thomas.

Montiero, L.A. (1979). *Cardiac patient rehabilitation: Social aspects of recovery*. New York: Springer.

Nagel, R., & Gargola, R. (1971). Factors influencing return to work after myocardial infarction. *Lancet*, 2, 454-459.

Navar, N. (1979). Leisure skill assessment process in leisure counseling. In D.J. Szymanske & G.L. Hitzhusen (Eds.), *Expanding horizons in therapeutic recreation*. Columbia: Curators.

O'Morrow, G.D. (1977). Recreation counseling, a challenge to rehabilitation. *Rehabilitation*, 31(8), 226-233.

Peterson, C.A. (1977). Contexts and concepts of leisure counseling. In D. Comptom & J. Goldstein (Eds.), *Perspectives of leisure counseling*. Arlington: National Recreation and Parks Association.

Siegel, D.G. (1969). A critique of studies of long term survivorship of patients with myocardial infarction. *American Journal of Public Health*, 58, 1348.

Totman, R.L. (1979). What makes life events stressful? *Journal of Psychosomatic Research*, 23(3), 193-201.

Wenger, N.K. (1971). Physical conditioning after myocardial infarction: An early intervention program. *Circulation, 44*(2), 119.

Wenger, N.K., & Hellerstein, H.D. (1978). *Rehabilitation of the coronary patient*. New York: John Wiley and Sons.

Wishnie, H.A. (1971). Psychological hazards of convalescence following myocardial infarction. *Journal of the American Medical Association, 215*(8), 1292-1296.

Chapter 11

Behavioral Medicine and Cardiac Rehabilitation: Introduction and Overview

Michael J. Asken

The idea that both behavior and health and psychology and physiology are intimately related is not new. It is probably as old as medicine itself and extends back at least as far as the early Greek civilizations (Kaplan, 1975; U.S. Department of Health, Education, and Welfare [DHEW], 1979; Matarazzo, 1980). The early Greeks identified four humors in the human body, which were derived from the basic elements of air, water, fire, and earth. The humors were thought to circulate through the body and in either correct or incorrect proportions influence behavior. From this came such behavioral descriptors as sanguine, phlegmatic, melancholic, or choleric temperaments.

The concept of behavioral medicine, however, has a much more recent formal history. Although there may be some disagreement on this point, work in the 1960s at three or four major medical centers seemed to foreshadow the articulated field of behavioral medicine. At that time, researchers raised the question as to whether myocardial infarction and open-heart surgery might not have a *psychological* impact as well as a physiological impact on the patient (Abram, 1965, 1970a; Cassem & Hackett, 1971; Hackett, Cassem, & Wishnie, 1968; Kornfeld, Zimberg, & Malm, 1965). Concomitantly, the same issues were being raised about hemodialysis and renal transplantation (Abram, 1968, 1969, 1970b; Kaplan DeNour, & Czaczkes, 1968; Kaplan DeNour, Shaltier, & Czaczkes, 1968). Although not defined as behavioral medicine at that time, this work in spirit and content served as a harbinger of what was to emerge a decade later.

The hallmark for behavioral medicine was the Yale Conference held in 1977 (Schwartz & Weiss, 1978a). At that time, the *Journal of Behavioral*

Medicine was instituted and a definition for the field proposed. Participants accepted the following as the official definition (Schwartz & Weiss, 1978b):

> Behavioral medicine is the interdisciplinary field concerned with the development and integration of behavioral and biomedical science, knowledge and techniques relevant to health and illness and the application of this knowledge and these techniques to prevention, diagnosis, treatment and rehabilitation. (p. 250)

Also in that year, the National Institutes of Health, through the National Heart, Lung, and Blood Institute, formed a behavioral medicine branch (Matarazzo, 1980). In 1978, the National Academy of Sciences established the Academy of Behavioral Medicine Research, which comprised 150 eminent researchers in medicine and the behavioral sciences (Matarazzo, 1980). In addition, the Society of Behavioral Medicine was formed at that time. Since these events, behavioral medicine has grown, developed, and attracted even international interest (Gentry, 1980).

It should be noted that behavioral medicine is not the singular proponent of the psychological aspects of medicine, nor has there been unanimity in accepting the Yale Conference's definition. These discrepancies have lead to some confusion. For example, concomitant with the growth of behavioral medicine has been a reorientation of psychiatry toward the psychiatric aspects of medicine and the physiological aspects of psychiatry. This has been reflected in the growth of *consultation-liaison psychiatry*, which has developed significantly from general hospital psychiatry and the tradition of psychosomatic medicine (Cohen-Cole, Haggerty, & Raft, 1982; Lipowski, 1974). However, in addition to other differences, such as that behavioral medicine has a distinct interdisciplinary focus, consultation-liaison psychiatry has remained a psychiatric endeavor.

Health psychology and *behavioral health* are also terms for current developments and the cause of some of the current confusion. They might be seen as psychology's counterpart to consultation-liaison psychiatry. Health psychology has been defined as follows (Matarazzo, 1982):

> Health psychology is the aggregate of the specific educational, scientific, and professional contributions of the discipline of psychology to the promotion and maintenance of health, the prevention and treatment of illness, the identification of etiologic and diagnostic correlates of health, illness and related dysfunction and to the analysis and improvement of the health care system and health care policy formation. (p. 4)

Behavioral health has been defined as follows (Matarazzo, 1980):

> Behavioral health is an interdisciplinary field dedicated to promoting a philosophy of health that stresses individual responsibility in the

application of behavioral and biomedical science, knowledge and techniques to the maintenance of health and the prevention of illness and dysfunction by a variety of self-initiated individual or shared activities. (p. 4)

A last area of potential confusion and lingering controversy has been over the significance of the term *behavioral* in behavioral medicine. There are those who maintain that behavioral refers exclusively to the use of a specific set of behavior change techniques in medicine, that is, those derived from behavior modification and behavior therapy (Birk, 1973; Blanchard, 1977; Doleys, Meredith, & Ciminero, 1982; Matarazo, 1980; Pomerleau, 1979; Pomerleau & Brady, 1979). This position has been summarized by Pomerleau and Brady (1979): "Behavioral medicine as a clinical activity is an outgrowth of behavior modification and therapy, borrowing procedures and techniques as well as assessment and research strategies."

Although it is true that the behavioral orientation may be responsible for the genesis of behavioral medicine and accounts for the bulk of current intervention approaches (Schwartz & Weiss, 1978), the much broader Yale definition, which allows for any orientation to behavior change, remains the formal definition.

Unique Aspects of Behavioral Medicine

More important than analyzing these definitional differences, however, is identifying how behavioral medicine is conceptually different from traditional psychiatry and psychology. That is, how is it a unique endeavor? There are at least five unique aspects to behavioral medicine that suggest it is not just another term for psychology or psychiatry.

Behavioral Medicine Is Interdisciplinary

Behavioral medicine is not psychiatry or psychology (Doleys et al., 1982); it does not deal with neuroses or psychoses, nor does it deal with these only as they might affect physical health. Behavioral medicine attempts to involve the physician and other health care specialists as part of an interdisciplinary team. The notion of the mind-body split has retained primacy in medicine. This is often expressed in the idea that if there's nothing wrong in your body (which usually means that medical diagnostics are not sensitive or sophisticated enough to detect pathology), there must be something wrong in your head. Behavioral medicine rejects this dualistic conception as making little sense, either logically or biologically. Therefore, behavioral medicine is truly a psychophysiologic or biopsychosocial approach to medicine, which is striving for interdisciplinary collaboration, not fragmentation.

Treatment Goal Is Physical Health

In the dualistic approach to medicine, if a patient was sent for psychological treatment, the goal was often personality change. Change in health status was perhaps implicit, but generally not explicit, and usually incidental to the goals of the psychotherapy. For example, there were many obese individuals, who, as a result of therapy, had intricate explanations of their problems or even gains in ego strength, but still overindulged and remained overweight and at medical risk. The goal of intervention in behavioral medicine is to affect physical health, but to do so by behavioral and psychological means.

Data-Based and Short-Term Interventions

The heritage of behavioral medicine in behavioral psychology has bequeathed to it a methodological rigor heretofore absent in the behavioral sciences. Just as behavior therapy has made psychology self-conscious with respect to a valid data base, behavioral medicine has attempted to utilize only that knowledge and those procedures which have empirical validity. This is a significant change from the past and from some other current approaches to behavior and medicine (Agras & Berkowitz, 1980).

Intervention in behavioral medicine tends to be short-term. Before behavioral medicine, a referred medical patient was likely to find a recommendation for several years on the couch. In behavioral medicine, there is more likely to be a suggestion for ten sessions of biofeedback, although the option for more involved intervention remains open if needed. Such a time-limited and pragmatic orientation fits much better with the realities of hospital and medical practice, the expectations of physicians, and the tolerance of medical patients.

A Special Body of Knowledge

Behavioral medicine does not involve simply applying the theories derived from psychiatric populations to medical patients. In fact, this approach is likely to be clinically and interpersonally disastrous. What is known in behavioral medicine derives from the study of medical patients, not psychiatric patients. It is this evolution of new knowledge or reconstruction of older knowledge for this special population that leads to innovative and appropriate consultations and intervention in the medical sphere.

Emphasis on Prevention and Health Maintenance

Although they state it somewhat strongly, Ferguson and Taylor (1981) believe that there must be some agreement that, whereas technical advances in medicine are needed, welcome, and newsworthy,

> Many of the greatest strides in medical care have neither been glamorous nor made the front pages of the *New York Times*. They have been simple measures such as sanitation, immunization and provision of clean wholesome food. And even the more glamorous medical breakthroughs in techniques like heart transplants [and currently artificial hearts or previously revascularization] are often last-ditch responses to largely preventable medical problems that required a lifetime to develop.

The quote underscores what is now becoming a well-known fact: Disease patterns in the United States have changed dramatically. The germ theory of illness has lost some priority as many of its representative illnesses, such as smallpox, diptheria, pertussis, tetanus, polio, measles, tuberculosis, and influenza, have been adequately controlled through vaccines, antibiotics, or other public health measures (DHEW, 1979; Knowles, 1977).

There is a new aspect to the major causes of death in the United States—a major behavioral component. Heart disease, cancer, and accidents have major behavioral (lifestyle) and environmental components, which must be addressed. A cure is not likely to come from a pill or vaccine. Knowles (1974) has noted that "99% of us are born healthy and made sick as a result of personal misbehavior and environmental conditions." Further, it has been suggested that of the 10 leading causes of death, 7 could be substantially reduced by changes in diet, smoking, exercise, alcohol use, and medication compliance. In addition, 50% of the mortality in the United States in 1976 could be attributed to unhealthy lifestyles (DHEW, 1979). Behavior change is no longer a medical nicety, but a medical necessity—a reality that has been recognized in other nations as well (LaLonde, 1974). Behavioral medicine seeks to contribute to the overall picture of medical care by using behavioral interventions to keep illness from getting worse, to stave off recurrence, but predominantly to prevent occurrence in the first place through prevention and promotion of health-related behavior.

Why Behavioral Medicine Now?

It is important to ask why behavioral medicine should emerge and flourish at this particular point in time. After all, behavioral medicine's forerunner, psychosomatic medicine, never achieved the impact predicted (Agras, 1982; Katz & Zlutnick, 1975). Why behavioral medicine should be different is a complex question to answer, but there are several obvious indicators that reflect the relationship of behavior and medicine.

One reason is that behavioral medicine emerged at a time when the importance of behavior to medicine was being rediscovered. There has been some disenchantment with the strict medical model to explain health and illness (Doleys et al., 1982; Schofield, 1980). Psychiatry has moved towards a more integrated view of behavior (Karasu, 1979; Lipowski, 1974), and the biopsychosocial model (Engel, 1977) of health and illness has gained support in mainstream medicine as well (Asken & Strock, 1978; Benson, Katch, & Crassweller, 1977; Matarazzo, 1980; Peterson, 1977; Schwartz & Weiss, 1978; Seyle, 1976). Seyle (1976) has made the study of stress a respectable endeavor and by doing so has further highlighted psychosocial factors in physical disorders. Psychology, too, has sought to contribute to the understanding of health and illness and has done so with a formalization of these efforts (American Psychological Association [APA] Task Force on Health Research, 1976; Matarazzo, 1982; Pomerleau, 1979; Stachnik, 1980). Thus an impetus for serious consideration of behavioral factors in medicine has come from many different arenas.

A second reason is the recognition and supporting data of the extent of psychosocial problems and concerns among medical patient populations (Schwab, Bell, Warheit, Schwab, & Traven, 1978-79). The growth of the primary care medical specialties, especially family medicine, with an emphasis on comprehensiveness of care, has served to highlight psychosocial concerns. Brown and Rieger (1977) have suggested that 60% of patients with mental disorders receive treatment exclusively in the primary care sector. More important for behavioral medicine, however, are reports indicating the need for training in behavioral science including behavioral medicine for family physicians because of the frequency of these types of problems (Maguire & Asken, 1978; Shienvold, Asken, & Cincotta, 1979).

The prevention focus is an independent variable that also has favored behavioral medicine, and in turn has been supported by the emergence of primary care specialists. The behavioral component of the major sources of death in the United States has already been mentioned, but a summary comment by a past Secretary of the Department of Health, Education and Welfare (DHEW, 1979) reiterates that point:

> We are killing ourselves by our own careless habits. We are killing ourselves by carelessly polluting our environment. We are killing ourselves by permitting harmful social situations to persist—conditions

like poverty, hunger and ignorance—which destroy health, especially for infants and children. (p. viii)

The rise of consumerism in medical care may also help sustain behavioral medicine to the degree that this signifies that individuals are willing to take some responsibility for their own health. People now appear to want to do something about their physical status rather than having things done to them. At a minimum, there is an interest in knowledge about medical matters. For example, a medical information telephone service has averaged just under 100,000 calls per year over a 5-year period ("Tel-Med Plan," 1983).

Another factor that has favored behavioral medicine is the growing concern over health care costs. Although much is made of the cost of medical care and the health industry, it is recognized less often how much of the nation's economy and gross national product goes into making people sick. Knowles (1977) has noted that struggling attempts at a healthy lifestyle may be mitigated by "a culture whose economy depends on high production and high consumption." In contrast "to the promotion of the use of tobacco, ingestion of alcohol, high fat-high sugar diets, high speed automobiles, and the exclusion of exercise and rest to faster forms of the good life," stand the behavioral medicine change strategies.

Health care costs remain a target for increasing scrutiny and regulation. Long before the establishment of current economic restraints on health care expenses, however, behavioral medicine asked of its interventions if they were not only effective but cost-effective (Olbrisch, 1977). Limited, cautious, but optimistic studies have now emerged, which suggest that attentiveness to the psychological and behavioral aspects of medicine can have positive effects in terms of appropriate health care resource utilization and, therefore, health care costs. Knowles (1977) reported that a program for diabetic self-care at the University of Southern California yielded a 50% drop in emergency room visits, a decrease in the number of patients experiencing diabetic coma, and an avoidance of 2,300 visits for medication. The estimated 2-year savings was $1.7 million. Rosen and Wiens (1979) reported that the use of psychological services in a medical population resulted in a decrease in outpatient visits, emergency room visits, diagnostic services, and prescriptions. The same kind of results have been reported in a health maintenance organization (HMO) setting, (Olbrisch, 1977), and monetary savings have been projected in a federal Blue Cross/Blue Shield plan (Schlesinger, Mumford, Glass, Patrick & Scharfstein, 1983). It has also been reported that in an industrial setting, an alcohol treatment program yielded a return of $5.83 for every dollar spent on its psychotherapy program (Olbrisch, 1977).

Another reason for the sustained development of behavioral medicine has been government support through the National Institutes of Health and the National Heart, Lung, and Blood Institute (Matarazzo, 1980). In an uncharacteristic manner, government has not ignored the groundswell of behavioral medicine, but has fostered it, no doubt because of many of the factors cited previously.

Finally, behavioral medicine has gained acceptance due to the characteristic that probably can be traced to its roots in behavioral psychology: the commitment to empirical validation and efficacy. Whereas previous attempts to blend psychiatry and medicine (i.e., psychosomatic medicine) tended to focus on descriptions and explanations (often in esoteric and confusing concepts and jargon), behavioral medicine has taken a pragmatic and interventive approach, which has been backed by demonstrated efficacious therapies (Agras, 1982; Katz & Zlutnick, 1975; Surwit, Feinglos, & Scovern, 1983). Biofeedback, or the operant conditioning of physiological responses, is a good example of a thoroughly researched and data-supported intervention (Schofield, 1980). Behavioral medicine has provided a discipline that is syntonic with the requirements and realities of medical practice.

The Content of Behavioral Medicine

Behavioral medicine denotes much more than the confusing definition offered earlier. It would be impossible to describe the entire content of behavioral medicine, for its scope is as broad as medicine itself. However, before I discuss the role of behavioral medicine in cardiac health and cardiac rehabilitation, some representative endeavors may be instructive. They will be divided into those that have become somewhat standard and those that reflect innovative and exciting frontiers in behavioral medicine.

Psychophysiologic problems, under the more popular term of *stress disorders*, form the area of behavioral medicine that is perhaps most readily recognizable. The life stress scale is now well known (Holmes & Rahe, 1967), although it has been recently suggested that daily hassles and uplifts (DeLongis, Coyne, Dakof, Folkman, & Lazarus, 1982; Kanner, Coyne, Schaefer, & Lazarus, 1981) may be more important in terms of health and illness than major life changes. The treatment of chronic pain is another standard area with treatments ranging from the more operant approaches (Fordyce, 1976) to new cognitive interventions (Turk, Meichenbaum, & Genest, 1983). Success has been demonstrated repeatedly in dealing with headaches (Blanchard & Andrasik, 1982) and other disorders amenable to biofeedback (Olton & Noonberg, 1980). The psychological aspects of chronic conditions and illnesses for adults (e.g., cancer [Wellisch, 1981], mastectomy [Asken, 1975], etc.) and for children (Drotar, 1981) (e.g., leukemia [Eiser, 1979], diabetes [Johnson, 1980], asthma [King, 1980], etc.) have been addressed. The Psychological preparation of individuals for hospitalization (Roberts, Wartele, Boone, Ginther, & Elkins, 1981) and for surgery (Peterson & Shigetomi, 1982; Wilson, 1981) is another typical area of activity. The whole issue of compliance with medical regimens, from glucose testing in diabetic children (Carney, Schechter, & Davis, 1983) to exercise in rheumatoid arthritis patients (Waggoner & LeLieuvre, 1981) to dialysis treatment in adults (Cummings, Becker, Kirscht, & Levin, 1981) as well as other areas, has been reviewed (Masur, 1981). The psychological aspects (or stresses) of health care providers such as physicians (Walker, 1980), residents (Asken & Raham, 1983), and critical care nurses (Asken, 1979) are also within the purview of behavioral medicine. Finally, in part from the emergence of behavioral medicine, there have been attempts to influence health behavior at the worksite in the area of industrial behavioral medicine (Wolinsky, 1983).

More innovative contributions are represented by recent work which has trained young children to recognize and make emergency telephone calls (Jones & Kazdin, 1980) and taught them fire escape skills (Jones, Kazdin, & Haney, 1981). Also in line with the prevention perspective has been work to increase the use of seat belts in general and car seats for children in particular (Christopherson & Gyulay, 1981; Geller, Patterson, & Talbott, 1982). An outgrowth of the psychological preparation of surgical patients has been work in preparing patients for short-term invasive procedures such as heart catheterization (Anderson & Masur, 1983) or sigmoidoscopy (Kaplan, Atkins, & Lenhard, 1982). Behavioral medicine interventions have had success in counterconditioning the nausea that frequently accompanies cancer chemotherapy (Lyles, Burish, Krozely, & Oldham, 1982; Morrow & Morrell, 1982). Behavioral medicine has addressed the psychological needs of special medical populations (Carrillo, 1980; Mahon, 1980; True, 1980) including such things as weight reduction programs for retarded individuals (Ratatori, Fox, & Mauser, 1981). There has been movement to recognize the psychological aspects of previously ignored areas such as the emergency room (Wustman, 1980). In a true blend of behavior and medicine and a rational extension of psychosomatics, there is exciting work now being done in the area of psychoimmunology (Locke, 1982).

Behavioral Medicine in Cardiac Health and Rehabilitation

It is clear that, because behavior is such a crucial determinant of cardiac status, behavioral medicine has a major role to play in cardiac health and cardiac rehabilitation. Blumenthal, Califf, Williams, and Hindman (in press) state that cardiac rehabilitation is a new frontier for behavioral medicine. Blackburn (1980) noted the following:

> Of all the recent developments in cardiovascular research, probably none is more important than the clear demonstration that cultural patterns, lifestyles and personal characteristics carry different degrees of risk of eventual heart attack or stroke. The full recognition and implementation of this knowledge could potentially be the most significant measure effecting the collective health of North Americans today. (p. 2)

Whether the behavioral medicine interface with cardiac health is considered prevention or rehabilitation is really a matter of timing and diagnosis: If no coronary event or diagnosis has been made, the label is prevention; if an event has occurred, it is rehabilitation. The goals of behavior change remain medical, however, and are to maximize function, to retard disease, and to prevent further complications.

Behavioral Medicine and Cardiac Health

Of the 10 major risk factors for coronary artery disease and myocardial infarction, at least 7 may be significantly influenced by behavioral means. Whereas little may be done about age, sex, or family history, interventions for smoking, obesity, dietary prudence, exercise, hypertension, and stress or the Type A behavior pattern are becoming well known.

Behavioral interventions with obesity have a long history dating from the classic works of Stuart and Davis (1971) and Stunkard (1972) and have been refined over the years (Brownell, 1982). Encouraging success has been the rule, including more recent data indicating that behavioral treatment is superior to even anorectic drugs in the maintenance of weight loss (Cohen & Stunkard, 1983). In an even more direct relationship to cardiac health, there have also been attempts to encourage overall nutrition and manage hyperlipidemia (Carmody, Fey, Pierce, Connor, & Matarazzo, 1982).

Smoking is a health threat without equal. Research continues to show harmful cardiac effects from smoking. Smokers have increased mortality rates from myocardial infarction and increased rates for initial cardiac events when compared to nonsmokers (Blackburn, 1980). One recent study has suggested smoking to be a primary factor in heart attacks occurring before the age of 36 (Glover, Kuber, Warren, & Vieweg, 1982). Smoking termination approaches have been developed and refined using behavioral techniques, many of which are now well known (Danaher & Lichtenstein, 1978; Pomerleau & Pomerleau, 1977).

Hypertension is another risk factor. The role of stress, the importance of adherence or compliance with medical regimen, and the use of relaxation and biofeedback techniques represent behavioral aspects to the management of hypertension (Shapiro & Goldstein, 1982).

Exercise has received attention in the behavioral medicine sphere as well. Factors that lead to compliance and reduce the dropout rate for exercise programs, self-management strategies, cognitive statements, and imagery to enhance participation have been addressed (Dishman, 1982; Dishman & Ickes, 1981; Dubbert, Martin, Raczynski, & Smith, 1982; Martin & Smith, 1981) as well as the effect of exercise on behaviors such as the Type A style (Blumenthal, Williams, & Wallace, 1980).

Finally, the role of stress and the Type A or coronary-prone behavior pattern has produced voluminous research in literature. This behavioral style has been reviewed in terms of assessment of the pattern (Jenkins, Zyzanski, & Rosenman, 1979; Rosenman, Friedman, & Straus, 1964) its cardiac effects (Dembroski, Weiss, Shields, Haynes, & Feinleib, 1978; Friedman & Rosenman, 1974), and potential interventions (Roskies, Spevack, Surkis, Cohen, & Gilman, 1978; Suinn, 1981; Suinn & Bloom, 1978). Of current interest is the role of cardiovascular hyperactivity to stress that is found in some normal individuals and its relationship to Type A behavior as a biological substrate or synergist (Buell & Eliot, 1980; Dembrowski, MacDougall, Shields, Pettito, & Lushene, 1978; Jorgensen & Houston, 1981; Krantz, Arabian, Davia, & Parker, 1982). The presence of Type A behavior and coronary risk in children has lead to increasing work in this area as well (Coates & Perry, in press; Matthews & Angulo, 1980).

Behavioral Medicine and Cardiac Rehabilitation

The role of behavioral medicine in cardiac rehabilitation is a reflection, extension, and continuance of the prevention focus. However, by virtue of a coronary event or cardiac diagnosis, the situation is different, and some new issues are raised and some modifications required.

A major new area is that of psychological response to the heart attack or open heart surgery, the coronary care unit, and the recuperative process. An extensive literature now exists beginning with those studies that predated behavioral medicine (Abram, 1965; Hackett, Cassem, & Wishnie, 1968; Kornfeld, Zimberg, & Malm, 1965) to the present on such matters as psychological response to the cardiac experience (Cassem & Hackett, 1977, 1978), management of behavior problems in the coronary care unit (such as AMA sign-outs [Baile, Brinker, Wachspress, & Engel, 1979]), and the effects of psychological interventions on outcomes (Mumford, Schlesinger, & Glass, 1982) and group therapy (Kolman, 1983) for adjustment to life-style changes. A recent important study looked at the neuropsychological effects of myocardial infarction and cardiac arrest resuscitation (Ergood & Tarter, 1983).

Exercise programs can only have an effect if patients participate. Thus, there has been increasing work to identify reasons for dropout from programs and means to increase compliance (Carmody, Senner, Malinow, & Matarazzo, 1980). For example, Andrew et al. (1981) found that the main categories associated with the high dropout rate included convenience aspects of the exercise center, perceptions of the exercise program, and family life-style factors. Standard behavioral techniques, such as the use of behavioral contracts, have been used with some success to increase adherence in exercise rehabilitation programs (Oldridge & Jones, 1983). The psychological effects of exercise on the cardiac patient have been assessed as well (Stein & Cleary, 1981).

Sexual adjustment after myocardial infarction is a crucial issue raised prominently by Hellerstein and Fried (1970). The nature of sexual response and adjustment after heart attack has been addressed (Masur, 1979; Mehta & Krop, 1979) as have suggestions for counseling programs to promote a healthy sexual adjustment (McLane, Krop, & Mehta, 1980).

Finally, although much of the Type A intervention work has been done with at-risk populations rather than patient groups, several studies have looked at the effects of intervention with coronary patients. In general, results have been encouraging (Suinn, 1975, 1982).

Structuring Behavioral Medicine and Cardiac Rehabilitation

There is an obvious, significant, dramatic, and important role for behavioral medicine to play within cardiac rehabilitation; however, the means of implementing this aspect are more obscure. To have a fully developed intervention program would require considerable time, a sizable staff, and consequently significant expense. Certainly, specific aspects of behavior change could be targeted as a more limited but in-depth approach, although meeting the needs of the broader cardiac rehabilitation population then becomes problematical.

One method to provide a broad behavioral medicine exposure to a broad segment of the target population is to use a quasi-educational approach.

This method has been successfully implemented at the Cardiac Rehabilitation Center of the Polyclinic Medical Center in Harrisburg, Pennsylvania, and will be discussed in some detail.

The program de-emphasizes actual behavioral change in favor of education, although homework assignments, exercises, and experiential components are utilized. One of the goals is to acquaint participants with the wide range of behavioral medicine interventions that are available. In line with the concept of having phases to cardiac rehabilitation, this is an initial step that allows the patient to choose and more fully pursue those options that are most appropriate to him or her after completion of the introductory phase.

The behavior and health component of the Cardiac Rehabilitation Center at Polyclinic Medical Center is an educational program designed to acquaint participants with the importance of behavioral and psychological factors in cardiac health and disease. Discussed are coronary risk factors that may be affected by behavioral change strategies, as well as more general psychological aspects of preventing or adjusting to cardiac problems. As mentioned, the purpose of the program is to present these relevant risk factors and to introduce a broad spectrum of means for behaviorally reducing such risks, which may then be pursued further by each individual at his or her own discretion.

The behavior and health component is not psychotherapy or a group therapy experience. It is an educational-informational forum. At individual request, however, recommendations can be made for referral to professional counseling. Content of the sessions is prepared in cooperation with the cardiac nurse therapist, the director of the center, and the cardiologists and consulting medical staff of the program. Sessions are held on a rotating 10-week schedule. Individuals may join at any time and may attend a missed session on the next rotation. The sessions are led by the health psychologist at the cardiac rehabilitation center. The cardiac nurse therapist attends the sessions as well. This provides a sense of familiarity and comfort for the participants, a visible stamp of validation of the importance of this component of the rehabilitation program, and a means for the cardiac nurse therapist to have continuing and comprehensive interactions with the patients in the program.

The general objectives of the program are as follows:

- To provide information, knowledge, and support related to normal psychological/behavioral concerns in adapting to cardiac disease.
- To help facilitate coping and prevent untoward and exaggerated problems in the rehabilitation and adaptation process.
- To demonstrate the universality of concerns and to remove stigma from such matters.

- To help facilitate the development of behavior to maintain positive health changes and emotional adjustment to contribute to an increased quality and quantity of life.
- To help monitor the psychological adjustment process, provide a point of contact for patients who may be having excessive difficulties, and provide feedback to attending physicians for their intervention or appropriate referral.

The content and goals for the weekly sessions are outlined in Table 11.1.

In general, such an approach has been well received by those individuals in the cardiac rehabilitation program. Data on patient satisfaction is presented in Table 11.2.

The true impact of the program is yet to be addressed; it is well known that education by itself does not ensure behavior change. The goals of the current approach are not to provide significant changes in behavior as much as to shape individuals toward pursuing more intensive programs through such a desensitizing introduction to the various possibilities. Whether participants do indeed follow through needs to be evaluated.

Anecdotal experience suggests increased interest, questions, and some referrals on the part of the participants. Additionally, the sessions have served as a stimulus for certain patients to approach the cardiac nurse therapist in a more open manner to pursue topics on an individual basis. Thus, although the data are not yet in, and although this quasi-educational approach is only a partial representation of the potential of behavioral medicine for cardiac rehabilitation, the initial experience has been positive.

Table 11.1 Content and Goals of Weekly Sessions of the Behavioral Medicine Component

Week 1	Introduction and overview
	Content: Rationale for behavioral medicine component Definition of behavioral medicine Distinction from psychiatry, psychology, psychotherapy Overview of modifiable cardiac risk factors
	Goal: To present basis and rationale for behavioral medicine component; to explain how it differs from psychotherapy; and to show the relationship between behavior and coronary risk factors.
Week 2	Psychological aspects of myocardial infarction (MI)
	Content: Psychological aspects of experiencing an MI Psychological aspects of CCU Psychological aspects of posthospital adjustment Psychological aspects of family adjustment to MI

(Cont.)

Goal: To present the common feelings and emotions associated with the experience of MI or revascularization; to demonstrate that such responses are normal adaptive processes; to demonstrate that health care providers are aware of these aspects and available to help; to assist in preventing exaggerated reactions.

Weeks 3 & 4   Stress and relaxation

Content: Definition of stress
Areas of stress (occupational)
Recognizing stress
Health effects of stress
Relaxation—coping with stress
Biofeedback applications

Goal: To help patients understand the concept of stress; to acquaint patients with means of reducing stress and its impact on health; to recognize personal areas of stress and genesis of stress.

Weeks 5 & 6   Type A behavior and intervention

Content: Definition of Type A behavior
Relationship of Type A behavior to coronary risk factors
Changing Type A behavior

Goal: To help patients understand the relationship of Type A behavior to coronary disease, recognize Type A behavior in themselves, and understand potential interventions for changing Type A behavior.

Weeks 7 & 8   Cognitive factors in coronary-related behavior

Content: General description of cognitions and relation to stress and emotion
Description of cognitions related to depression
Description of cognitions related to frustration/anger

Goal: To help patients understand how cognitive behavior (thoughts, thinking) can increase or decrease stress, depression, anger

Week 9   Sexuality and the Cardiac Patient

Content: General description of sexual anatomy and physiology
General description of sexual response
Discussion of typical sexual concerns of cardiac patients and spouses
Discussion of sexual activity in cardiac patients

Week 10   Conclusion and summary

Content: Catch-up and review questions

Goal: Classification or explanation of any areas of interest.

Table 11.2   Patient Response to Behavioral Medicine Component

Item	Patient	Spouse	Total
1. Content useful?	4.2	4.3	4.2
2. Content important?	4.6	4.3	4.5
3. New information?	3.6	4.0	3.7
4. Easily understood?	4.3	4.2	4.3
5. Well-organized?	4.3	4.2	4.3
6. Leader kept interest?	4.7	4.6	4.5
7. Leader encouraged participation?	4.5	4.2	4.4
8. Leader knew material?	4.6	4.8	4.7
9. Leader able to answer questions?	4.7	4.3	4.4
10. Recommend to a friend?	4.5	4.2	4.4
11. Useful to non-heart attack people?	4.3	4.4	4.4
12. Positive impact?	4.2	4.0	4.1

Summarized from ratings in which 5 = strongly agree; 4 = agree; 3 = no comment; 2 = disagree; 1 = strongly disagree. N = 20.

Summary

In conclusion, two cautions are in order. The first is that the enthusiasm for behavioral medicine should remain geared to its *contributions* and not to its predictions or potential. This is a caveat that has been raised repeatedly by several of the primary figures in the development of behavioral medicine (Katz & Zlutnick, 1975; Matarazzo, 1980; Pomerleau & Brady, 1979). Although behavioral medicine provides exciting opportunities for interdisciplinary collaboration, innovative developments, and enhancement of quality of care, promise is not fulfillment. As Agras (1982) has insightfully noted, new approaches such as those in behavioral medicine are only as valid as their supporting data and only as useful as their applications.

This leads to the final comment as to what behavioral medicine is not. Behavioral medicine is neither wellness nor holistic health. Although these concepts may be part of behavioral medicine, they are, unfortunately, often comprised of bandwagon fads and philosophies with little or no empirical validation. Behavioral medicine is a cooperative scientific endeavor. In a bit of an ironic twist, the philosophy of behavioral medicine might be succinctly summarized by paraphrasing the words of Traffert, who recently used them to describe *wellness*.

While [behavioral medicine] is receiving welcome emphasis, we must be sure we do not, in our enthusiasm and evangelism, simply add a new set of wivestales to the burdensome lore of old ones. [Behavioral medicine] is an attempt to substitute data for slogans and facts for beliefs. [Behavioral medicine] should not be just a welcome emphasis, but a credible science.

That is the spirit and promise of behavioral medicine.

References

Abram, H. (1965). Adaptation to open heart surgery: A psychiatric study of response to the threat of death. *American Journal of Psychiatry*, **122**, 659.

Abram, H. (1968). The psychiatrist, the treatment of chronic renal failure, and the prolongation of life—I. *American Journal of Psychiatry*, **124**, 1351.

Abram, H. (1969). The psychiatrist, the treatment of chronic renal failure, and the prolongation of life—II. *American Journal of Psychiatry*, **126**, 157.

Abram, H. (1970a). Psychological reactions to cardiac operations: An historical perspective. *International Journal of Psychiatry in Medicine*, **1**(4), 277.

Abram, H. (1970b). Survival by machine: Psychological aspects of chronic hemodialysis. *International Journal of Psychiatry in Medicine*, **1**, 37.

Agras, W. (1982). Behavioral medicine in the 1980's: Non-random connections. *Journal of Consulting and Clinical Psychology*, **50**(6), 797.

Agras, W., & Berkowitz, R. (1980). Clinical research and behavior therapy: Halfway there? *Behavior Therapy*, **11**, 472.

American Psychological Association Task Force on Health Research. (1976). Contributions of psychology to health research. *American Psychologist*, **31**(4), 263.

Anderson, K., & Masur, F. (1983). Psychological preparation for invasive medical and dental procedures. *Journal of Behavioral Medicine*, **6**(1), 1.

Andrew, G., Oldridge, N., Parker, J., Cunningham, D., Rechnitzer, P., Jones, N., Buck, C., Kavanaugh, T., Shephard, R., Sutton, J., & McDonald, W. (1981). Reasons for drop-out from exercise program in postcoronary patients. *Medicine and Science in Sports and Exercise*, **13**(3), 164.

Asken, M. (1975). Psychoemotional aspects of mastectomy: Review of recent literature. *American Journal of Psychiatry*, **132**(1), 56.

Asken, M. (1979). Psychological stress in ICU affects both patients, staff. *Pennsylvania Medicine*, **82**(11), 40.

Asken, M., & Raham, D. (1983). Resident performance and sleep deprivation: A review. *Journal of Medical Education*, **58**(5), 382.

Asken, M., & Strock, B. (1978). The family physician as medical-psychological counselor. *Primary Care,* **5**(1), 111.

Baile, W., Brinker, J., Wachspress, J., & Engel, B. (1979). Sign-outs against medical advice from a coronary care unit. *Journal of Behavioral Medicine,* **2**(1), 85.

Benson, H., Kotch, J., & Crassweller, K. (1977). The relaxation response: A bridge between psychiatry and medicine. *Medical Clinics of North America,* **61**(4), 929.

Birk, L. (Ed.). (1973). *Biofeedback: Behavioral medicine.* New York: Grune and Stratton.

Blackburn, H. (1980). Risk factors and cardiovascular disease. In The American Heart Association (Ed.), *Heart book.* New York: E.P. Dutton.

Blanchard, E. (1977). Behavioral medicine: A perspective. In R. Williams, Jr., & W. Gentry (Eds.), *Behavioral approaches to medical treatment.* Cambridge, MA: Ballinger.

Blanchard, E., & Andrasik, F. (1982). Psychological assessment and treatment of headache: Recent developments and emerging issues. *Journal of Consulting and Clinical Psychology,* **50**(6), 859.

Blumenthal, J., Califf, R., Williams, R., & Hindman, M. (in press). Cardiac rehabilitation: A new frontier for behavioral medicine. *Journal of Cardiac Rehabilitation.*

Blumenthal, J., Williams, R., & Wallace, A. (1980). Effect of exercise on the type A (coronary prone) behavior pattern. *Psychosomatic Medicine,* **42**(2), 289.

Brown, B., & Rieger, D. (1977). How NIMH views primary care practitioners. *Practical Psychology for Physicians,* **4**, 12.

Brownell, K. (1982). Obesity: Understanding and treating a serious, prevalent and refractory disorder. *Journal of Consulting and Clinical Psychology,* **50**(6), 820.

Carmody, T., Fey, S., Pierce, D., Connor, W., & Matarazzo, J. (1982). Behavioral treatment of hyperlipidemia: Techniques, results and future directions. *Journal of Behavioral Medicine,* **5**(1), 91.

Carmody, T., Senner, J., Malinow, M., & Matarazzo, J. (1980). Physical exercise rehabilitation: Long-term drop-out rate for cardiac patients. *Journal of Behavioral Medicine,* **3**(2), 163.

Carney, R., Schechter, K., & Davis, T. (1983). Improving adherence to blood glucose testing in insulin-dependent diabetic children. *Behavior Therapy,* **14**, 247.

Carrillo, C. (1980). Overcoming barriers to the treatment of the hispanic patient. In N. Jospe, J. Nieberding, & B. Cohen (Eds.), *Psychological factors in health care: A practitioner's manual.* Lexington: Lexington Books.

Cassem, N., & Hackett, T. (1971). Psychiatric consultation in a coronary care unit. *Annals of Internal Medicine*, **75**, 9.

Cassem, N., & Hackett, T. (1977). Psychological aspects of myocardial infarction. *Medical Clinics of North America*, **61**(4), 711.

Cassem, N., & Hackett, T. (1978). The setting of intensive care. In T. Hackett & N. Cassem (Eds.), *Massachusetts general hospital handbook of general hospital psychiatry*. St. Louis: C.V. Mosby.

Christopherson, E., & Gyulay, J. (1981). Parental compliance with car seat usage: A positive approach with long-term follow-up. *Journal of Pediatric Psychology*, **6**(3), 301.

Coates, T., & Perry, C. (in press). Multifactor risk reduction with children and adolescents: Taking care of the heart in behavioral group therapy. In D. Upper & S. Ross (Eds.), *Behavior group therapy: An annual review*. Champaign, IL: Research Press.

Cohen, R., & Stunkard, A. (1983). Behavior therapy and pharmacotherapy of obesity: A review of the literature. *Behavioral Medicine Update*, **4**(3), 7.

Cohen-Cole, S., Haggerty, J., & Raft, D. (1982). Objectives for residents in consultation psychiatry: Recommendations of a task force. *Psychosomatics*, **23**(7), 699.

Cummings, K., Becker, M., Kirscht, J., & Levin, N. (1981). Intervention strategies to improve compliance with medical regimens by ambulatory hemodialysis patients. *Journal of Behavioral Medicine*, **4**(1), 111.

Danaher, B., & Lichtenstein, E. (1978). *Become an ex-smoker*. Englewood Cliffs, NJ: Prentice-Hall.

DeLongis, A., Coyne, J., Dakof, G., Folkman, S., & Lazarus, R. (1982). Relationship of daily hassles, uplifts and major life events to health status. *Health Psychology*, **1**(2), 119.

Dembroski, T., Weiss, S., Shields, J., Haynes, S., & Feinleib, M. (Eds.). (1978). *Coronary prone behavior*. New York: Springer-Verlag.

Dembroski, T., MacDougall, J., Shields, J., Pettito, J., & Lushene, R. (1978). Components of type A coronary-prone behavior pattern and cardiovascular response to psychomotor performance challenge. *Journal of Behavioral Medicine*, **1**(2), 159.

Dishman, R. (1982). Compliance/adherence in health related exercise. *Health Psychology*, **1**(3), 237.

Dishman, R., & Ickes, W. (1981). Self motivation and adherence to therapeutic exercise. *Journal of Behavioral Medicine*, **4**(4), 421.

Doleys, D., Meredith, R., & Ciminero, A. (1982). Introduction and overview. In D. Doleys, R. Meredith, & A. Ciminero (Eds.), *Behavioral medicine: Assessment and treatment strategies*. New York: Plenum Press.

Drotar, D. (1981). Psychological perspectives in chronic childhood illness. *Journal of Pediatric Psychology*, **6**(3), 211.

Dubbert, P., Martin, J., Raczynski, J., & Smith, P. (1982, March). *The effects of cognitive behavioral strategies in the maintenance of exercise*. Paper presented at the Third Annual Meeting of the Society of Behavioral Medicine, Chicago, IL.

Eiser, C. (1979). Psychological development of the child with leukemia: A review. *Journal of Behavioral Medicine, 2*(2), 141.

Engel, G. (1977). The need for a new medical model: A challenge for biomedicine. *Science, 196*, 129.

Ergood, J., & Tarter, R. (1983). Neuropsychologic measurement of encephalopathy after myocardial infarction. *Journal of Cardiac Rehabilitation, 3*, 368.

Ferguson, J., & Taylor, C. (1981). Preface. In J. Ferguson & C. Taylor (Eds.), *The comprehensive handbook of behavioral medicine* (Vol. 1). New York: S.P. Medical Scientific Books.

Fordyce, W. (1976). *Behavioral methods for chronic pain and illness*. St. Louis: C.V. Mosby.

Friedman, M., & Rosenman, R. (1974). *Type A behavior and your heart*. Greenwich, CT: Fawcett.

Geller, E., Patterson, L., & Talbott, E. (1982). A behavioral analysis of incentive prompts for motivating seat belt use. *Journal of Applied Behavior Analysis, 15*(3), 403.

Gentry, W. (1980). Behavioral medicine abroad. *International Journal of Mental Health, 1*(1-2), 197.

Glover, M., Kuber, M., Warren, S., & Vieweg, W. (1982). Myocardial infarction before age 36: Risk factors and arteriographic analysis. *American Journal of Cardiology, 49*(5), 1600.

Hackett, T., Cassem, N., & Wishnie, H. (1968). The coronary care unit: An appraisal of its psychological hazards. *New England Journal of Medicine, 279*, 1365.

Hellerstein, H., & Fried, E. (1970). Sexual activity and the post-coronary patient. *Archives of Internal Medicine, 125*(6), 987.

Holmes, T., & Rahe, R. (1967). The social adjustment rating scale. *Journal of Psychosomatic Research, 11*, 213.

Jenkins, C., Zyzanski, S., & Rosenman, R. (1979). *Jenkins activity survey manual*. New York: The Psychological Corporation.

Jones, R., & Kazdin, A. (1980). Teaching children how and when to make emergency telephone calls. *Behavior Therapy, 11*(4), 509.

Jones, R., Kazdin, A., & Haney, J. (1981). Social validation and training of emergency fire safety skills for potential injury and life saving. *Journal of Applied Behavior Analysis, 14*(3), 249.

Johnson, S. (1980). Psychosocial factors in juvenile diabetes: A review. *Journal of Behavioral Medicine, 3*(1), 95.

Jorgensen, R., & Houston, B. (1981). Family history of hypertension, gender and cardiovascular reactivity in stereotyping during stress. *Journal of Behavioral Medicine, 4*(2), 175.

Kanner, A., Coyne, J., Schaefer, C., & Lazarus, R. (1981). Comparison of two modes of stress management: Daily hassles and uplifts vs. major life events. *Journal of Behavioral Medicine, 4*(1), 1.

Kaplan, H. (1975). History of psychophysiological medicine. In A. Freedman, H. Kaplan, & B. Sadock (Eds.), *Comprehensive textbook of psychiatry* (Vol. 2). Baltimore: Williams and Wilkins.

Kaplan, R., Atkins, C., & Lenhard, L. (1982). Coping with stressful sigmoidoscopy: Evaluation of cognitive and relaxation procedures. *Journal of Behavioral Medicine, 5*(1), 67.

Kaplan DeNour, A., & Czaczkes, J. (1968). Emotional problems and reactions of the medical team in a chronic hemiodialysis unit. *Lancet, 2,* 987.

Kaplan DeNour, A., Shaltier, J., & Czaczkes, J. (1968). Emotional reactions of patients on chronic hemodialysis. *Psychosomatic Medicine, 35,* 521.

Karasu, T. (1979). Psychotherapy of the medically ill. *American Journal of Psychiatry, 136*(1), 1.

Katz, R., & Zlutnick, S. (1975). *Behavior therapy and health care.* Elmsford, NY: Pergamon Press.

King, N. (1980). The behavioral management of asthma and asthma-related problems in children: A critical review of the literature. *Journal of Behavioral Medicine, 3*(2), 169.

Knowles, J. (1977). The responsibility of the individual. In J. Knowles (Ed.), *Doing better and feeling worse: Health in the United States.* New York: W.W. Norton.

Kolman, P. (1983). The value of group psychotherapy after myocardial infarction: A critical review. *Journal of Cardiac Rehabilitation, 3,* 360.

Kornfeld, D., Zimberg, S., & Malm, J. (1965). Psychiatric complications of open heart surgery. *New England Journal of Medicine, 273*(6), 287.

Krantz, D., Arabian, J., Davia, J., & Parker, J. (1982). Type A behavior and coronary artery bypass surgery: Intraoperative blood pressure and perioperative complications. *Psychosomatic Medicine, 44*(3), 273.

LaLonde, M. (1974). A new perspective on the health of Canadians. Ottawa, Canada: Ministry of Health and Welfare.

Lipowski, Z. (1974). Consultation-liaison psychiatry: An overview. *American Journal of Psychiatry, 131*(6), 623.

Locke, S. (1982). Stress, adaptation and immunity: Studies in humans. *General Hospital Psychiatry, 4,* 49.

Lyles, J., Burish, T., Krozely, M., & Oldham, R. (1982). Efficacy of relaxation training and guided imagery in reducing the aversiveness of cancer chemotherapy. *Journal of Consulting and Clinical Psychology,* 50(4), 509.

Maguire, P., & Asken, M. (1978). Psychological problems in family practice: Implications for training. *Journal of Child Clinical Psychology,* 7(1), 13.

Mahon, R. (1980). Psychological factors in providing health care to blacks. In N. Jospe, J. Nieberding, & B. Cohen (Eds.). *Psychological factors in health care: A practitioner's manual.* Lexington: Lexington Books.

Martin, J., & Smith, P. (1981). *Factors predicting exercise adherence: A two-year evaluation.* Paper presented at the Fifteenth Annual Meeting of the Association of the Advancement of Behavior Therapy, Toronto, Canada.

Masur, F. (1979). Resumption of sexual activity following myocardial infarction. *Sexuality and Disability,* 2(2), 98.

Masur, F. (1981). Adherence to health care regimens. In C. Prokop & L. Bradley (Eds.), *Medical psychology: Contributions to behavioral medicine.* New York: Academic Press.

Matarazzo, J. (1980). Behavioral health and behavioral medicine: Frontiers for a new health psychology. *American Psychologist,* 35(9), 807.

Matarazzo, J. (1982). Behavioral health's challenge to academic, scientific and professional psychology. *American Psychologist,* 37(1), 1.

Matthews, K., & Angulo, J. (1980). Measurement of the type A behavior pattern in children: Assessment of children's competitiveness, impatience-anger, and aggression. *Child Development,* 51, 466.

McLane, N., Krop, H., & Mehta, J. (1980). Psychosocial adjustment and counseling after myocardial infarction. *Annals of Internal Medicine,* 92, 514.

Mehta, J., & Krop, H. (1979). The effect of myocardial infarction on sexual function. *Sexuality and Disability,* 2(2), 115.

Morrow, G., & Morrell, C. (1982). Behavioral treatment for anticipatory nausea and vomiting induced by cancer chemotherapy. *New England Journal of Medicine,* 307(12), 1476.

Mumford, E., Schlesinger, H., & Glass, G. (1982). The effects of psychological intervention on recovery from surgery and heart attacks: An analysis of the literature. *American Journal of Public Health,* 72(2), 141.

Olbrisch, M. (1977). Psychotherapeutic intervention and physical health: Effectiveness and economic efficiency. *American Psychologist,* 32(9), 761.

Oldridge, N., & Jones, N. (1983). Improving patient compliance and cardiac exercise rehabilitation: Effects of written agreement and self-monitoring. *Journal of Cardiac Rehabilitation,* 3, 257.

Olton, D., & Noonberg, A. (1980). *Biofeedback: Clinical applications in behavioral medicine.* Englewood Cliffs, NJ: Prentice-Hall.

Peterson, H. (1977). Who'll sponsor a biopsychosocial model of disease? *Patient Care*, **5**, 8.

Peterson, L., & Shigetomi, C. (1982). One year follow-up of elective surgery child patients receiving preoperative preparation. *Journal of Pediatric Psychology*, **7**(1), 43.

Pomerleau, O. (1979). Behavioral medicine: The contribution of the experimental analysis of behavior to medical care. *American Psychologist*, **34**(8), 654.

Pomerleau, O., & Brady, J. (1979). Introduction: The scope and promise of behavioral medicine. In O. Pomerleau & J. Brady (Eds.), *Behavioral medicine: Theory and practice*. Baltimore: Williams and Wilkins.

Pomerleau, O., & Pomerleau, C. (1977). *Break the smoking habit: A behavioral program for giving up cigarettes*. Champaign, IL: Research Press.

Roberts, M., Wartele, S., Boone, R., Ginther, L., & Elkins, P. (1981). Reduction of medical fears by use of modeling: A preventive application in a general population of children. *Journal of Pediatric Psychology*, **6**(3), 293.

Rosen, J., & Wiens, A. (1979). Changes in medical problems and use of medical services following psychological intervention. *American Psychologist*, **34**(5), 420.

Rosenman, R., Friedman, M., & Straus, R. (1964). A predictive study of coronary heart disease: The Western Collaborative Group study. *Journal of the American Medical Association*, **189**, 15.

Roskies, E. (1978). Changing the coronary prone (type A) behavior pattern in a non-clinical population. *Journal of Behavioral Medicine*, **1**, 201.

Rotatori, A., Fox, R., & Mauser, A. (1981). Validation of the weight reduction treatment package for the retarded. *Journal of Behavioral Medicine*, **4**(2), 231.

Schlesinger, H., Mumford, E., Glass, G., Patrick, C., & Scharfstein, S. (1983). Mental health treatment and medical care utilization in a fee-for-service system: Outpatient mental health treatment following the onset of chronic disease. *American Journal of Public Health*, **73**(4), 422.

Schofield, W. (1980). Forward. In N. Jospe, J. Nieberding, & B. Cohen (Eds.), *Psychological factors in health care: A practitioner's manual*. Lexington: Lexington Books.

Schwab, J., Bell, R., Warheit, G., Schwab, R., & Traven, N. (1978-79). Some epidemiologic aspects of psychosomatic medicine. *International Journal of Psychiatry in Medicine*, **9**(2), 147.

Schwartz, G., & Weiss, S. (1978a). Yale conference on behavioral medicine: A proposed definition and statement of goals. *Journal of Behavioral Medicine*, **1**(1), 3.

Schwartz, G., & Weiss, S. (1978b). Behavioral medicine revisited: An amended definition. *Journal of Behavioral Medicine*, **1**, 249.

Selye, H. (1976). Forty years of stress research: The principle remaining problems and misconceptions. *Canadian Medical Association Journal,* **115,** 53.

Shapiro, D., & Goldstein, I. (1982). Biobehavioral perspectives on hypertension. *Journal of Consulting and Clinical Psychology,* **50**(6), 841.

Shienvold, A., Asken, M., & Cincotta, J. (1979). Family practice residents' perceptions of behavioral science: Needs and relevancy. *Journal of Family Practice,* **8**(1), 97.

Stachnik, T. (1980). Priorities for psychology in medical education and health care delivery. *American Psychologist,* **35**(1), 8.

Stern, M., & Cleary, P. (1981). National exercise and heart disease project: Psychosocial changes observed during a low level exercise program. *Archives of Internal Medicine,* **141,** 1463.

Stuart, R., & Davis, B. (1971). *Slim chance in a fat world.* Champaign, IL: Research Press.

Stunkard, A. (1972). New therapies for the eating disorders. *Archives of General Psychiatry,* **26,** 391.

Suinn, R. (1975). Intervention with type A behaviors. *Journal of Consulting and Clinical Psychology,* **50**(6), 933.

Suinn, R. (1981). Pattern A behaviors and heart disease: Intervention approaches. In J. Ferguson & C. Taylor (Eds.), *The comprehensive handbook of behavioral medicine* (Vol. 1). New York: S.P. Medical and Scientific Books.

Suinn, R. (1982). The cardiac stress management program for type A patients. *Cardiac Rehabilitation,* **5**(4), 13.

Suinn, R., & Bloom, L. (1978). Anxiety management training for type A behavior. *Journal of Behavioral Medicine,* **1**(1), 25.

Surwit, R., Feinglos, M., & Scovern, A. (1983). Diabetes and behavior: A paradigm for health psychology. *American Psychologist,* **38**(3), 255.

Tel-Med plan is five years old. (1983, May 2). *The Patriot Evening News.*

Traffert, D. (1982). Rustproofing people: Wellness in perspective. *Postgraduate Medicine,* **71**(1), 179.

True, R. (1980). Health care issues for Asian Americans. In N. Jospe, J. Nieberding, & B. Cohen (Eds.), *Psychological factors in health care: A practitioner's manual.* Lexington: Lexington Books.

Turk, D., Meichenbaum, D., & Genest, M. (1983). *Pain and behavioral medicine: A cognitive behavioral approach.* New York: Guilford Press.

U.S. Department of Health, Education, and Welfare. (1979). *Healthy people: The Surgeon General's report on health promotion and disease prevention* (DHEW Publication No. PHS 79-55071). Washington, DC: U.S. Government Printing Office.

Waggoner, C., & LeLieuvre, R. (1981). A method to increase compliance to exercise regimens in rheumatoid arthritis patients. *Journal of Behavioral Medicine,* **4**(2), 191.

Walker, J. (1980). Prescription for the stressed physician. *Behavioral Medicine, 9,* 12.

Wellisch, D. (1981). Intervention with the cancer patient. In C. Prokop & L. Bradley (Eds.), *Medical psychology: Contributions to behavioral medicine.* New York: Academic Press.

Wilson, J. (1981). Behavioral preparation for surgery: Benefit or harm? *Journal of Behavioral Medicine, 4*(1), 79.

Wolinsky, J. (1983). Companies find wellness pays, but it's hard to assess costs. *APA Monitor,* **14**(6), 17.

Wustman, E. (1980). Psychological factors in emergency medical services. In N. Jospe, J. Nieberding, & B. Cohen (Eds.), *Psychological factors in health care: A practitioner's manual.* Lexington: Lexington Books.

Chapter 12

Biofeedback: A Viable Intervention in the Management of the Cardiac

K. Zirkel

There is an increasing recognition of the important role of behavioral and psychological factors in both the prevention and treatment of cardiovascular disease, and in the rehabilitation of patients who have experienced myocardial infarctions and other circulatory disorders. Such publications as *HeartCare* by the American Medical Association (AMA, 1982) present a strong case for the significant influence of behavioral and lifestyle variables in the development of cardiovascular disorders.

Biofeedback is one component in the treatment of cardiovascular disorders from a behavioral medicine perspective. Indeed, one of the first uses of the term *behavioral medicine* appeared with the publication of *Biofeedback: Behavioral Medicine* (Birk, 1973). This chapter will present an overview of the applications of biofeedback for the management of cardiovascular disorders and symptoms, and will cover not only rehabilitation but also preventive aspects. In this respect, biofeedback is akin to exercise or diet management strategies of which, although these are crucial elements of effective rehabilitation programs, their best use is in prevention.

In many respects, biofeedback applications remain in early stages of development. As is the case with many innovative treatment approaches, biofeedback was initially greeted as a cure-all for a wide variety of symptoms and disorders. This initial enthusiasm has given way to the more reasoned acceptance of biofeedback as a legitimate medical methodology with particular applications for specific types of symptoms. Thousands of research studies have been conducted during the past 10 years dealing with the applications of biofeedback to specific clinical problems, exploring the mechanisms behind its effects, and investigating fascinating questions of basic research regarding the self-regulation of autonomic nervous system functioning. Several journals, such as *Biofeedback and Self-Regulation* and the *American Journal of Clinical Biofeedback*, are devoted entirely to research in the field. The remainder of this chapter will present a model for understanding the process of biofeedback, several common modalities of biofeedback, and specific application of biofeedback to management of stress; treatment of peripheral vascular disease, cardiac arrhythmias, and essential hypertension; and potential use in cardiac rehabilitation programs. Finally, future trends of application of biofeedback to treatment of cardiovascular dysfunction will be discussed.

Definition of Biofeedback

Basmajian (1983) defines *biofeedback* as the "techniques of using equipment (usually electronic) to reveal to human beings some of their internal physiological events, normal and abnormal, in the form of visual and auditory signals, in order to teach them to manipulate these otherwise involuntary or unfelt events by manipulating the displayed signals" (p. 1). Advances in technology have greatly assisted the growth of biofeedback—sensitive instruments which can detect microvolt level changes in muscle tension, or detect differences of a hundredth of a degree of skin temperature, are presently in common use. "Internal physiological events" may include changes in muscle tension, cardiac output, peripheral vasodilation, brain waves, intestinal motility, or changes in electrical potential of the skin. The central point in biofeedback is that once an individual can become aware of changes in any physiological event, the potential exists for exerting voluntary control over that event.

A Behavioral Model

Figure 12.1 presents a simple model for assisting in the conceptualization of biofeedback as an example of *biobehavioral systems theory*. This new conception of human behavior lies at the foundation of behavioral medicine and arises from a joint application of cybernetics theory and general systems theory (Shapiro, 1981). The model portrays the complex, circular interaction between events, cognitions, feelings and physiological reactions, and behavior. In Figure 12.1, Arrow 1 illustrates the input from the external environment, which is perceived by sensory organs. Based on the cognitive appraisal process, or interpretation, the body is mobilized to react to the environmental event Via arrow 2. The ensuing physiological reaction is biologically designed to motivate the most appropriate behavior (Arrow 3) for coping with the event (Arrow 4). In sum, a feedback loop, represented by Arrows 1, 2, 3, and 4, operates to keep the organism in harmony with the constantly varying demands of the environment. For example: I smell smoke (Arrow 1), which I interpret as potentially threatening my survival. I respond with a fear reaction, represented by a number of physiological responses, including increased heart rate and blood pressure; increased muscle tone; rapid, shallow breathing; and so on (Arrow 2). This reaction is intended to mobilize my behavior to gain safety and flee the threat (Arrow 3), which in effect removes me from the originally threatening event (Arrow 4).

MIND-BODY INTERACTION

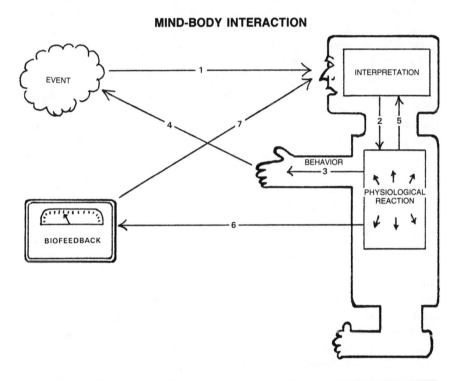

Figure 12.1.   A biobehavioral model for understanding biofeedback.

There is an *internal* feedback loop that operates on several levels. Outside of our immediate awareness, various transducers within the body are constantly monitoring our physiological reactions. These baroreceptors and chemoreceptors loop back to the hypothalamus to control vital functions such as breathing, internal temperature, heart rate, and blood pressure.

At another level, one more available to our awareness, we are able to sense internal events (Arrow 5) such as muscle tension, pain, heart beat, heat, and posture and to make adjustments more or less consciously, in conjunction with the body's own continual internal adjustments noted above. We also tend to affix *labels* of various kinds to these varying internal sensations—we may label muscle tension and elevated heart rate as excitement or anxiety depending upon a number of factors, which in turn affects the physiological sensation being monitored. For example, one individual may label an occasional extrasystole as a serious sign that something is dreadfully wrong with the heart, with a resultant increase in heart rate and a likelihood that the extra beats will continue or even increase. Another individual may interpret these sensations in a less threatening manner, believing that everyone experiences this from time to time, so it's nothing to get worried about. This different interpretation will have quite different effects upon the individual's mental and physical reaction, with corresponding differences in behavior. The point to keep in mind is that when any part of these feedback loops becomes broken or attenuated, the smooth regulation of internal homeostasis fails and disorder occurs, usually resulting in a breakdown of some sort. For example, we may choose to ignore internal signals (i.e., Arrow 5 is broken or otherwise weakened) such as tension in the neck, churning stomach, and palpitations to the point at which increasing disregulation occurs, usually resulting in an acute breakdown such as a heart attack, ulcer, or muscle spasm. The point is that the internal feedback loop, represented by Arrows 2 and 5, is attenuated or broken, with resulting disregulation and disorder.

Biofeedback is the addition of an *external* feedback loop (Arrows 6 and 7) to supplement or retrain the inner loop so that increased regulation can occur. For example, many individuals experience tension or muscle-contraction headaches resulting from locally sustained contractions of the muscles of the head and neck. Many of these sufferers are unable to notice the slowly increasing levels of tension during the day (Arrow 5 is attenuated) and no signals are perceived by the individual until the intensity of the signals is excessive, whereupon it is too late to reverse the muscle tension and associated pain. The addition of the external loop via use of muscle tension biofeedback enables the individual to recover the sensitivity potentially available via Arrow 5, and hence gives the individual *control* over the varying levels of muscle tension which do occur. As such, increased awareness over internal biological changes results in the potential for increased control over these changes in a healthful direction. What is more impressive is that the physiological responses to be modified were heretofore thought to be involuntary. Such physical parameters as peripheral blood flow, blood pressure, heart rate, visceral activity, and gastric secretion can all be brought under voluntary control with the addition of the appropriate external feedback loop.

Biofeedback Modalities

There are three different types of biofeedback demonstrating clinical utility for individuals with cardiovascular disorders. Electromyographic (EMG) or muscle tension feedback is normally used for helping individuals to become more aware of varying levels of muscle tension. Biofeedback provides an external signal loop for providing feedback to the patient regarding levels of muscle tension. Sensors are placed over the muscle site, which can detect changes in myoelectric potential. These signals are magnified and converted to varying sounds or needle movements on an indicator. The individual is then able to observe the varying levels of tension produced and, armed with this information, is able to reduce these levels to extremely low values. EMG biofeedback finds its major use in stress management. Symptoms that have proven amenable to biofeedback treatment include muscle contraction headaches, bruxism, chronic pain syndromes, and muscle rehabilitation.

The second mode of biofeedback in current clinical practice is thermal biofeedback. This type of biofeedback utilizes a sensitive thermistor, which senses extremely small differences in skin temperature. Changes in surface skin temperature are thought to be a function of changes in blood volume in the peripheral vasculature. It is a widely observed clinical phenomenon that one reaction to stress or anxiety is reduced blood flow to the surface of the skin, whereas relaxation or reduced sympathetic outflow is marked by vasodilation. Thermal biofeedback has found its greatest use in assisting individuals to control vascular headaches and peripheral vascular disorders, and has recently been found to be effective in teaching individuals to control hypertension.

The final type of biofeedback is called skin potential response biofeedback (SPR) and is based on the electrodermal activity of the skin in response to stress. This type of biofeedback senses fluctuations in skin electrical potential, which are physiological indications of underlying variations in level of arousal experienced by the individual. SPR biofeedback is useful in helping patients gain control over anxiety reactions and for teaching patients how to relax during stressful medical procedures or tests. This type of biofeedback is very sensitive to transient states of anxiety or increased sympathetic arousal, and is fairly easy for the individual to learn to control within a few sessions.

It should be noted that a fourth type of biofeedback training, EEG or brain-wave feedback, has found limited use, mainly in helping individuals learn control over certain types of seizure activity. The much-heralded *alpha-training* of the early seventies appears to have limited clinical value, given the controversy in the field over what alpha waves really represent.

Applications in Cardiovascular Dysfunction

In this section, five different types of cardiovascular dysfunctions will be discussed, followed by an analysis of the associated biofeedback strategies that have shown promise as adjunctive treatments.

Type A Personality

The Type A or cardiac-prone personality, first described by Friedman and Rosenman (1974), has been found to be a strong predictor of recurring heart attacks among a list of risk factors including smoking and hyper-cholesterolemia (Jenkins, Rosenman, & Zyzanski, 1974). In addition, the Review Panel of Coronary-Prone Behavior and Coronary Heart Disease (Suinn, 1982) has stated that Type A behavior is an independent risk factor of the same magnitude as that associated with age, serum cholesterol, systolic blood pressure, and smoking.

For many Type A individuals, many events are interpreted as threats. As such, these individuals experience elevated sympathetic nervous system arousal, which, if maintained over long periods of time, is likely to have irreversible effects on all aspects of the cardiovascular system. As with most treatments directed towards symptoms displaying a strong lifestyle component, intervention must occur on four different levels (see Figure 12.2). At the level of the *event*, the individual is guided to re-structure the environment (at work or at home) to reduce the perceived threats to loss of control. This may involve reduction of activities that mobilize the hostile-competitive elements of the Type A personality, or even deciding to terminate a career position that is too threatening for the Type A to handle effectively. At the level of the *interpretation*, the in-dividual may be guided to change the meanings he or she attributes to events that occur in the environment in order to reduce their perceived threat value (Roskies, 1983). At the level of *physiological* intervention, efforts may be made to reduce directly the physiological and emotional upheaval experienced by the individual in response to threat, utilizing perhaps medication, relaxation training, meditation, and biofeedback training. Finally, the level of *behavioral outcome* lends itself to training the individual to utilize new skills in coping with his or her environment, such as effective time-management skills or communication skills.

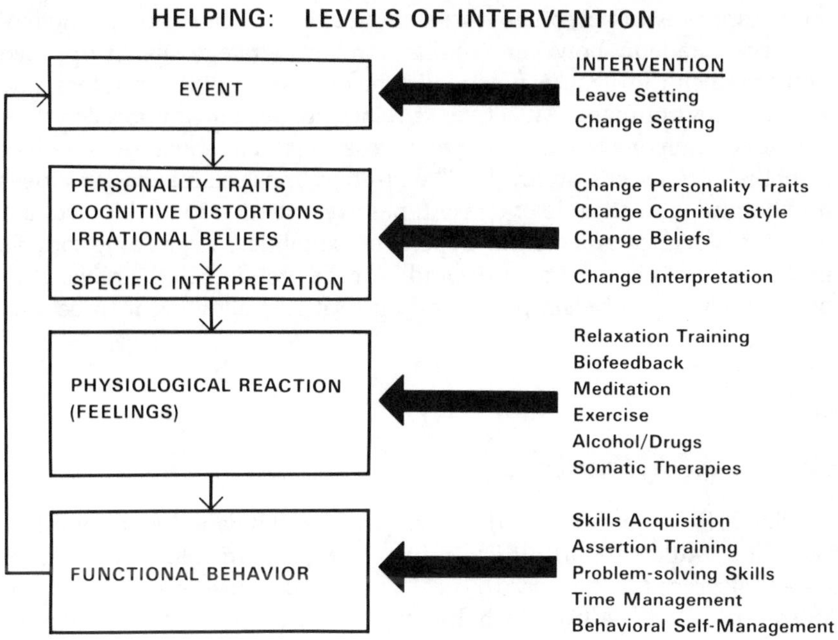

HELPING: LEVELS OF INTERVENTION

INTERVENTION

EVENT

Leave Setting
Change Setting

PERSONALITY TRAITS
COGNITIVE DISTORTIONS
IRRATIONAL BELIEFS

Change Personality Traits
Change Cognitive Style
Change Beliefs

SPECIFIC INTERPRETATION

Change Interpretation

PHYSIOLOGICAL REACTION
(FEELINGS)

Relaxation Training
Biofeedback
Meditation
Exercise
Alcohol/Drugs
Somatic Therapies

FUNCTIONAL BEHAVIOR

Skills Acquisition
Assertion Training
Problem-solving Skills
Time Management
Behavioral Self-Management

Figure 12.2.   Four levels of intervention.

Biofeedback can be a useful addition to relaxation training in general in that Type A individuals report extreme difficulty simply sitting still and relaxing. The addition of a biofeedback monitor provides a specific focus for the individual's attention beyond asking him or her simply to observe sensations of relaxation that may be occurring. A specific instruction of "see how long you can keep the green light on" (when the green light is contingent upon a level of muscle tension below a particular threshold) provides the client with a concrete goal in addition to giving specific feedback as to the progress being attained. Additional research is needed in order to assess these types of biofeedback strategies in teaching Type A personalities healthier coping strategies. Adler (1983) discusses the advantages of training Type A individuals with biofeedback. In learning control of pulse rates, such an individual gains a sense of mastery over his or her own internal functioning in a positive and healthful direction by utilizing a strategy which itself is an important skill to master.

There is a lack of controlled studies investigating the relative efficacy of biofeedback as a treatment tool in helping Type A individuals change their responses to potentially threatening events. The nature of the bio-feedback paradigm, however, requires a training strategy directly opposed to that which the Type A personality has always utilized in interacting with the environment. An active, striving, goal-oriented approach does not work when one is attempting to increase digital temperature or reduce frontalis muscle tension levels. The strategy most biofeedback trainees find helpful is an attitude of relaxed, passive attention to the biofeedback monitor, which is unusual for Type A personalities. Type A individuals find themselves in a therapeutic bind—for the first time in their lives they must reach a goal by simply attending to it and allowing it to occur.

Cardiac Arrhythmias

Cardiac arrhythmias are hard to treat from a behavioral standpoint as many individuals report difficulty in sensing a particular physiological state that precedes their occurrence. There is promise, however, in the utilization of biofeedback in helping patients reduce the frequency of several types of arrhythmias (Pinkerton, Hughes, & Wenrich, 1982). The earliest studies have used beat-to-beat heart rate feedback for teaching patients with supraventricular arrhythmias to lower their heart rate (Engel & Bleeker, 1974; Scott, Blanchard, Edmundson, & Young, 1978). Engel and Baile (1983) report success with patients experiencing paroxysmal atrial tachycardia and intermittent Wolff-Parkinson-White syndrome. One of their patients was able to learn to control her cardiac conduction pattern through both increasing and inhibiting aberrantly-conducted beats. Bleeker and Engel (1973) report success with a small sample of patients with fixed atrial fibrillation. These patients learned to increase and decrease their ventricular rates reliably. The most success has been reported in teaching patients to control ventricular ectopic beats. Pickering and Miller (1977) reported results in training patients to reduce the frequency of premature ventricular contractions mainly by learning to lower their ventricular rates via heart rate feedback. Engel reports that such biofeedback studies have the potential of improving the assessment of the efficacy of various pharmacotherapies or diagnosing potential toxicity to certain drugs used to control arrhythmias.

Most research investigating the utility of biofeedback for controlling arrhythmias has been conducted with very small patient samples. Larger, controlled, clinical trials remain necessary before reliable conclusions can be drawn regarding the efficacy of biofeedback in the management of cardiac arrythmias.

Angina Pectoris

Although the most significant behavioral treatment for angina remains precise control of exercise regimes, control of hypertension, diet management, and cessation of smoking, Hartman reports success in training three VA patients in hand warming using thermal biofeedback. All these patients learned to control the frequency and intensity of their angina episodes. Steiner (personal communication, 1984) reports success in training a patient suffering from Prinzmetal's angina, which is characterized by spasm of the coronary vessels, to control her symptoms by learning biofeedback-assisted hand warming. The physiological mechanisms responsible for these initial results remain open to question, and further research is being conducted in an effort to discover these mechanisms as well as devise more specific interventions for angina patients.

Peripheral Vascular Disorders

One of the most successful uses to date of biofeedback has been in the treatment of Raynaud's disease (Sedlacek, 1983). This disease is characterized by a severe reduction in peripheral blood flow, resulting in a blanched and cyanotic appearance of the fingers. In severe cases, amputation of a finger or toe has been carried out. Primary Raynaud's disease can be precipitated by physical (cold) or emotional stress, and thermal biofeedback has been found to be a major treatment modality for this disease. Treatment involves approximately 10-30 sessions of thermal biofeedback training, and most treatment packages include home practice with hand warming, general relaxation training, and mental imagery. The vast majority of patients who have undergone biofeedback training gain control over their vasospastic episodes, and many have found that the biofeedback and stress management have carried over into other areas of their lives, resulting in improved physical health and more positive attitudes in general.

Intermittent claudication refers to ischemic leg pain experienced by individuals upon exercise. This disorder is thought to be due to arterial spasm or, in more advanced cases, arteriosclerosis. Biofeedback has been used as an adjunctive treatment for patients with ischemic leg pain. Patients who are taught foot warming techniques using thermal biofeedback training have been shown to significantly increase daily walking distances after about 20 sessions of training (Cox & Lefevre, 1981). Although it is not certain what underlying mechanisms are responsible for these results, it is thought that volitional increase of peripheral blood flow to the extremities somehow correlates with increased blood flow to the muscle vasculature.

Hypertension

In the late sixties, researchers at the Harvard Psychology Department and Medical School demonstrated that individuals have the ability to increase or decrease systolic and diastolic blood pressure when given feedback of blood pressure changes on a beat-to-beat basis (Shapiro, Tursky, Gershon, & Stern, 1968). A large number of studies have been conducted since that time which indicate that individuals do have the capacity to significantly decrease both systolic and diastolic blood pressures as a result of biofeedback training programs (Blanchard, Haynes, Kallman, & Harkey, 1976; Erbeck, Elfner, & Driggs, 1983; Goebel, Viol, Lorenz, & Clements, 1980; Patel, 1977; Shapiro, Schwartz, Ferguson, Redmond, & Weiss, 1977). Initial success with such behavioral interventions for controlling hypertension is exciting in that many patients are able to terminate antihypertensive medications, many of which have undesirable or dangerous side effects.

One of the most successful biofeedback-based programs for teaching control of hypertension is located at the Menninger Foundation in Topeka, Kansas (Green, Green, & Norris, 1980). This program utilizes thermal biofeedback to assist patients in learning hand and foot warming, which produces lasting and significant changes in systolic and diastolic blood pressure as well as EMG feedback to reduce chronic muscle tension. In addition, patients are taught more effective stress-management techniques such as altering cognitive interpretations of stressors, learning time-management skills, and practicing more effective communication skills. Other training elements include learning diaphragmatic breathing, educating patients regarding the physiological mechanisms underlying treatment, self-monitoring and charting of blood pressures, and transferring learned skills to home or office. Treatment personnel at the Menninger Foundation report that 88% of their patients with diagnosed hypertension become normotensive while eliminating medication. The average patient achieved normotensive levels within 20 weeks after beginning treatment. Results indicate that the treatment is effective for both severe and mild cases of hypertension, whether chronic or labile. Clearly, biofeedback offers another potent treatment for those who suffer from hypertension, and does so without the potentially harmful side effects of other medical interventions.

Cardiac Rehabilitation

Although research data exploring the utility of biofeedback treatment for a variety of cardiovascular disorders continues to accumulate, the use of biofeedback for other symptoms that typically are experienced by cardiac patients is well established. Biofeedback remains a primary modality for helping patients control excessive anxiety symptoms and can augment the positive benefits obtained from exercise and relaxation therapies. Biofeedback also reinforces an increased sense of internal locus of control and self-responsibility on the part of the patient, which counteracts the development of the familiar *cardiac cripple* syndrome. Biofeedback training can also help the patient learn improved ability to discriminate internal physiological events and thus reduce misattribution of symptoms, which often occurs. For example, many patients mistakenly assume that myofascial pain in the pectoral region means they are having another infarction, further increasing anxiety levels that are already elevated. Electromyographic feedback of these muscles helps inform the patient as to the true source of his or her pain, which alleviates anxiety. Finally, biofeedback interventions can help reduce other stress-related symptoms, including muscle-contraction and vascular headaches, gastrointestinal disorders, insomnia, and the vasoconstrictive disorders noted above.

Future Trends

Coming years will see biofeedback become an increasingly integral component of both prevention and rehabilitation programs involving cardiovascular dysfunction. Initial single-case research studies are now giving way to large-scale clinical trials investigating the utility of biofeedback in either primary or adjunctive roles in the treatment of peripheral vascular disease, cardiac arrhythmias, essential hypertension, and angina pectoris. Computerization of biofeedback display and of data collection and charting is providing biofeedback practitioners with more efficient methods of treatment. The development of impedance cardiography (Mohapatra, 1981), a noninvasive technique for monitoring and providing feedback for a number of cardiac functions such as stroke volume, heart rate, myocardial contractility, and ventricular ejection time, offers exciting possibilities for training individuals in self-control of patterns of specific cardiac functions (Wilson, Albright, & Steiner, 1983). In conclusion, the promise of biofeedback is based on the observation that any physiological process that can be monitored and fed back to the individual offers the individual the capability of learning increased control over that process. Research investigations have not yet discovered the practical limits to this ability, and the next 10 years should see an expanding use of biofeedback in the prevention and treatment of cardiovascular disease.

Further information related to biofeedback training programs can be obtained from the Biofeedback Society of America, 4301 Owens Street, Wheat Ridge, CO 80033. Tel. (303) 420-2889.

References

Adler, C.P. (1983). Biofeedback and psychosomatic disorders. In J. Basmajian (Ed.), *Biofeedback: Principles and practice for clinicians* (2nd ed.). Baltimore: Williams and Wilkins.

American Medical Association. (1982). *Heartcare*.

Basmajian, J. (1983). *Biofeedback: Principles and practice for clinicians* (2nd ed.). Baltimore: Williams and Wilkins.

Birk, L. (Ed.). (1973). *Biofeedback: Behavioral medicine*. New York: Grune and Stratton.

Blanchard, E. G., Haynes, M.R., Kallman, M.D., & Harkey, L.S. (1976). A comparison of direct blood pressure feedback and electromyographic feedback on the blood pressure of normotensives. *Biofeedback and Self-Regulation*, 1, 445-451.

Bleeker, E.R., & Engel, B.T. (1973). Learned control of ventricular rate in patients with atrial fibrillation. *Psychosomatic Medicine*, 35, 161-175.

Cox, D., & Lefevre, R.C. (1981). Thermal biofeedback in the treatment of intermittent claudication of diabetic patients. *Proceedings of the 12th Annual Meeting of the Biofeedback Society of America*.

Engel, B., & Baile, W. (1983). Behavioral applications in the treatment of patients with cardiovascular disorders. In J. Basmajian (Ed.), *Biofeedback: Principles and practice for clinicians* (2nd ed.). Baltimore: Williams and Wilkins.

Engel, B., & Bleeker, E.R. (1974). Application of operant conditioning techniques to the control of the cardiac arrhythmias. In P.A. Obrist (Ed.), *Cardiovascular psychophysiology: Current issues in response mechanisms, biofeedback, and methodology*. Chicago: Aldine.

Erbeck, J.R., Elfner, L.F., & Driggs, D.F. (1983). Reduction of blood pressure by indirect biofeedback. *Biofeedback and Self-Regulation*, 8(1), 63-72.

Friedman, M., & Rosenman, R. (1974). *Type A behavior and your heart*. Greenwich: Fawcett/Crest.

Goebel, M., Viol, G.W., Lorenz, G.J., & Clements, J. (1980). Relaxation and biofeedback in essential hypertension: A preliminary report of a six year project. *American Journal of Clinical Biofeedback*, 3(1), 20-29.

Green, E., Green, A., & Norris, P. (1980). Self-regulation training of hypertension: An experimental method for restoring or maintaining normal blood pressure. *Primary Cardiology*, 6.

Hartman, C.H. (1979). The response of anginal pain to hand-warming. *Biofeedback and Self-Regulation*, 4, 4.

Jenkins, C., Rosenman, R., & Zyzanski, S. (1974). Prediction of clinical coronary heart disease by a test for the coronary-prone behavior pattern. *New England Journal of Medicine*, 290, 1271-1275.

Mohapatra, S.N. (1981). *Non-invasive cardiovascular monitoring by electrical impedance techniques*. London: Pitman Medical.

Patel, C.H. (1977). Biofeedback-aided relaxation and meditation in the management of hypertension. *Biofeedback and Self-Regulation, 2*, 1-41.

Pickering, T.G., & Miller, N.E. (1977). Learned voluntary control of heart rate and rhythm in two subjects with premature ventricular contractions. *British Heart Journal, 39*, 152-159.

Pinkerton, S., Hughes, H., & Wenrich, W.W. (Eds.). (1982). *Behavioral medicine: Clinical applications*. New York: Wiley.

Roskies, E. (1983). Stress management for Type A individuals. In D. Meichenbaum & M.E. Jaremko (Eds.), *Stress reduction and prevention*. New York: Plenum Press.

Scott, R.W., Blanchard, E.B., Edmundson, E.D., & Young, L.D. (1978). A shaping procedure for heart-rate control in chronic tachycardia. *Perceptual Motor Skills, 37*, 327-338.

Sedlacek, K. (1983). Biofeedback treatment of primary raynaud's disease. In J. Basmajian (Ed.), *Biofeedback: Principles and practice for clinicians* (2nd ed.). Baltimore: Williams and Wilkins.

Shapiro, D. (Ed.). (1981). *Biofeedback and behavioral medicine 1979-80: Therapeutic applications and experimental foundations*. Chicago: Aldine.

Shapiro, A.P., Schwartz, G.E., Ferguson, D.C.E., Redmond, D.P., & Weiss, S.M. (1977). Behavioral methods in the treatment of hypertension. *Annals of Internal Medicine, 86*, 626-636.

Shapiro, D., Tursky, B., Gershon, E., & Stern, M. (1968). Effects of feedback and reinforcement of the control of human systolic blood pressure. *Science, 163*, 588-590.

Suinn, R. (1982). Intervention with Type A behaviors. *Journal of Consulting and Clinical Psychology, 50-56*, 933-949.

Wilson, B.L., Albright, G.L., & Steiner, S.S. (1983). Cardiac dynamics accompanying stress induced blood pressure changes: Two replications. *Proceedings of the 14th Annual Meeting of the Biofeedback Society of America*.

Part III

Exercise Testing

Chapter 13

Protocols

Linda K. Hall

Selecting the appropriate protocol for a stress test appears to be a foregone conclusion in a number of laboratories across the nation. The Bruce Protocol is the one that is chosen more often than not for several reasons: (a) It is the most widely used in research and therefore has the most documentation, (b) it has been found to be a reliable and valid tool for estimation of energy cost, and (c) it crosses a broad spectrum of fitness levels as a testing method with reliable results. However, it is becoming more and more apparent that, as the uses of graded exercise testing (GXT) broaden to encompass more areas of the disease spectrum, the Bruce Protocol has some shortcomings and should not always be the protocol of choice.

This chapter will present a broad spectrum of possible protocols for the many uses of the GXT and give a rationale for the different choices. I hope that reading this chapter will give you the courage to try new and different methods for testing in the GXT laboratory.

Preliminary Informational Needs

Before selecting a GXT, criteria for test selection and the patient's exercise history need to be considered.

Uses of the GXT

The graded exercise test has evolved over the past 20 years to be more than an assessor of maximal aerobic ability or a tool for diagnosis. As more studies make use of the GXT in a myriad of ways, it is proving to be an economical as well as a fairly reliable informational tool in a number of roles in health as well as disease. As the uses for the GXT become defined, so also does the type of protocol chosen. The list of current uses of the GXT is as follows (I expect that this list will grow in the near future):

1. Health risk screening. In this instance the GXT is used to identify people with latent coronary artery disease (CAD) and other diseases that are regarded as health hazards.
2. Diagnosis of atypical chest pain. This is considered by a number of physicians to be an economical as well as a less traumatic test for the patient complaining of atypical chest pain. It is a diagnostic test to either rule out coronary heart disease (CHD) or diagnose its presence.
3. Assessment of functional aerobic capacity. This is a test to determine the maximal amount of aerobic work a person is capable of doing with the absence of symptoms and/or physiologically measured detrimental parameters such as hypotension, ST depression, arrhythmias, and so on. This is the GXT from which the best exercise prescription can be determined.
4. Detection of treatable exercise-induced arrhythmias. This is a GXT utilized to force the heart into arrhythmic patterns that are suspected or have been noticed by the patient.
5. Evaluation of interventional therapy. This is a multiple purpose GXT used to evaluate drug therapy, exercise therapy, angioplasty, and surgical intervention and to see whether they have been efficacious in their results.
6. Prognostic testing. This uses the GXT to aid in determining prognosis and management of the early recovery from acute myocardial infarction (MI) and bypass surgery.

Each of these uses has the possibility of requiring a different protocol to make sure that the most significant amount of information is derived from the GXT. It is essential for the exercise technician and the supervising physician to evaluate the reasons for doing the test and then to select the appropriate protocol.

Patient History

Patients undergoing the GXT should be interviewed for an exercise history immediately upon arrival at the lab. The fact that this procedure is infrequently done explains why inappropriate protocols are selected, which give results that are masked by fatigue, produce isolated pain in specific muscles untrained for the protocol, or give false positive ST responses. A thorough interview of the prospective exerciser relative to his or her exercise history is essential:

1. Is he or she a regular exerciser?
2. How often?
3. What modality (e.g., swimming, running, cycling, etc.)?
4. How long has the individual been exercising (years, months, number of times per day)?
5. Is the modality used (e.g., swimming, running, cycling) primarily a leg activity, arm activity, or both?
6. When was the last time the person exercised? Was it on a regular basis?
7. How fast does the individual do his or her exercise (at what percentage of maximum ability)? What speed in mi/hr, min/mi, HR/min?
8. What does the individual want to do for exercise when and if it is prescribed?

In order to assure the best possible test administration, the test-giver should know a number of other things about the test-taker prior to selection of the appropriate protocol. For example, it has been my experience that a number of women between the ages of 30 and 50 are tested in the laboratory after complaining of nonspecific chest pain, fatigue, and general apathy. In most instances they are considerably underfit and have a general MET level of between 7 and 10 METs. Consider the following example: A woman is to be tested who does no regular exercise, did not participate in athletics in high school or college, has no special exercise activities that she does on weekends or even leisurely, but has informed you that she is about 40 years old; her potential is 8 METs (see Table 13.1). If you selected the Bruce Protocol as the method of testing, it is likely that this woman would manifest ST-segment depression in the first stage and the test would be declared positive. This ST-segment depression may be due to the fact that the woman was not warmed up properly.

Table 13.1 Prediction Equations for $\dot{V}O_2$max for Healthy Men and Women

---

Active men = 69.7 − .612(age)

Sedentary men = 57.8 − .445(age)

Active women = 42.9 − .312(age)

Sedentary women = 42.3 − .356(age)

Note. From "Principles of Exercise Testing" by R.A. Bruce, 1973, in J.P. Naughton and H.K. Hellerstein (Eds.), *Exercise Testing and Exercise Training in Coronary Heart Disease* (p. 53), New York: Academic Press. Copyright 1973 by Academic Press. Reprinted by permission.

My colleagues and I have found that excellently trained runners manifest ST-segment depression if they have not been warmed up properly; in separate test situations, these same runners do not manifest ST-segment problems if they have warmed up beforehand. If the ST depression that the 40-year-old woman manifested was due to an improper or nonexistent warm-up, it is likely that this is a false positive test. This is because the first stage of the Bruce Protocol is 4.2 METs, which is a work load of 50% of her predicted maximal capacity and is not an appropriate warm-up; the result is coronary myocardial ischemia and thus ST-segment depression (Caso, Greenberg, & Ellestad, 1979). In addition, the test might not give the desired results in terms of functional capacity because the first stage is 4.2 METs, the second stage is 7.2 METs, and the third stage 10.2 METs (Bruce, Blackman, Jones, & Strait, 1963). The woman in the example, most likely would be able to finish the second stage but would be unable to complete the third stage. The resulting analysis would indicate that she had a capacity of 7.2 METs when in fact she had a capacity between 7.2 and 10.2 METs. This incorrect analysis would occur because of the large area between the second and third stages in which the woman would fall in terms of her ability to work at a functional maximal capacity. For such a person, the Bruce Protocol should be adapted from increments of 3 METs to increments of 1-1 1/2 METs and from an initial capacity of 4.2 METs to 2 METs: These adaptations will likely produce more diagnostic and useful results.

The above example emphasizes the need to be aware of the many aspects of the individual's background in exercise habits before testing. In addition, careful quizzing of the participant will allow you to detect whether the exercise habits described are true. For example, you should question the information of an individual who claims to walk 4 mi in 25 minutes on a daily basis. A number of daily joggers would be happy to be doing 4 mi in 33 minutes after a number of years of jogging; to walk at that speed would put your respondent in the Olympics as a fairly competitive racewalker.

Careful quizzing of the subject to be tested also allows for selection of the appropriate testing modality. If the subject has arthritis of the hip, a leg injury, or some problem which makes weight-bearing exercise difficult, a weight-supported method, such as bicycle ergometer or arm cranking, is the modality of choice. If the purpose of the GXT is to set an exercise prescription, it is appropriate to know what activity the subject plans to do for the exercise program so that the modality of the test fits the prescribed exercise program. For example, if the person wants to swim for the exercise program, test him or her in a swimming flume or by using a tethered swimming protocol. Because few laboratories are equipped to do that type of protocol, the person writing the exercise prescription must determine the differences in stroke volume relative to upright versus supine exercise and adjust the prescription accordingly.

The more detailed the reasons are for selecting a modality and protocol, the more specific and exact will be the results. With careful attention to the above considerations, the physician and exercise prescriber may be able to have greater assurance of the quality and reliability of the prescription and results.

Test Modalities

Often laboratories are not equipped financially to have a large number of modalities to select from when conducting GXTs. If this situation is familiar to you, the following information might be helpful in selecting the appropriate ergometer for doing test procedures.

The bicycle ergometer has been the mode of choice in most European laboratories (Caso et al., 1979). It has the advantages of being easy to maneuver and relatively inexpensive, with a minimal upkeep. In addition, it is easy to calibrate, and there are a number of substantial studies to validate the results (Åstrand & Rodahl, 1977; Atterhog, Jonsson, & Samuelson, 1979). The patient's body weight is supported, blood pressures are more easily taken, and the test appears less threatening. The results produce a maximal O_2 uptake from 7-10% lower than the treadmill and slightly higher blood pressures (Shephard, 1966, 1971).

The treadmill also has advantages: It elicits a higher max $\dot{V}O_2$, uses a larger muscle mass, and is a weight-bearing test. The treadmill is considered a better test than the bicycle ergometer because it elicits higher max heart rates and higher power (Sydney & Shephard, 1977). Wicks, Sutton, Oldridge, & Jones, (1978) found that there were no differences between electrocardiograph (ECG) changes and rate pressure products (RPP), yet a slightly higher blood pressure and lower max heart rate were produced on tests done on the bicycle when compared to the treadmill.

The arm crank is a test that can be done when it is impossible for the person to ambulate or use the legs. Often in these cases the test is conducted to elicit cardiorespiratory responses that would indicate the absence or presence of disease, to establish a baseline from which an exercise prescription can be made, or to gain prognostic information. By hooking a person up to an ECG machine and stressing his or her heart, it is possible to look at those very parameters. Arm cranking can be accomplished by placing a bicycle ergometer on a table and having the person sit in a chair and pedal from behind with the arms. The workload can be increased by varying resistance and increasing the tension on the fly wheel; alternatively, a specific arm-crank ergometer may be purchased.

There is no reason why a stress test cannot be conducted using other modalities such as a rowing machine, Schwinn Air-Dyne, or other ergometer. As was indicated above, the essential pieces of information in a stress test are heart rate (HR), heart rhythm, blood pressure (BP), perceived exertion, chest pain, ST response, claudication, skin response, and other symptoms such as dizziness and shortness of breath. These parameters can be obtained by using a 12-lead ECG and putting the heart at stress with ergometers.

Treadmill Protocols

There are several questions to consider when choosing the appropriate protocol for a particular stress test (Sheffield & Roitman, 1976):

1. Is the test single work load, or is it multistaged with progressive work loads?
2. Is the work load preselected from beginning to end or is it determined relative to the response of the test-taker?
3. Is it an intermittent test (periods of work intervened with periods of rest) or a continuous test (work loads progress as in an intermittent test but with no rest periods)?
4. Is the test to be a submaximal effort (85% and below) or a maximal effort?

Single work load tests usually are not of sufficient power to elicit the heart rate, RPP, BP, and ECG changes that are desired to make the test of value diagnostically, prognostically, and prescriptively. In this case, if the work load is hard enough to elicit a response and it appears to be positive, is it possible to determine whether it is a true or false positive? Because the work load has to be difficult enough in a single work load test to elicit the response, adequate warm-up is not possible and a false positive test results. In contrast, a progressively increasing work load provides an adequate warm-up with a slow progression to maximal stress and often a reasonably slow increase in symptom severity.

The ability to change the work load during the course of the test, as opposed to the inflexibility of working with a preselected protocol, makes it possible to tailor the test to the needs and abilities of the test-taker. Quite often the test-taker's abilities are overestimated, which causes the individual to progress too rapidly. In this instance, switching to a lower level of advancement in the middle of the test might allow the person to achieve a higher rate of oxygen exchange. This is the disadvantage of some of the newer, highly computerized ECG machines from which information is lost when a change occurs from automatic to manual control of the treadmill's speed and grade.

Research has shown that the true estimation of maximal oxygen uptake is best achieved by using an intermittent protocol (Åstrand, 1960). However, in the interest of time, expense, personnel, equipment, and patient comfort, continuous testing is a more prudent choice. There is no evidence that there is a loss of diagnostic accuracy when using the continuous versus the intermittent protocol (Sheffield & Roitman, 1976).

Several studies have been done to identify the optimal protocol by comparing one protocol to another (Falls & Humphrey, 1973; Froelicher, Rammell, Davis, Stewart, & Lancaster, 1974; Pollock et al., 1976). Essentially all of the studies showed that the tests correlated highly with one another, there were no significant differences between estimations of maximal oxygen uptake from one protocol to the other, and no protocol could be singled out as producing significantly better results than the others. Table 13.2 is a compilation of guidelines for protocol selection from several studies and associations (American College of Sports Medicine [ACSM], 1980; Bruce, 1974). Following these guidelines will facilitate the process of eliciting a good test response.

Table 13.2   Guidelines for Construction of GXT Protocols

1. No special training or skill is required by the individual to be able to take the test.
2. Utilization of large muscle groups is required wtih the avoidance of isometric muscle contraction.
3. Progressive work should be utilized starting with submaximal work loads and continuing until fatigue or signs and symptoms that would terminate the test.
4. The test-taker should feel safe and unthreatened by the test.
5. The protocols should be multistaged.
6. The beginning load should be no greater than 3 METs.
7. The work load should gradually increase from 1 to 2 METs at each stage.
8. The length of time in each stage should be at least 1 min.

Sullivan and Froelicher (1983) state that the standard design of the GXT protocol is one of progressively increasing work until maximal effort is achieved. The time at each work load should be sufficient to reach a steady state in $\dot{V}O_2$ because estimations of $\dot{V}O_2$ are made from the steady state concepts. Margaria, Mangili, Luttica, and Ceretelli (1965) as well as diPrampero, Davies, Ceretelli, and Margaria (1970) have shown that steady state is achieved after approximately two minutes into the work load. A study by Whipp and Wasserman (1972) indicated that at higher work loads (moderately heavy to heavy), steady state $\dot{V}O_2$ can take as long as 4-10 min to be achieved. In this case if you were testing someone in the laboratory and kept advancing the protocol every 2 min, there is a strong likelihood that an overprediction of the actual MET capacity of the person would occur (Wasserman, VanKessel, & Burton, 1967).

Tables 13.3-13.9 are treadmill protocols in current use across the country. After interviewing the test-taker and determining the type of test to be done, you can choose the appropriate protocol from one that is already developed. Tables 13.10 and 13.11 are compilations of estimated MET costs for progressing speeds and elevations, which allow for the construction of an individualized protocol specific to the test-taker.

Table 13.3   The Modified Bruce and the Bruce Protocols

Stage	Speed (mph)	% Grade	Duration (min)	METs
0	1.7	0	3	1.7
1/2	1.7	5	3	2.9
1	1.7	10	3	4.7
2	2.5	12	3	7.1
3	3.4	14	3	10.2
4	4.2	16	3	13.5
5	5.0	18	3	17.3
6	5.5	20	3	24.6
7	6.0	22	3	28.4

Note. From ''Principles in Exercise Testing'' by R.A. Bruce, 1973, in J.P. Naughton and H.K. Hellerstein (Eds.), *Exercise Testing and Exercise Training in Coronary Heart Disease* (p. 45-61), New York: Academic Press. Copyright 1973 by Academic Press. Reprinted by permission.

Table 13.4   **Balke Standard Treadmill Test**

Stage	Speed (mph)	% Grade	Duration (min)	METs
1	3.0	2.5	2	4.3
2	3.0	5.0	2	5.4
3	3.0	7.5	2	6.4
4	3.0	10.0	2	7.4
5	3.0	12.5	2	8.5
6	3.0	15.0	2	9.5
7	3.0	17.5	2	10.5
8	3.0	20.0	2	11.6
9	3.0	22.5	2	12.6
10	3.0	25.0	2	13.6
11	3.0	27.5	2	14.7
12	3.0	30.0	2	15.7

Note. From "An Experimental Study of Physical Fitness of Air Force Personnel" by B. Balke and R.W. Ware, 1959, *U.S. Armed Forces Medical Journal*, **10**, pp. 675-688. Copyright 1959 by *U.S. Armed Forces Medical Journal*. Reprinted by permission.

Table 13.5   **Ellestad Treadmill Test**

Stage	Speed (mph)	% Grade	Duration (min)	METs
1	1.7	10	3	4.7
2	3	10	2	7.4
3	4	10	2	9.6
4	5	10	2	11.7
5	5	15	2	15.2
6	6	15	3	22.6

Note. From *Stress Testing: Principles and Practice* (p. 155) by M. H. Ellestad, 1980, Philadelphia: F.A. Davis. Copyright 1980 by F.A. Davis. Reprinted by permission.

Table 13.6   Kattus Treadmill Test

Stage	Speed (mph)	% Grade	Duration (min)	METs
1	1.5	10	3	4.2
2	2.0	10	3	5.3
3	2.5	10	3	6.4
4	3.0	10	3	7.4
5	3.5	10	3	8.5
6	4.0	10	3	9.6
7	4.0	14	3	11.8
8	4.0	18	3	14.0
9	4.0	22	3	16.2

Note. From "Physical Training and Beta Adrenergic Blocking Drugs in Modifying Coronary Insufficiency" by A.A. Kattus, 1967, in G. Marchetti and B. Toccardi (Eds.), *Coronary Circulation and Energetics of the Myocardium* (pp. 302-317), New York: Karger. Copyright 1967 by Karger. Reprinted by permission.

Table 13.7   Balke Substandard Treadmill Test

Stage	Speed (mph)	% Grade	Duration (min)	METs
1	2.0	0	2	2.5
2	2.0	2.5	2	3.2
3	2.0	5.0	2	3.9
4	2.0	7.5	2	4.6
5	2.0	10.0	2	5.3
6	2.0	12.5	2	6.0
7	2.0	15.0	2	6.7
8	2.0	17.5	2	7.4
9	2.0	20.0	2	8.1
10	2.0	22.5	2	8.7

Note. From "An Experimental Study of Physical Fitness of Air Force Personnel" by B. Balke and R.W. Ware, 1959, *U.S. Armed Forces Medical Journal, 10*, pp. 675-688. Copyright 1959 by *U.S. Armed Forces Medical Journal.* Reprinted by permission.

Table 13.8   Naughton Treadmill Test

Stage	Speed (mph)	% Grade	Duration (min)	METs
1	1.0	0	2	1.8
2	2.0	0	2	2.5
3	2.0	3.5	2	3.5
4	2.0	7.0	2	4.5
5	2.0	10.5	2	5.4
6	2.0	14.0	2	6.4
7	2.0	17.5	2	7.4

Note. From "Refinements in Methods of Evaluation and Physical Conditioning Before and After Myocardial Infarction" by J. B. Naughton, B. Balke, and F. Nagle, 1964, *American Journal of Cardiology,* **14**, p. 837. Copyright 1964 by *American Journal of Cardiology.* Reprinted by permission.

Table 13.9   Sivarjian Low-Level Treadmill Test

Stage	Speed (mph)	% Grade	Duration (min)	METs
1	1.2	0	3	2.1
2	1.2	3	3	2.4
3	1.2	6	3	2.7
4	2.0	3.5	3	3.5
5	2.0	7.0	3	4.5
6	2.0	10.5	3	5.4
7	2.5	12.0	3	6.4

Note. From "Progressive Ambulation and Treadmill Testing of Patients With Acute Myocardial Infarction During Hospitalization" by E.S. Sivarajan, J. Leerman, L.W. Mansfield, and R.A. Bruce, 1977, *Archives of Physical Medicine and Rehabilitation,* **58**, p. 241. Copyright 1977 by *Archives of Physical Medicine and Rehabilitation.* Reprinted by permission.

Table 13.10 Approximate Relative Energy Expenditures in METs During Walking Treadmill Tests

Grade %		Speed of Walking							
	km/h	2.7	3.2	4.0	4.8	5.5	5.6	6.4	6.8
	mph	1.7	2.0	2.5	3.0	3.4	3.5	4.0	4.2
0		1.7	2	2.5	3	3.4	3.5	4.6	5
2.5		2.3	2.7	3.3	4	4.5	4.7	6	6.5
5.0		2.9	3.4	4.2	5	5.7	5.9	7.3	7.9
7.5		3.4	4	5	6	6.9	7.1	8.7	9.3
10.0		4	4.7	5.9	7	8	8.3	10	10.8
12.0		4.5	5.3	6.6	7.9	9	9.2	11.1	11.9
12.5		4.6	5.4	6.8	8	9.2	9.5	11.4	12.2
14.0		4.9	5.8	7.3	8.7	10	10.2	12.2	13
15.0		5.2	6.1	7.6	9	10.3	10.7	12.8	13.6
16.0		5.4	6.4	8	9.5	10.8	11.1	13.3	14.2
17.5		5.8	6.8	8.5	10	11.5	11.8	14.1	15
20.0		6.3	7.5	9.3	11	12.7	13	15.5	16.5

Table 13.11 Approximate Relative Energy Expenditures in METs During Running Treadmill Tests

Grade %		9.7	11.3	12.9	14.5
	km/h	9.7	11.3	12.9	14.5
	mph	6.0	7.0	8.0	9.0
0		10	11.5	12.8	14.2
2.5		11.4	12.7	14.1	15.4
5.0		12.7	14	15.4	16.7
7.5		13.9	15.3	16.6	18
10.0		15.2	16.5	17.9	19.3
12.5		16.5	17.8	19.2	20.5

Note. A commonly-used test is to have the subject walk at 3 mph with 2.5% grade increments utilized each 2 min. To convert from mph to km/h, multiply by 1.6093.

Choosing the Protocol to Fit the Test

At the beginning of this chapter I provided a list of reasons why a test would be administered. The reasons are as numerous as the protocols that should be used to do the tests.

If tests are done for a single reason (e.g., diagnostic), without sideline requirements such as writing an exercise prescription, then the Bruce Protocol should be selected, which is the most time-efficient and easiest test to administer. If, besides diagnostic and prognostic information, an analysis of the person's functional capacity is desired, however, then thought should be given to designing a protocol that is appropriate to the individual test-taker, moves him or her through moderately progressing MET stages for each level (1–1-1/2 METs), and warms him or her up properly.

If the test is required for health risk screening purposes or as a diagnostic tool then a protocol that moves the person through stages of taxing effort, such as the Bruce Protocol, is the most appropriate. Table 13.3 presents a modification of the Bruce Protocol as well as the true Bruce Protocol, which does not start until Stage 1 is reached. This modification makes the protocol more applicable to those people in the population who are so deconditioned that to start them at Stage 1 would not give them an adequate warm-up. This reemphasizes the fact that an interview of the test-taker prior to the test is efficacious in selecting the appropriate starting point. A woman who jogs 3-4 mi per day, 5 days per week would be able to handle Stage 1 with no difficulty. For a man who has been sedentary for the past 15 years, holds an office job, is a two-pack-a-day smoker, and is 20 lb overweight, a more appropriate starting point would be at Stage 1/2.

If the test is required for assessment of functional aerobic capacity then careful consideration of the staging of the protocol must be given. Often my colleagues and I will combine two or three protocols in order to achieve one that will assess the aerobic capacity fairly accurately. For example, the same woman who jogs 3–4 mi per day, 5 days per week, will likely max at between 10 and 14 METs. Using the first three stages of the original (unmodified) Bruce would be appropriate. Using the regular Bruce with her, you would find that she would finish Stage 3 and not be able to complete Stage 4, which would functionally underassess her at 10.2 METs. Suppose that at Stage 4 the treadmill were increased to 4 mph and the grade decreased by 2 to 12% equalling an 11.1 MET work load. If the stage were completed then Stage 5 could be the return of the grade to 14% equalling 12.2 METs, thus allowing test-takers to progress more slowly as they approach their maximal ability. Because the assessment of aerobic capacity determines the type of exercise prescription, an underassessment would mean an underprescription, and progress in conditioning might be too slow, leading to frustration. In addition a functional protocol would probably be the one to choose for evaluating therapy because the objective of the evaluation is to determine at which level the therapy has enabled the person to function.

Detecting treatable arrhythmias would require a protocol that would put the myocardium at stress. In this case the Bruce Protocol or any progressive protocol would suffice because the test is easy to administer and of sufficient power to induce the arrhythmias.

The last reason for conducting a test is a relatively new use for a GXT in many laboratories across the nation. Although the use of the GXT at discharge or immediately after discharge from the hospital following an acute MI or coronary artery bypass surgery (CABS) is frightening to some medical professionals, evidence has shown that it is not only safe, with no increases in morbidity and mortality from the normal application of the GXT, but is also an excellent prognosticator of future events and an indicator of further interventional techniques (Debusk & Haskell, 1980a, 1980b; DeFeyter, Van Eenige, Machiel, Dignton, & Roos, 1983; Haskell & DeBusk, 1979; Madsen & Gilfin, 1983; Moss, 1983; Weld, 1985; Winer, 1983). Studies have varied showing different cutoff points, 3-5 METs, percentage of age predicted max HR, time, symptoms, to using a symptom-limited test. Starling, Crawford, and O'Rourke (1982) compared a discharge HR-limited and Symptom-Limited (SLM) Naughton test at a mean of 14 days post-MI to a SLM Naughton and regular Bruce 6 weeks later. There were no changes in morbidity or mortality in either testing situation. The SLM Naughton predicted significantly better than the HR-limited at discharge (21/29 vs. 12/29), and the Bruce predicted significantly better after 6 weeks than the Naughton (20/31 vs. 13/31). The study showed that the more difficult stress test gives a better prognostic effect with no greater risk. Included in the listing of GXT protocols are several that can be held to low MET values if you want to limit the exercise by heart rate or MET capacity. The Naughton and/or Bruce are provided if you choose to go with a symptom-limited test.

Bicycle Protocols

As noted above, bicycle tests have been the primary modality of choice in Europe. More recently the YMCA has developed protocols for men and women, which are used widely in the United States in the *Y's Way to Fitness* program (YMCA, 1982) (see Figures 13.1, 13.2, 13.3). The practical reasons for using the bicycle were enumerated earlier. Andersen, Shephard, Denolin, Varnauskas, & Masironi (1971) state that there are a number of physiological reasons for preferring the use of the bicycle ergometer to the treadmill.

1. There is less variability in physiological response.
2. The subject is in the same posture before, during, and after the test is done.
3. The bicycle is less alarming and gives a greater sense of security to the person being tested.
4. Minimum arm, torso, and total body movement makes data collection much easier.
5. The bicycle is quiet, small, and as a result produces a less stressful atmosphere for the patient.

There are two main types of bicycles, mechanical and electrical. The mechanical bicycle uses a friction force against the wheel developed either by an outside source (weighted belt) or within the wheel. The work performed is a product of the amount of force applied (kilograms) times the circumference of the wheel times the number of revolutions per minute. Electrically braked bicycles use a magnetic or electromagnetic field to provide the resistance against the wheel (Mellerowicz & Smodlaka, 1981).

The bicycle has developed into a variable modality because it allows tests to be given in three postures: standing and arm cranking, sitting and pedaling, and supine lying and pedaling. The most common form for regular exercise testing is the upright sitting position. However, as the use of radionucleid Technetium 99 studies becomes more prevalent, the supine pedaling test will become more popular.

Building a Bicycle Protocol

Essentially, a GXT done on a bicycle is a weight-supported stress test. Energy requirements are related not to the weight of the subject but to the amount of work required to move the wheel of the bicycle against a resistance. Energy requirements are also related to the spinning speed in revolutions per minute (RPM). There is a formula for the prediction of energy cost utilizing the bicycle ergometer manufactured by Monarch (ACSM, 1986).

kg of resistance × 6 m (circumference of the wheel) × RPM = kilogram-meters/minute.

Energy cost in mls/min = kg-m/min × 2 + 300.

Example: A 70-kg man rides at 80 RPM, 2.5 kg resistance.
    80 × 6 × 2.5 = 1200 kg-m/min
    1200 × 2 + 300 = 2,700 mls/min
    2,700 ÷ 70 = 38.6 mls/kb-min
    38.6 ÷ 3.5 (1 MET) = 11.0 METs

Table 13.12　Scale Settings and Work Loads for Monarch Bicycle (50 RPM)

Scale setting	kg-m/min	Scale setting	kg-m/min
.5 kg	150	4.0 kg	1200
1.0 kg	300	4.5 kg	1350
1.5 kg	450	5.0 kg	1500
2.0 kg	600	5.5 kg	1650
2.5 kg	750	6.0 kg	1800
3.0 kg	900	6.5 kg	1950
3.5 kg	1050	7.0 kg	2100

Table 13.13　Energy Costs for 70-Kg Person: 50 RPM

kg-m	mls/min	METs
150	600	2.5
300	900	3.7
450	1200	5.0
600	1500	6.0
750	1800	7.5
900	2100	8.5
1050	2400	10.0
1200	2700	11.0
1350	3000	12.0
1500	3300	13.5
1650	3600	14.5
1800	3900	16.0
1950	4200	17.0

Table 13.12 gives the scale settings and work loads found on the Monarch bicycle ergometer.

Table 13.13 gives the approximate energy costs for pedaling at 50 RPM by a 70-kg person.

It is possible to increase the work loads that are found in Table 13.13 by increasing or decreasing the spinning speed. This would either increase or decrease the energy cost. Generally an increase of 1/2 kg of resistance gives an increase of 1 MET.

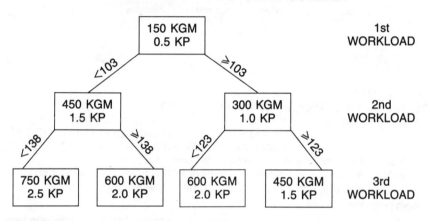

GUIDE TO SETTING WORKLOADS
FOR FEMALES ON THE BICYCLE ERGOMETER

DIRECTIONS
1. Set the first workload to 150 kgm/min (.5 KP).
2. If steady-state heart rate is < 103, set 2nd load at 450 kgm/min (1.5 KP).
   If steady-state heart rate is ≥ 103, set 2nd load at 300 kgm/min (1.0 KP).
3. Follow this same pattern for setting the third and final load.
4. NOTE: If the 1st workload elicits an HR of 110 or more, it is used on the graph, and only ONE more workout will be necessary.

FOOTNOTES
i. *The Y's Way to Physical Fitness* bicycle test is for healthy individuals who have been cleared by a physician to exercise. This test measures cardiorespiratory fitness and is *not* a medical screening test.
II. This aid to setting workloads is only a guide; common sense should also be used. Always be conservative. Use lower workloads for borderline scores.
III. The two plot points should be in the linear portion of the curve (approximately 100–150 bpm). It is better to have the two points toward the low end of this linearity.

Figure 13.1. *The Y's Way to Physical Fitness* guide to setting workloads for females on the bicycle ergometer.

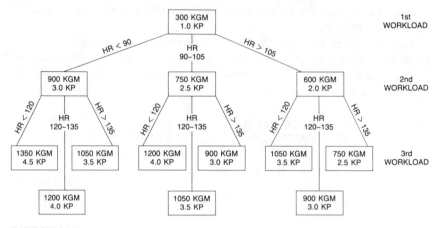

**GUIDE TO SETTING WORKLOADS
FOR MALES ON THE BICYCLE ERGOMETER**

DIRECTIONS
1. Set the 1st workload at 300 kgm/min (1.0 KP)
2. If HR in 3rd min is: Less than (<) 90, set 2nd load at 900 kgm (3 KP)
   Between 90 and 105, set 2nd load at 750 kgm (2.5 KP)
   Greater than (>) 105, set 2nd load at 600 kgm (2.0 KP)
3. Follow the same pattern for setting 3rd and final load.
4. NOTE: If the 1st workload elicits an HR of 110 or more, it is used on the graph, and only ONE more workload will be necessary.

FOOTNOTES
I. The *Y's Way to Physical Fitness* bicycle test is for healthy individuals who have been cleared by a physician to exercise. This test measures cardiorespiratory fitness and is *not* a medical screening test.
II. This aid to setting workloads is only a guide; common sense should also be used. Always be conservative. Use lower workloads for borderline scores.
III. The two plot points should be in the linear portion of the curve (approximately 10–150 bpm). It is better to have the two points toward the end of this linearity.

Figure 13.2. *The Y's Way to Physical Fitness* guide to setting workloads for males on the bicycle ergometer.

Another type of bicycle protocol was developed by the YMCA to test men and women. This protocol is supposedly a submaximal test; however, it has been my experience that very unfit men and women perceive the work load as an 18 or 19 on the Borg Scale when they are in the last work load (Borg, 1962), which is an indication of maximal work. It is possible that this is because a small mass of muscles is doing work with which it is unfamiliar and for which there has been no practice. The tests for men and women are designed as branching protocols. Thus advancements in work are done as a result of heart rate response to exercise; the lower the heart rate response, the larger the work load added in the next stage. These protocols may be done by recording heart rate and blood pressure only or by recording ECGs. After the data have been collected predictions of maximal capacity are made by doing appropriate calculations and graphing. Figures 13.1 and 13.2 depict the protocols and Figure 13.3 gives the graph and directions for doing the calculations necessary to make the prediction (YMCA, 1982). Table 13.14 presents a chart of energy expenditures in METs for various weights and work loads (ACSM, 1960).

If the bicycle is chosen as the modality to be used for the GXT, then the reasons for the test need to be examined, after which the protocol can be determined or even constructed to fit the person. Usually the stages of the protocols on a bicycle test are 3 min in duration.

Arm Ergometry

Occasionally in the exercise testing situation the patient is unable to walk on the treadmill or ride a bicycle due to arthritis, hip and/or knee replacements, paralysis, or other reasons. If this is the case it means neither that a test can't be given, nor that the individual is unable to exercise. Arm ergometry has been explored by a number of researchers and found to

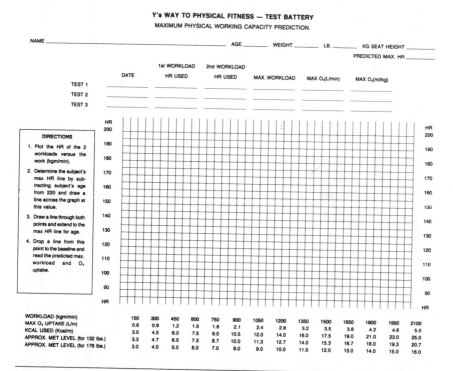

Figure 13.3. *The Y's Way to Physical Fitness test battery.*

Table 13.14 Energy Expenditure During Bicycle Ergometry Exercise

Body Weight		Work rate on bicycle ergometer (kg-m/min and watts)													
(kg)	(lb)	75	150	300	450	600	750	900	1050	1200	1350	1500	1650	1800	(kg-m/min)
		12	25	50	75	100	125	150	175	200	225	250	275	300	(watts)
20	44	4.0	6.0	10.0	14.0	18.0	22.0								
30	66	3.4	4.7	7.3	10.0	12.7	15.3	17.9	20.7	23.3					
40	88	3.0	4.0	6.0	8.0	10.0	12.0	14.0	16.0	18.0	20.0	22.0			
50	110	2.8	3.6	5.2	6.8	8.4	10.0	11.5	13.2	14.8	16.3	18.0	19.6	21.1	
60	132	2.7	3.3	4.7	6.0	7.3	8.7	10.0	11.3	12.7	14.0	15.3	16.7	18.0	
70	154	2.6	3.1	4.3	5.4	6.6	7.7	8.8	10.0	11.1	12.2	13.4	14.0	15.7	
80	176	2.5	3.0	4.0	5.0	6.0	7.0	8.0	9.0	10.0	11.0	12.0	13.0	14.0	
90	198	2.4	2.9	3.8	4.7	5.6	6.4	7.3	8.2	9.1	10.0	10.9	11.8	12.6	
100	220	2.4	2.8	3.6	4.4	5.2	6.0	6.8	7.6	8.4	9.2	10.0	10.8	11.6	
110	242	2.4	2.7	3.4	4.2	4.9	5.6	6.3	7.1	7.8	8.5	9.3	10.0	10.7	
120	264	2.3	2.7	3.3	4.0	4.7	5.3	6.0	6.7	7.3	8.0	8.7	9.3	10.0	

(example; body weight, 80 kg, 176 lb; work rate, 900 kb-m/min, 150 watts; energy expenditure, 8 METs [28.0 ml/kg-min as 1 MET = 3.5 ml/ kg-min])

Note. From "Guidelines for Exercise Testing and Prescription," ACSM, 1975, Philadelphia: Lea and Febiger. Copyright 1975 by Lea and Febiger. Reprinted by permission.

Table 13.15 Means and Standard Deviations of MET Levels During the Three Arm-Cranking Protocols

Workload (kpm)	3-min stages Mean S.D.		4-min stages Mean S.D.		5-min stages Mean S.D.	
90	2.99	.39	3.09	.39	2.93	.29
180	3.89	.53	3.93	.43	3.74	.37
270	4.71	.65	4.73	.55	4.65	.53
360	5.56	.70	5.76	.65	5.89	.89
450	6.86	1.21	6.97	.90	7.12	1.16

Note. From "MET Levels for Various Workloads Using the Arm Ergometer" by W. Boles and G. Porter, 1982, unpublished master's thesis (p. 33), University of Wisconsin-La Crosse.

be safe, usable, and predictive in terms of eliciting heart rate, blood pressure, and ECG responses (Schwade, Blomquist, & Shapiro, 1977; Shaw et al., 1974; Wahren & Bygolman, 1971). The difficulty is in evaluating the energy requirements or the cost of arm work. Boles and Porter (1982) produced a formula for predicting oxygen costs of arm cranking with the Monarch arm-crank ergometer.

$$\text{mls/kg/min} = \frac{\text{kg-meter} \times 2.9 + 510}{\text{Body weight}}$$

Included in Table 13.15 are relative MET costs for arm cranking at different work loads in 3-, 4-, & 5-min stages. Arm cranking will produce higher heart rates and blood pressures for the same work load as done on the treadmill. This is because of the smaller muscle mass. Also the rate of perceived exertion will be higher for arm work alone at the same work load. The work is perceived as more difficult because of the size of the muscle mass asked to do the work (Mostardi, Gandee, & Norris, 1981).

Conclusion

In this chapter, I have not attempted to demonstrate every possible protocol available, for there are many more than time or pages will allow. The main thrust of this chapter is to present the idea that creativity, specificity, and knowledge of the test-taker are required when devising the mode, protocol, and method for doing a graded exercise test. It would be necessary, if one were doing a research project, to maintain standardization and remove variability by either using the same protocol or matching energy costs for work loads as well as stage duration. The literature has shown that no one treadmill protocol is better than another for eliciting response, and that bicycle and arm ergometry are safe and valid modalities for the GXT.

References

American College of Sports Medicine. (1983). *Exercise specialist training notebook.* Indianapolis: Author.

American College of Sports Medicine. (1986). *Guidelines for graded exercise testing and exercise prescription.* Philadelphia: Lea and Febiger.

Andersen, K.L., Shephard, R.J., Denolin, H., Varnausakas, E., & Masironi, R. (1971). *Fundamentals of exercise testing.* Geneva: World Health Organization.

Åstrand, I. (1960). Aerobic work capacity in men and women with special reference to age. *Acta Physiologica Scandinavica* (Suppl. 169), 1-92.

Åstrand, P.O., & Rodahl, K. (1977). *Textbook of work physiology.* New York: McGraw-Hill.

Atterhog, J.H., Jonsson, B., & Samuelson, R. (1979). Exercise testing in Sweden: A survey of procedures. *Scandinavian Journal of Clinical Laboratory Investigations, 39,* 87-92.

Balke, B., & Ware, R.W. (1959). An experimental study of physical fitness of Air Force personnel. *U.S. Armed Forces Medical Journal, 10,* 675-688.

Boles, W., & Porter, G. (1982). *MET levels for various workloads using the arm ergometer.* Unpublished master's thesis, University of Wisconsin, La Crosse.

Borg, G.A.V. (1962). *Physical performance and perceived exertion.* Lund, Sweden: Gleerup.

Bruce, R.A. (1973). Principles of exercise testing. In J.P. Naughton & H.K. Hellerstein (Eds.), *Exercise testing and exercise training in coronary heart disease* (pp. 45-61). New York: Academic Press.

Bruce, R.A. (1974). Methods of exercise testing. *The American Journal of Cardiology, 33,* 715-720.

Bruce, R.A., Blackman, J.R., Jones, J.W., & Strait, G. (1963). Exercise testing in adult normal subjects and cardiac patients. *Pediatrics,* 742-756.

Caso, R., Greenberg, P.S., & Ellestad, M.H. (1979). Stress testing: New and established clinical concepts. *Primary Cardiology, 5,* 25-32.

DeBusk, R.F., & Haskell, W.L. (1980a). Heart-rate limited exercise testing soon after myocardial infarction. *Circulation, 61,* 738-743.

DeBusk, R.F., & Haskell, W.F. (1980b). Symptom limited versus heart rate limited exercise testing after myocardial infarction. *Circulation, 61,* 1179-1181.

DeFeyter, P.J., Van Eenige, M.J., Machiel, J., Dignton, D.H., & Roos, J.P. (1983). Exercise testing soon after myocardial infarction. *Chest,* **83,** 853-859.

diPrampero, P.E., Davies, C.T.M., Ceretelli, P., & Margaria, R. (1970). An analysis of O₂ debt contracted in submaximal exercise. *Journal of Applied Physiology,* **29,** 547-551.

Ellestad, M.H. (1980). *Stress testing: Principles and practice.* Philadelphia: F.A. Davis.

Falls, H.B., & Humphrey, D.L. (1973). A comparison of methods for evaluating maximal oxygen uptake from college women during treadmill walking. *Medicine and Science in Sports,* **5**(4), 239-241.

Froelicher, V.F., Rammell, H., Davis, G., Stewart, A., & Lancaster, M.C. (1974). A comparison of the reproducibility and physiologic response to three maximal treadmill exercise protocols. *Chest,* **68,** 331-336.

Haskell, W.L., & DeBusk, R.F. (1979). Cardiovascular responses to repeated treadmill testing soon after myocardial infarction. *Circulation,* **60,** 1247-1251.

Kattus, A.A. (1967). Physical training and beta adrenergic blocking drugs in modifying coronary insufficiency. In G. Marchetti and B. Toccardi (Eds.), *Coronary circulation and energetics of the myocardium* (pp. 302-317). New York: Karger.

Madsen, E.B., & Gilfin, E. (1983). How much prognostic information do exercise test data add to clinical data after acute myocardial infarction? *International Journal of Cardiology,* **4,** 15-27.

Margaria, R., Mangili, F., Luttica, F., & Ceretelli, P. (1965). The kinetics of oxygen consumption at the onset of muscular exercise in man. *Ergonomics,* **8,** 49-54.

Mellerowicz, H., & Smodlaka, V.N. (1981). *Ergometry, basics of medical exercise testing.* Baltimore: Urban and Schwarzenberg.

Moss, A.J. (1983). Prognosis after myocardial infarction. *American Journal of Cardiology,* **52,** 667-669.

Mostardi, R.A., Gandee, R.N., & Norris, W.A. (1981). Exercise training using arms and legs versus legs alone. *Archives of Physical Medicine and Rehabilitation,* **62,** 332-335.

Naughton, J.B., Balke, B., & Nagle, F. (1964). Refinements in methods of evaluation and physical conditioning before and after myocardial infarction. *American Journal of Cardiology,* **14,** 837-843.

Pollock, M.L., Bahannon, R.L., Cooper, K.H., Ayres, J.J., Ward, A., White, S.R., & Linnerud, A.C. (1976). A comparative analysis of four protocols for maximal treadmill stress testing. *American Heart Journal,* **92**(1), 39-46.

Schwade, J., Blomquist, C.G., & Shapiro, W. (1977). A comparison of the response to arm and leg work in patients with ischemic heart disease. *American Heart Journal,* **94,** 203-208.

Shaw, D.J., Crawford, M.H., Karliner, J.S., Dedonna, G., Carleton, R.M., Ross, J., & O'Rourke, R.A. (1974). Arm-crank ergometry: A new method for the evaluation of coronary artery disease. *American Journal of Cardiology,* **33,** 801-805.

Sheffield, L.T., & Roitman, D. (1976). Stress testing methodology. *Progress in Cardiovascular Disease,* **19,** 33-49.

Shephard, R.J. (1971). Standard tests of aerobic power. In R.J. Shephard (Ed.), *Frontiers of fitness.* Springfield, IL: Charles C Thomas.

Shephard, R.J. (1966). The relative merits of the step test, bicycle ergometer and treadmill in the assessment of cardio-respiratory fitness. *International Zeit Angew Physiolol,* **23,** 219-230.

Sivarajan, E.S., Lerman, J., Mansfield, L.N., & Bruce, R.A. (1977). Progressive ambulation and treadmill testing of patients with acute myocardial infarction during hospitalization. *Archives of Physical Medicine and Rehabilitation,* **58,** 241.

Starling, M.R., Crawford, M.H., & O'Rourke, R.A. (1982). Superiority of selected treadmill exercise protocols predischarge and six weeks post-infarction for detecting ischemic abnormalities. *American Heart Journal,* **104,** 1054-1060.

Sullivan, M., & Froelicher, V. (1983). Maximal oxygen uptake and gas exchange in coronary heart disease. *Journal of Cardiac Rehabilitation,* **3,** 549-560.

Sydney, K., & Shephard, R.J. (1977). Maximal and submaximal exercise tests in men and women in the seventh, eighth, and ninth decades of life. *Journal of Applied Physiology,* **43,** 280-287.

Wahren, J., & Bygdeman, S. (1971). Onset of angina pectoris in relation to circulatory adaptation during arm and leg exercise. *Circulation,* **44,** 432-441.

Wasserman, K., VanKessel, A.L., & Burton, G. (1967). Interaction of physiological mechanisms during exercise. *Journal of Applied Physiology,* **22,** 71-85.

Weld, F.M. (1985). Exercise testing early after myocardial infarction. *Journal of Cardiac Rehabilitation,* **5,** 20-27.

Whipp, B.J., & Wasserman, K. (1972). Oxygen uptake kinetics for various intensities of constant-load work. *Journal of Applied Physiology,* **33,** 351-356.

Wicks, J.R., Sutton, J.R., Oldridge, N.B., & Jones, N.L. (1978). Comparison of the electrocardiographic changes induced by maximum exercise testing with treadmill and cycle ergometer. *Circulation,* **57,** 1066-1070.

Winer, D. (1983). Prognostic value of exercise testing early after myocardial infarction. *Journal of Cardiac Rehabilitation,* **3,** 114-122.

YMCA. (1982). *Y's way to physical fitness: YMCA exercise testing manual.* Chicago: National Board of YMCA.

Chapter 14

Sudden Death and the GXT

Carl Foster

Graded exercise testing (GXT) is a technique of accepted value for the evaluation of patients with known or suspected cardiovascular disease. It represents the frontline, noninvasive technique for the evaluation of patients with exertional chest pain, is useful in the provocation of occult cardiovascular disease, and provides the objective basis for exercise prescription. Because one of the primary purposes of GXT is the provocation of abnormalities of cardiovascular physiology, the risk for life-threatening cardiovascular events is inherent to the technique. The purpose of this chapter is to define the acute risk of cardiovascular emergencies during GXT. In addition, the ability of the GXT to identify patients at high risk of death will be reviewed.

Acute Risk of GXT

Five contemporary clinical series have examined the acute risk of complications during GXT. Rochmis and Blackburn (1971) reported that GXT was associated with a mortality rate of 1 per 10,000. Nonfatal complications occurred at a rate of 2.4 per 10,000. The combined complication rate was about 4 per 10,000 tests. Mortality was unrelated to the type or severity of exercise. More recently Stuart and Ellestadt (1980) have demonstrated a mortality rate of 0.5 per 10,000. Serious, nonfatal complications occurred in 4.8 per 10,000 tests. The series reported by Irving and Bruce (1977) contained no fatal events. Serious, nonfatal complications occurred in 4.8 per 10,000 tests. The series reported by Irving and Bruce (1977) contained no fatal events. Serious, nonfatal complications were observed at a rate of 6 per 10,000 tests. Kaltenbach, Scherer, and Dowinsky (1982) reported a fatal complication rate of only 0.24 per 10,000 tests. Nonfatal complications occurred in 1.2 per 10,000 tests. Tests conducted with apparently healthy individuals have a much lower incidence of complications. Kaltenbach et al. (1982) observed no serious complications among 353,638 tests performed by apparently healthy young athletes. Gibbons, Meyer, Pollock, and Cooper (1981) observed only one complication, a nonfatal, subendocardial myocardial infarction, in 7,057 maximal tests in a group of essentially healthy middle-aged men. In contrast to American studies, which primarily utilize treadmill testing, the series by Kaltenbach et al. (1982) reported on studies primarily using bicycle ergometry or arm-assisted step testing. They reported a much higher rate of pulmonary edema following supine bicycle exercise as opposed to upright bicycle ergometry. In agreement with the findings of Rochmis and Blackburn (1971), Kaltenbach et al. (1982) observed no increase in complications when GXT was maximal as opposed to submaximal. The apparently declining complication rate during exercise testing from the early report of Rochmis and Blackburn to the recent report by Kaltenbach et al. may be attributed to better recognition of contraindications for exercise testing, improved monitoring capabilities, a better understanding of basic exercise physiology, and improved resuscitation methods. In summary, the risk of fatal complications during GXT ranges from 0.24 to 1 per 10,000 tests. They are apparently not more common during maximal versus submaximal testing. Nonfatal complications may be expected to occur at a rate ranging from 0.7 to 6 per 10,000 tests.

Identification of High-Risk Patients

As demonstrated, the acute risk of morbidity/mortality during GXT is very low. GXT may be very useful, however, in the identification of patients at high risk for future clinical episodes. Bruce, DeRouen, and Blake (1977) demonstrated that the rate of sudden death among 10,000 asymptomatic men is 0.05% per year. Patients with positive GXT had a rate of primary cardiovascular events seven times that observed in patients with a negative stress test. More recently, Bruce, Hossack, De Rouen, and Hofen (1983) reported on the results of 10 years' experience with the Seattle Heart Watch. They demonstrated that the combination of any one conventional risk factor plus a positive GXT was much more predictive of future clinical events than positive GXT observed in patients without primary risk factors. This suggests a potentially cost-effective approach to the application of GXT in asymptomatic individuals, which will allow identification of high-risk patients. The findings of Bruce et al. (1983) are in basic agreement with the suggestion of Uhl and Froelicher (1983) that GXT should only be undertaken in asymptomatic individuals when risk factor analysis indicates a 5- to 6-year risk for primary cardiovascular events in excess of 5%.

In patients with known cardiovascular disease GXT results may be very powerful relative to identifying patients at high risk for further clinical episodes and may serve to identify patients needing coronary arteriography and surgical management. McNeer et al. (1978) have demonstrated that survival in medically treated patients with coronary artery disease is strongly related to a variety of exercise predictors including exercise tolerance and maximum heart rate attained. Patients with a positive test and an exercise duration of less than 6 min on the Bruce protocol had a 4-year survival rate of only 60% as compared to 95% in patients with a negative test and exercise duration greater than 9 min or a maximum heart rate in excess of 160 bpm. In patients with a strongly positive exercise electrogram (Dagenais, Ronleau, Christen, & Fabia, 1982; Podrid, Graboy, & Lown, 1981) survival is highly related to exercise tolerance. Patients attaining Stage 4 of the Bruce Protocol have excellent survival even in the presence of greater than 2 mm ST depression. In patients with very low exercise tolerance sudden death is the usual cause of the mortal event. Weiner (1981) has demonstrated that a markedly positive GXT including 2 mm ST depression beginning in Stage 1, lasting 6 min into recovery and occurring in at least five leads, had a 74% predictive value for either left main or three vessel disease. Blumenthal, Weiss, Mellits, and Gerstenblith (1981) have shown that the GXT could predict left main coronary artery disease even in asymptomatic patients. GXT results including (a) early ST changes, (b) < 2 mm ST depression, (c) downsloping ST depression, (d) exercise-induced hypotension, (e) prolonged ST changes during recovery, and f) multiple areas of ST depression occurring in concert were highly predictive of left main coronary artery disease. Gibbons et al. (1981) reported that ECG abnormalities occurring early in patients incapable of achieving at least 85% of the age predicted maximum heart rate had a much less favorable prognosis than individuals with either normal tests or late abnormalities.

The prognostic significance of GXT soon after myocardial infarction is well established (Sami, Kraemer, & DeBusk, 1979; Theroux, Waters, Halphen, Debaiseux, & Mizgala, 1979). Patients with ST depression at hospital discharge have a mortality rate 13 times greater during the first postinfarction year than those without ST changes (Theroux et al., 1979). Exercise-induced ischemia 3 weeks after myocardial infarction predicts early fatal events, whereas ventricular arrhythmia on serial testing predicts late nonfatal events (Sami, Kraemer, & DeBusk, 1979). Exercise-induced dysrhythmias are predictive of future clinical events, particularly when they are associated with ST-segment depression (Udall & Ellestad, 1977). Patients with the combination of ST depression and exercise-induced dysrhythmias had an annual incidence rate seven times higher than patients without ischemic changes or dysrhythmias. Exercise-induced dys-rhythmias may also serve as a marker for patients with multivessel coronary artery disease (Goldschlager, Cake, & Cohn, 1973).

GXT may also identify patients at risk for fatal or nonfatal events during exercise training. Several studies have reported on cardiovascular compli-cations during exercise-based rehabilitation programs (Haskell, 1978; Hossack & Hartwig, 1982; Mead, Pyfer, Trembold, & Frederick, 1976). The overall complication rate for a multicenter survey was one nonfatal event for every 34,673 participant-hr and one fatal event for every 116,402 participant-hr. Complications were lower in programs that continuously monitored the ECG during exercise and were markedly lower if the pre-1970 experience was excluded. Significant cardiovascular complica-tions have been shown to be associated with violation of target heart guidelines (Hossack, 1982; Mead et al., 1976), particularly in patients with evidence of exercise-induced myocardial ischemia (Hossack, 1982).

In summary abnormal GXT results have been shown to be powerful predictors of patients who are at risk for clinically significant endpoints including death. In patients with exercise-induced myocardial ischemia, survival is strongly related to effort tolerance and to the presence/absence of ventricular dysrhythmias. Following acute myocardial infarction, ST-segment depression is significantly predictive of future angina, recurrent myocardial infarction, and death. During exercise programs the likelihood of significant complications is related to the violation of heart rate limits designed to protect against exercising with an ischemic myocardium.

Practical Implications

As demonstrated GXT may significantly predict future clinical events at a very low acute risk. Because the acute risk of exercise testing is apparently not increased during maximal testing (Kaltenbach et al., 1982; Rochmis & Blackburn, 1971) and because the yield of exercise testing is significantly enhanced by maximal testing (Cumming, 1972; Gibbons et al., 1981; Starling, Crawford, & O'Rourke, 1982), the logic for maximal testing is clear. Stated differently, one of the goals of exercise testing should be to make every effort to provoke abnormalities inducible by exercise. The risk of dealing with an acute emergency in a well-equipped laboratory must be considerably less than giving the patient a false sense of security by conservative testing, particularly given the increased difficulty in deal-ing with emergencies in the gymnasium. This may be particularly perti-nent today in prevention programs. Given the wide use of beta adrenergic blocking agents, the prevalence of surgically treated patients, and the extensive use of monitoring in contemporary cardiac rehabilitation programs, the likelihood of exercising a patient with an ischemic myocardium must be lower than that when complication rates in rehabilitation programs were surveyed 5 years ago (Haskell, 1978). However, many adult fitness programs do not routinely use GXT prior to entry, even in participants with identifiable primary risk factors. Given the danger of exercising with ischemia (Hossack & Hartwig, 1982), the potential for significant complications in these programs must be considerable. The safety of exercise programs with prior exercise testing has been demonstrated (Gibbons, Cooper, & Meyer, 1979). Because both Bruce et al. (1983) and Uhl and Froelicher (1983) have demonstrated the increased yield of exercise testing in asymptomatic individuals with primary risk factors, it seems reasonable to suggest preliminary exercise testing for these patients as a cost-effective technique for improving the safety of preventive exercise programs. In view of observations by several investigators that patients at high risk for subsequent clinical episodes may be identified by a constellation of abnormal findings rather than by the mere presence/absence of ST-segment changes, the desirability of a multifaceted approach to the interpretation of GXT is clear. Such utilization of GXT results should allow for more aggressive medical and surgical therapy of patients with cardiovascular disease and serve to reduce mortality.

References

Blumenthal, D.S., Weiss, J.L., Mellits, E.D., & Gerstenblith, G. (1981). The predictive value of a strongly positive stress test in patients with minimal symptoms. *American Journal of Medicine, 70*, 1005-1010.

Bruce, R.A., De Rouen, T.A., & Blake, B. (1977). Maximal exercise predictors of coronary heart disease events among asymptomatic men in Seattle Heart Watch. *Circulation, 56* (Suppl.), 111-115.

Bruce, R.A., Hossack, K.F., De Rouen, T.A., & Hofen, V. (1983). Enhanced risk assessment for primary heart disease events by maximal exercise testing: 10 years experience of Seattle Heart Watch. *Journal of the American College of Cardiology, 2*, 565-573.

Cumming, G.R. (1972). Yield of ischemic exercise electrocardiograms in relation to exercise intensity in a normal population. *British Heart Journal, 34*, 919-923.

Dagenais, G.R., Ronleau, J.R., Christen, A., & Fabia, J. (1982). Survival of patients with a strongly positive electrocardiogram. *Circulation, 65*, 452-456.

Gibbons, L., Cooper, K., & Meyer, B. (1979). The acute risk of strenuous exercise. *Medicine and Science in Sports, 11*, 111.

Gibbons, L., Meyer, B.M., Pollock, M.L., & Cooper, K.H. (1981). The value of maximal versus submaximal treadmill testing. *Journal of Cardiac Rehabilitation*, 1, 362-368.

Goldchlager, N., Cake, D., & Cohn, K. (1973). Exercise induced ventricular arrhythmias in patients with coronary artery disease. *American Journal of Cardiology*, 31, 434-444.

Haskell, W.L. (1978). Cardiovascular complications during exercise training of cardiac patients. *Circulation*, 57, 920-924.

Hossack, K.F., & Hartwig, R. (1982). Cardiac arrest associated with supervised cardiac rehabilitation. *Journal of Cardiac Rehabilitation*, 2, 402-408.

Irving, J.B., & Bruce, R.A. (1977). Exertional hypotension and post-exertional ventricular fibrillation in stress testing. *American Journal of Cardiology*, 39, 849-851.

Kaltenbach, M., Scherer, D., & Dowinsky, S. (1982). Complications of exercise testing: A survey of three German-speaking countries. *European Heart Journal*, 3, 199-202.

McNeer, J.F., Margolis, J.R., Lee, K.L., Kisslo, J.A., Peter, R.H., Kong, Y., Behan, V.S., Wallace, A.G., McCants, C.B., & Rosati, R.A. (1978). The role of the exercise test in the evaluation of patients for ischemic heart disease. *Circulation*, 57, 64-70.

Mead, W.F., Pyfer, H.R., Trombold, J.C., & Fredrick, R.C. (1976). Successful resuscitation of two near simultaneous cases of cardiac arrest with a review of fifteen cases occurring during supervised exercise. *Circulation*, 53, 187-189.

Podrid, P.H., Graboy, T.B., & Lown, B. (1981). Prognosis of medically treated patients with coronary artery disease with profound ST segment depression during exercise testing. *New England Journal of Medicine*, 305, 1111-1116.

Rochmis, P., & Blackburn, H. (1971). Exercise tests: A survey of procedures, safety and litigation experiences in approximately 170,000 tests. *Journal of the American Medical Association*, 217, 1061-1066.

Sami, M., Kraemer, H., & DeBusk, R.F. (1979). The prognostic significance of serial exercise testing after myocardial infarction. *Circulation*, 60, 1238-1246.

Starling, M.R., Crawford, M.H., & O'Rourke, R.A. (1982). Superiority of selected treadmill exercise protocols predischarge and six weeks post infarction for detecting ischemic abnormalities. *American Heart Journal*, 104, 1054-1060.

Stuart, R., & Ellestad, M. (1980). National survey of exercise stress testing facilities. *Chest*, 77, 94-97.

Theroux, P., Waters, D.D., Halphen, C., Debaiseux, J.C., & Mizgala, H.F. (1979). Prognostic value of exercise testing soon after myocardial infarction. *New England Journal of Medicine*, 301, 341-345.

Udall, J.A., & Ellestad, M.H. (1977). Predictive implications of ventricular premature contractions associated with treadmill stress testing. *Circulation, 56*, 985-989.

Uhl, G.S., & Froelicher, V.F. (1983). Screening for asymptomatic coronary artery disease. *Journal of the American College of Cardiology, 1*, 946-955.

Weiner, D.A. (1981). Exercise testing for the diagnosis and severity of coronary disease. *Journal of Cardiac Rehabilitation, 1*, 438-444.

Chapter 15

Diagnostic, Discharge, and Symptom-Limited GXTs: Why, When, and How in the Rehabilitation Continuum

Glen H. Porter

Graded exercise testing (GXT) continues to be one of the most valuable noninvasive studies available to the physician in evaluating the presence and/or severity of coronary artery disease (CAD). In most cases the data obtained from the GXT outperform the clinical assessment obtained in the more traditional manner (Froelicher, 1983). The possible clinical applications of GXT include the following:

- Diagnose atypical chest pain
- Determine severity of coronary artery disease
- Determine prognosis
- Screen for latent coronary artery disease in asymptomatic patients
- Detect treatable exercise-induced dysrhythmias
- Aid in the management of the early recovery period from acute cardiac events
- Evaluate the intervention therapy (medical, surgical, percutaneious transluminal coronary angioplasty)
- Determine functional aerobic capacity
- Aid in writing an individualized exercise prescription that can guide rehabilitation efforts

Depending upon its specific purpose, the GXT can be further classified into one of the following three types: (a) a diagnostic GXT (DGXT), (b) a low-level graded exercise test completed prior to hospital discharge (LL-GXT), or (c) a symptom-limited functional capacity graded exercise test (FGXT).

Diagnostic Graded Exercise Testing

The usefulness of the DGXT continues to be hotly debated because of the less than perfect sensitivity and specificity of the test (Froelicher, 1983). Chapter 16 by Murphy in this text discusses in greater detail this specific problem and points out how the use of Bayes' Theorem of Probability can be beneficial in making appropriate probability statements about the presence of CAD based on the GXT data. The DGXT has the following purposes (Sketch & Aronow, 1983): (a) to estimate the probability of significant CAD, (b) to estimate the degree of severity of CAD or specifically estimate the number of coronary vessels involved, and (c) to estimate the risk of future morbidity and mortality as a result of having CAD. Stone (1983) pointed out that the greatest value of the DGXT may be in predicting the severity of the CAD and thus estimating the subsequent prognosis of patients with suspected CAD. The DGXT data can separate patients into groups of high and low risk. Members of the high-risk group become candidates for further noninvasive (i.e., radionuclide) GXTs or invasive coronary arteriography.

Because of the wealth of data that has been collected by Bruce and his colleagues using the Bruce GXT Protocol, the Bruce Protocol continues to be the most often utilized DGXT procedure (Bruce, Kusumi, & Hosmer, 1973). The great majority of studies completed by other investigators have interpreted their data on the basis of the responses to particular stages of the Bruce Treadmill Protocol. Some have modified the original protocol by adding an early stage or changing the later stages slightly to accommodate an older or orthopedically limited population. Others have used their own personal protocols, but most personal modifications have striking similarities (Froelicher, 1983).

The DGXT is useful in the diagnosis of CAD because patients begin to develop abnormal responses to progressively increasing work demands placed upon the myocardium (Goldschlager, Selzer, & Cohn, 1976). These abnormal responses can be interpreted as an ischemic myocardial response and thus CAD can be inferred if other possible causes of myocardial ischemia have been eliminated by clinical study. The most important indicators of an ischemic myocardial response are (a) electrocardiographic changes, (b) hemodynamic changes, and (c) the onset of symptoms. Table 15.1 presents these common abnormal responses in more detail.

Table 15.1 Abnormal Responses to Graded Exercise Testing

Electrocardiographic
  ST-segment changes
    Time of onset
    Magnitude of ST-segment change
    Configuration of ST-segment change
    Duration of ST-segment change
  Exercise-induced arrhythmias
    Atrial
    Ventricular
    A-V block
Hemodynamic
  Heart rate
    Excessive tachycardia
    Bradycardia
    Failure of heart rate to increase
  Blood pressure
    Failure of systolic blood pressure to increase
    Progressive decline in systolic blood pressure
Symptomatic
  Angina pectoris
  Inappropriate dyspnea
  Claudication-type pain
  Signs
    Cyanosis, pallor
    Cold sweats
    Gallop heart sounds

The current state-of-the-art interpretation of DGXT data requires that not only the electrocardiographic ST-segment displacement be used to interpret the presence and/or severity of the CAD, but that the several variables be combined and used collectively to make a sound probability statement about the likelihood of existing CAD (Porter & Allen, 1981). The interpretation and statement must be made in light of knowing the history and clinical data of a particular patient. With these approaches, patients can be separated into high- and low-risk groups (Froelicher, 1983; McNeer, et al., 1978). For example, McNeer and colleagues (1978) at Duke University followed two groups of patients separated into a high- and low-risk group for a 4-year period. The high-risk group had a 35% mortality in 4 years whereas the low-risk group had a 4% mortality in the same 4-year period. On the DGXT the high-risk group had ST-segment depression and an exercise duration of less than Stage 2 (about 6.6 METs) on the standard Bruce Protocol. The low-risk group had no ST-segment change, an exercise duration of Bruce Stage 4 or greater, or a maximal heart rate of 160 bpm or greater.

Who should receive a DGXT is an important question to ask. Economics, feasibility, and manpower considerations do not allow for the testing of the masses of asymptomatic people. Froelicher (1983) recommended that patients with one or more of the following risk factors are the best candidates: (a) family history of CAD, (b) hypertension, (c) smoking history, and (d) hypercholesterolemia. In addition, the patient with atypical chest discomfort is a desirable candidate for GXT.

Graded Exercise Testing in the Rehabilitation Continuum

In the patient types just mentioned, the DGXT often gets the patient into the rehabilitation process because an abnormal GXT culminates with subsequent coronary artery bypass surgery (CABGS) or percutaneous transluminal coronary angioplasty (PTCA). In addition the patient who has suffered a myocardial infarction (MI) as a first symptom or has had the MI before other invasive intervention was accomplished becomes part of the rehabilitation process. The GXT is an important part of the overall cardiac rehabilitation process for several reasons, which will be discussed below in some detail. Figure 15.1 presents the placement of GXTs in the cardiac rehabilitation continuum as we see the overall program using the typical Phase I, II, III, and IV nomenclature. Indicated at about 2 weeks following an acute hospitalization is the LL-GXT completed prior to hospital discharge. Currently in the CABGS patient, this LL-GXT may be completed as early as 6–7 days postsurgery, and 1–2 days following PTCA. Symptom-limited functional capacity GXTs occur at 10 and 22 weeks (Figure 15.1). This type of GXT may be repeated at 6-month to yearly intervals in the Phase III and IV rehabilitation program.

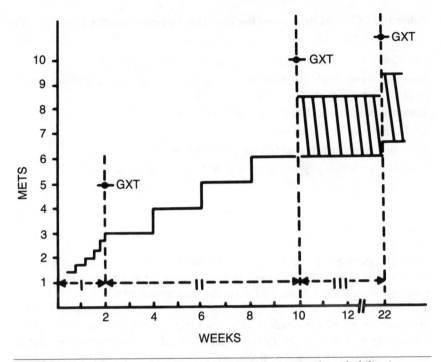

Figure 15.1. The placement of graded exercise tests in the rehabilitation continuum. This is an example of the exercise intensity prescription over the phases of cardiac rehabilitation. I = Phase I time frame, II = Phase II time frame, and III = Phase III time frame. The shaded area in the Phase III time frame represents an exercise intensity of 60–85% functional MET capacity. *Note.* From "General Concepts and a Specific Approach to Phase II Exercise Programming" by G.H. Porter, 1984, in L.K. Hall, G.C. Meyer, and H.K. Hellerstein (Eds.), *Cardiac Rehabilitation: Exercise Testing and Prescription* (p. 205), New York: SP Medical and Scientific Books.

Low-Level Graded Exercise Testing

The LL-GXT, completed before hospital dismissal, has several clinical benefits (see Table 15.2). As Froelicher (1983) pointed out, the LL-GXT can be the first step in the cardiac rehabilitation process. The LL-GXT can be therapeutic in itself: The test can lead to an increase in activity at home and a self-rehabilitation program after the patient is encouraged and reassured by completion of the LL-GXT.

Table 15.2   Clinical Benefits of the Low-Level Graded Exercise Test (LL-GXT)

Provides a more precise definition of safely tolerated activity

Identifies those capable of more rapid progress and those needing closer surveillance and/or a modified rehabilitation program

Provides prognosis (identifies residual ischemia)

Elicits treatable abnormalities

Identifies those needing additional medical therapy

Provides a positive psychological benefit to the patient and family

---

For the post-MI group the LL-GXT has been shown to be a safe procedure and it does provide good prognostic information. In general, ST-segment displacement, angina pectoris, a drop in systolic blood pressure, and/or poor exercise duration during the LL-GXT are strong indicators of a poor prognostic outlook (Madsen & Gilpin, 1983; Weiner, 1983; Weld, Chu, Bigger, & Rolnitzky, 1981). Exercise duration in most studies stands out as a powerful indicator probably because of its close relationship to the onset of left ventricular failure with progressive, low-level exercise (Weld et al., 1981). Weiner's (1983) summary article of five studies dealing with the MI population supports the above statements. Weiner and colleagues, by combining the data of five studies, followed a population of 881 patients for an average of 15 months. ST-segment displacement on the LL-GXT separated out a high-risk group that had a 10% risk of death versus only 4% for the group with no ST-segment displacement. These investigators found that the total treadmill time was also a very important predictor of subsequent coronary events. The inability to maintain an appropriately increasing systolic blood pressure response was also a significant predictor of subsequent high risk. The onset of angina pectoris and exercise-induced arrhythmias was not as helpful because the reproducibility of these findings were often poor. The onset of angina pectoris with the LL-GXT did correlate with angina pain at home and therefore the finding was important in terms of possible medication changes, which should be made following the LL-GXT.

The usefulness of the LL-GXT in CABGS patient groups has been studied a good deal less. Data are really not available to indicate that the LL-GXT completed prior to hospital discharge provides good prognostic information. The other clinical benefits (Table 15.2) and the safety aspects of the LL-GXT in this specific group have been documented (Hartman, Bartel, Call, McCracken, & Burroughs, 1981; Rod, Squires, Pollock, Foster, & Schmidt, 1982). Rod and colleagues (1982) studied 86 patients with GXT about 11 days post-CABGS. The GXT procedure was referred to as a symptom-limited test, but the average exercise capacity attained was 4 to 5 METs. Fatigue was the major reason for test termination (88% of the patients). Seven percent of the GXTs were terminated because of failure of the systolic blood pressure to increase, and 9% were terminated because of ventricular couplets. Rod et al. (1982) found considerably fewer problems in the CABGS group than in the MI group. There was a lack of ST-segment depression and angina pectoris. They concluded that the LL-GXT performed during this time frame was of little value for predicting residual ischemia and bypass graft patency. Hartman et al. (1981) using an LL-GXT performed 3–4 weeks after CABGS, again found no serious complications. They did report that 9% of the patients had ST-segment displacement. Based on their test results, Hartman et al. (1981) stated that 33% of the patients needed medical therapy alterations. The long-term meaning and impact of these alterations in therapy are not known.

Most CABGS patients currently remain in the hospital only 7 to 10 days, and the LL-GXTs are completed at the end of approximately 1 week. Our experience with this approach the past 3 to 4 years has been that the LL-GXT can be completed safely and does provide the above-stated clinical benefits.

The PTCA patients present a very new group of patients, and data on them are only now being accumulated and interpreted. These patients are completing an LL-GXT the day after PTCA in some cases. Those having PTCA performed from a femoral approach are generally held for an additional day before the LL-GXT is done. In our opinion the data obtained are again beneficial for the reasons previously stated (see Table 15.2). Prognostic information provided by the LL-GXT at this time frame in this population is not clear.

Regardless of the specific population being tested prior to hospital discharge, the test protocols being used are modifications of the Bruce or Naughton Protocols (Naughton & Haider, 1973; Sivarajan, Lerman, Mansfield, & Bruce, 1977). This means that the initial starting MET level is usually 1.5–2.0 METs, and the incremental increase per stage is 0.5–1.0 MET. Although some investigators are using so-called symptom-limited GXTs, most physicians in the clinical setting are still using an endpoint of 5.0–6.0 METs if significant signs/symptoms do not occur first. A priori absolute heart rate cutoff endpoints do not seem appropriate. An endpoint to volitional fatigue, if signs/symptoms are lacking, seems safe and appropriate.

Symptom-Limited Functional Capacity Graded Exercise Test

The symptom-limited functional capacity GXT, completed 4–8 weeks post-hospital discharge and then again as a periodic follow-up, provides a number of possible benefits (see Table 15.3). At a time when the patient is in a state of better physical condition, and when the myocardium can be safely pushed to more traditional maximal limits, the FGXT gives a good indication of a patient's functional status postrecovery and post-intervention. A good estimate of the amount of myocardium in jeopardy, if any, can be made. An indication of the myocardial reserve is possible. In this regard, exercise radionuclide thallium and ventriculography studies may be very helpful (Froelicher, 1983).

Again, exercise duration before signs/symptoms and the systolic blood pressure response to the GXT provide valuable information about left ventricular function and performance (Bruce et al., 1977). An important consideration to be made concerns the use of medications by the patients completing this FGXT. In cases where the specific purpose is to get prognostic information and to follow the disease progression, it may be necessary to have particular medications discontinued before the FGXT (Froelicher, 1983).

The FGXT can be particularly useful in making comparisons pre- and post-therapeutic intervention. For example, if a GXT was completed before antianginal medication or before CABGS, the FGXT completed after intervention can give data to document any changes that resulted. Particularly important is the comparison of the following: functional capacity (MET capacity), functional aerobic impairment (Bruce, 1973), and the rate pressure product (heart rate times systolic blood pressure) at angina pectoris.

Table 15.3   Benefits of Symptom-Limited Functional Capacity Graded Exercise Testing (FGXT)

Provides an extension of the physical examination

Provides prognosis (may be the best time to determine long-term prognosis)

Helps make decisions about returning patient to work

Provides clearance for recreational activities

Provides psychological benefit for patient and family

Documents the training effect

Provides the data to rewrite an appropriate exercise prescription

Provides data to follow the progression (regression ?) of the disease process with serial testing

---

As with the DGXTs, many physicians use the Bruce GXT Protocol for this functional evaluation. The protocol is adequate for this purpose. It is my opinion that a more slowly progressing protocol like a Naughton, Balke, or Naughton-Balke combination (Naughton & Haider, 1973) is better suited for the functional evaluation. The purpose of the FGXT is to get a good estimation of functional capacity and plot a slow, smooth progression of the heart rate and blood pressure responses throughout the range from low-level to volitional maximal exercise tolerance. This is important if the data are to be used in the activity prescription as well as for prognostic indications. Sometimes a large MET increment from stage to stage does not really allow the patient to terminate the GXT at an endpoint representative of his or her more realistic functional limitation.

Summary

When used appropriately, the GXT is a useful tool and is a significant part of the cardiac rehabilitation process. The GXT must be used for specific purposes within particular time frames. Appropriate interpretation of the GXT data necessitates knowing the particular patient and also utilizing all of the obtained data with a multifactorial approach.

References

Bruce, R.A. (1973). Principles of exercise testing. In J.P. Naughton & H.K. Hellerstein (Eds.), *Exercise testing and training in coronary heart disease* (pp. 45-61). New York: Academic Press.

Bruce, R.A., Kusumi, F., & Hosmer, O. (1973). Maximal oxygen intake and nomographic assessment of functional aerobic impairment. *American Heart Journal*, **85**, 546-562.

Bruce, R.A., DeRouen, T., Peterson, D.R., Irving, J.B., Chinn, N., Blake, B., & Hofer, V. (1977). Noninvasive predictors of sudden cardiac death in men with coronary disease: Predictive value of maximal stress testing. *American Journal of Cardiology*, **39**, 833-840.

Froelicher, V.F. (1983). *Exercise testing and training*. New York: Le Jacq.

Goldschlager, N., Selzer, A., & Cohn, K. (1976). Treadmill stress test as indicator of presence and severity of coronary artery disease. *Annals Internal Medicine*, **85**, 277-286.

Hartman, C.W., Bartel, A.G., Call, T.D., McCracken, J., & Burroughs, R. (1981). The safety and value of exercise testing soon after coronary artery bypass surgery. *Journal of Cardiac Rehabilitation*, **1**, 142-144.

Madsen, E.B., & Gilpin, E. (1983). Prognostic value of exercise test variables after myocardial infarction. *Journal of Cardiac Rehabilitation, 3*, 481-488.

McNeer, J.F., Margolis, J.R., Lee, K.L., Kisslo, J.A., Peter, R.H., Kong, Y., Beher, V.S., Wallace, A.G., McCants, C.B., & Rosati, R.A. (1978). The role of the exercise test in the evaluation of patients for ischemic heart disease. *Circulation, 57*, 64-70.

Naughton, J., & Haider, R. (1973). Methods of exercise testing. In J.P. Naughton & H.K. Hellerstein (Eds.), *Exercise testing and exercise training in coronary heart disease* (pp. 79-91). New York: Academic Press.

Porter, G.H., & Allen, T.J. (1981). Interpretation of diagnostic graded exercise tests on the basis of electrocardiographic, hemodynamic and symptomatic responses. In F.J. Nagle & H. Montoye (Eds.), *Exercise in health and disease* (pp. 235-249). Springfield, IL: Charles C Thomas.

Rod, J.L., Squires, R.W., Pollock, M.L., Foster, C., & Schmidt, D.H. (1982). Symptom-limited graded exercise testing soon after myocardial revascularization surgery. *Journal of Cardiac Rehabilitation, 2*, 199-205.

Sivarajan, E.S., Lerman, J., Mansfield, L.W., & Bruce, R.A. (1977). Progressive ambulation and treadmill testing of patients with acute myocardial infarction during hospitalization: A feasibility study. *Archives of Physical Medicine and Rehabilitation, 58*, 241-247.

Sketch, M.H., & Aronow, W.S. (1983). Diagnostic and prognostic value of exercise testing. *Journal of Cardiac Rehabilitation, 3*, 495-508.

Stone, P.H. (1983). Exercise testing in perspective. *Primary Cardiology, 9*, 111-138.

Weiner, D.A. (1983). Prognostic value of graded exercise testing early after MI. *Journal of Cardiac Rehabilitation, 3*, 114-122.

Weld, F.M., Chu, K.L., Bigger, J.T., Jr., & Ronitzky, L.M. (1981). Risk stratification with low-level exercise testing two weeks after acute myocardial infarction. *Circulation, 64*, 306-314.

Chapter 16

Application of Bayes' Theorem in Diagnostic Exercise Testing

Catherine Reith Murphy

In an era of increased concern about the values and costs of medical care, statistical inference has application in establishing the diagnostic impact, efficacy, safety, and benefits of therapeutic regimens. Medical statistics play a primary role in decision making. Unless a diagnostic test is 100% accurate, the probabilistic nature of the test must also be evaluated. Bayes' Theorem provides a form of mathematical reasoning for contemplating clinical decisions.

Historical Overview

In 1763, the Royal Society of London (Feinstein, 1977) published an "Essay Towards Solving a Problem in the Doctrine of Chances." The paper had been found posthumously among the writings of Reverend Thomas Bayes, a Presbyterian minister, who had died 2 years previously. The idea of Bayes remained dormant for nearly 2 centuries. Not until more recently have these ideas been used as the basis to develop new approaches both to statistical inference and to clinical reasoning (Feinstein, 1977).

Bayes' ideas were based on a reversal of the customary logic of thought in considering issues in conditional probability. In contrast to ordinary probability, which involves the occurrence of a single event, conditional probability involves two events, with the occurrence of the second event depending on the previous occurrence of the first. Conditional probability requires that a priori probabilities, or those established in advance, be used to estimate the occurrence of the final outcome. Bayes sought a

305

reversal of this form of a priori reasoning. In fact, he estimated probabilities after the outcome was known to have occurred (a posteriori probability) and from this was able to determine the accuracy of the final outcome. Bayes' great contribution was to develop a general algebraic expression for this process. The formula for a posteriori probability has been dignified with the name Bayes' Theorem, although in reality it is nothing more than a straightforward algebraic truism (Feinstein, 1977).

Ledley and Lusted (1959), recognizing the potential for clinical diagnostic reasoning, suggested the use of Bayes' Theorem in medical practice. Exercise electrocardiographers were the first to apply probability theory to cardiology in a routine way, particularly in the diagnosis of coronary artery disease. Rifkin and Hood (1977) introduced the use of Bayesian analysis in the interpretation of exercise electrocardiograms. It was recommended that the cardiologist consider the a priori probability of coronary artery disease based on the age and sex of the patient, the presence and type of chest pain, and other factors. The degree of ST-segment depression was then combined with the a priori probability to yield the a posteriori or final probability estimate of coronary artery disease (Wagner, 1982).

Diamond and Forrester (1979) expanded Bayes' Theorem in cardiology by combining the pretest likelihood of coronary artery disease based on age, sex, and symptoms with the data from four diagnostic tests. These tests included exercise electrocardiography, cardiomyography, thallium scintigraphy, and cardiac fluoroscopy. Since this time, Diamond and Forrester's program has been expanded to include other data such as gated blood pool imaging and has been incorporated into a commercially available microprocessor computer system that is inexpensive enough for use in the cardiologist's office (Diamond & Forrester, 1979b; Diamond & Hirsh, 1980).

In current diagnostic practice, the essence of Bayes' Theorem is that equal importance is given to the a priori probabilities and to the end results of tests. Each contributes to the estimation of the certainty of the final diagnosis (Wagner, 1982).

Terminology

Bayes' Theorem has clinically evolved in its application in the area of exercise tolerance testing. Exercise testing is used as a diagnostic tool for coronary artery disease and as a prognostic indicator of subsequent coronary events in patients with and without evidence of prior myocardial infarction. The results of exercise testing provide a probability statement rather than a definitive answer regarding the existence of coronary disease. To fully understand the application of Bayes' Theorem in exercise testing, there must be a complete understanding of terms and knowledge of calculations.

Sensitivity and Specificity

Sensitivity and *specificity* are the terms used to define how reliably a test distinguishes diseased from nondiseased individuals. Sensitivity is the percentage of times the test gives an abnormal result when those with the disease are tested. Specificity is the percentage of times the test gives a normal result when those without the disease are tested (Wilson, Fardy, & Froelicher, 1981). Methods of calculation are shown in Table 16.1.

The sensitivity and specificity of exercise-induced ST-segment depression can be determined by calculating the results of studies that have used exercise testing and coronary angiography to evaluate patients. As observed in Table 16.2, the exercise tolerance test approximates a 90% specificity for angiographically significant coronary artery disease. In other words, 90% of those without significant angiographic disease had a normal exercise test. These same studies revealed a 70% sensitivity of the exercise test for angiographic coronary artery disease. It is of interest to note that in many of these studies only a single lead was recorded and the criterion of 0.1 mV horizontally or down-sloping ST-segment depression was used to indicate an abnormal exercise test. When the study employed a greater number of coronary arteries, the sensitivity was greatly increased. Obviously, if additional criteria (e.g., exercise test symptomology, blood pressure response, heart rate, etc.) were utilized, sensitivity would have been enhanced (Wilson et al., 1981).

A reciprocal relationship exists between sensitivity and specificity. The more specific a test is (i.e., the more able it is to determine who is disease free) the less sensitive it is. By adjusting the criterion for abnormal, the values of sensitivity and specificity are altered. For example, when the criterion for an abnormal exercise-induced ST-segment response is altered from 0.1 mV to 0.2 mV depression to make it more specific for coronary artery disease, the sensitivity of the test can be cut in half. The specificity of the ST-segment response is decreased when the test is used in patients with ST-segment depression at rest or when used in women. The reasons for this are unknown (Wilson et al., 1981).

Sensitivity and specificity can also be altered by various factors that effect exercise tests. Table 16.3 lists potential conditions that can result in an exercise-induced abnormal ST-segment depression without the presence of coronary artery disease (false positive test) (Conklin & Froelicher, 1979). Possible causes of a false negative test are

1. inadequate exercise stress test,
2. too few leads monitored,
3. beta-blocking agents,
4. cancelling ST-segment vectors,
5. improper recording equipment,
6. failure to consider other abnormal end points, and
7. coronary lesions not causing ischemia.

Table 16.1 Definition and Calculation of Sensitivity and Specificity

$$\text{Sensitivity} = \frac{TP}{TP + FN} \times 100 \quad \text{Specificity} = \frac{TN}{FP + TN} \times 100$$

TP = True positives or those with abnormal test and with disease

FN = False negatives or those with normal test and with disease

TN = True negatives or those with normal test and no disease

FP = False positives or those with abnormal test and no disease

Table 16.2 Studies Evaluating the Diagnostic Value of the ECG Response to Exercise in Studies with Coronary Angiography as the Endpoint for Coronary Disease

Study	N	Specificity	Sensitivity			
			1-Vessel	2-Vessel	3-Vessel	Total
Kasselbaum	68	97%	25%	38%	85%	53%
Martin	100	89%	35%	67%	86%	62%
McHenry	166	95%	61%	91%	100%	81%
Helfant	63	83%	60%	83%	91%	79%
Bartel	609	94%	39%	62%	73%	63%
Goldschlager	410	93%	40%	63%	79%	64%
Mason	84	89%	—	—	—	78%
Roitman	100	82%	—	—	—	73%
Average	—	90%	43%	67%	86%	69%

Note. From "Applications of Exercise Testing" by P.K. Wilson et al., 1981, in P.K. Wilson, P.S. Fardy, and V.F. Froelicher (Eds.), *Cardiac Rehabilitation, Adult Fitness and Exercise Testing* (p. 314), Philadelphia: Lea and Febiger. Copyright 1981 by Lea and Febiger. Adapted by permission.

Table 16.3 Conditions That Can Possibly Result in an Exercise-Induced Abnormal ST-Segment Depression Without the Presence of Coronary Artery Disease (False Positive Exercise Test)

Valvular heart disease	Left ventricular hypertrophy
Congenital heart disease	WPW syndrome
Cardiomyopathies	Pre-excitation variants
Pericardial disorders	Mitral valve prolapse syndrome
Drugs	Vasoregulatory abnormality
Electrolyte abnormalities	Hyperventilation repolarization abnormalities
Nonfasting state	
Anemia	Hypertension
Sudden excessive exercise	Excessive double product
Inadequate recording equipment	Improper lead systems
Bundle branch block	Incorrect criteria
Improper interpretation	

Note. From "Value of the Exercise ECG Test for Screening Asymptomatic Subjects for Latent Coronary Artery Disease" by J. Conklin and V.F. Froelicher, 1979, in E.K. Chung (Ed.), *Exercise Electrocardiography Practical Approach* (p. 310), Baltimore: Williams and Wilkins. Copyright 1979 by Williams and Wilkins. Adapted by permission.

Relative Risk and Predictive Value

The terms *relative risk* and *predictive value* also assist in defining the diagnostic capabilities of an exercise test. Relative risk is the relative chance of having disease if the test is abnormal as compared to having disease if the test is normal. The predictive value of an abnormal test is the percentage of those with an abnormal test who have disease. Subtracting the predictive value from 100% yields the false positive rate. Predictive value and the false positive rate are dependent upon the prevalence of disease in the population tested. More false positive responses are evidenced when exercise testing is used in a population with a low prevalence of disease as compared to a population with a high prevalence of disease. This explains the greater number of false positive responses when testing is used as a screening procedure in asymptomatic individuals compared to when it is used as a diagnostic tool in patients with symptoms suggestive of coronary artery disease (Wilson et al., 1981). The calculation of relative risk and predictive value is

$$\text{Relative risk} = \frac{\dfrac{TP}{TP + FP}}{\dfrac{FN}{TN + FN}} \qquad \text{Predictive value} = \frac{TP}{TP + FP} \times 100$$

Figure 16.1, taken from the National Heart, Lung and Blood Institute (NHLBI) study, shows the predictive accuracy of the ST-segment response to exercise in patients who had typical angina pectoris or a history of prior myocardial infarction (Epstein, 1978). In these symptomatic patients, the level of predictive accuracy was extremely high. There was only one false positive test, resulting in a predictive accuracy of 95%.

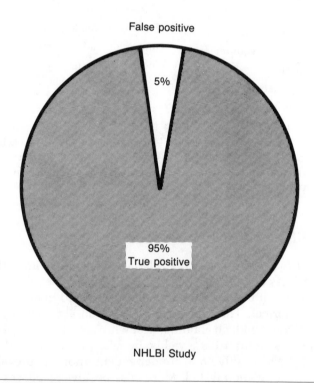

False positive

5%

95%
True positive

NHLBI Study

Figure 16.1.   Predictive accuracy of 1 mm or greater ST-segment depression in response to exercise in 20 subjects with angina pectoris, myocardial infarction, or both. *Note.* From "Value and Limitations of the Electrocardiographic Response to Exercise in the Assessment of Patients With Coronary Artery Disease" by S.E. Epstein, 1978, *American Journal of Cardiology,* **42,** p. 668. Copyright 1978 by *American Journal of Cardiology.* Adapted by permission.

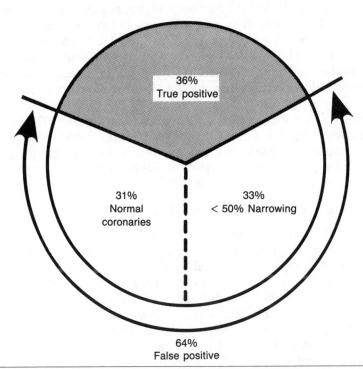

Figure 16.2.   Predictive accuracy of 1 mm or greater ST-segment depression induced by exercise in 39 asymptomatic subjects. *Note.* From "Value and Limitations of the Electrocardiographic Response to Exercise in the Assessment of Patients with Coronary Artery Disease" by S.E. Epstein, 1978, *American Journal of Cardiology*, **42**, p. 688. Copyright 1978 by *American Journal of Cardiology*.

Figure 16.2 illustrates the results obtained in the asymptomatic subjects of the NHLBI study. Approximately two-thirds of the test results were false positives. This reinforces the Bayesian concept that the diagnostic accuracy of the test is dependent upon the prevalence of disease in the population being tested (Epstein, 1978).

Table 16.4 illustrates the performance of an exercise test in a population with a 1% prevalence of disease, a sensitivity of 70%, and a specificity of 90% (Conklin & Froelicher, 1974). As demonstrated through previously mentioned studies, these values approximate the sensitivity and specificity of maximal or near maximal exercise tolerance testing. In reference to Table 16.5, because 1% of the 10,000 men have disease, 100 men have disease.

The middle column distinguishes the men with abnormal tests, and the far right column depicts the number with normal tests. Because the test is 70% sensitive, 70 of those with disease will have abnormal tests and are true positives. The remaining 30 have normal tests and are false negatives. Because the test is 90% specific, 90% of 9,900 without disease are true negatives, whereas the remainder are false positives. Calculation of predictive value is obtained by dividing the true positives by all of those with an abnormal test (Wilson et al., 1981).

Table 16.5 shows the performance of a test with the same 70% sensitivity and 90% specificity in a population with 50% prevalence of disease. The same calculations demonstrate that the use of an exercise test in a population with a greater disease prevalence reduces the false positive rate (Epstein, 1978; Wilson et al., 1981).

Likelihood Ratio and Bayes' Theorem

The most important information to the professional attempting to make a diagnosis is the likelihood of the patient having the disease once the test result is known. Such a likelihood cannot be accurately estimated from the test result and the diagnostic characteristics of the test alone. The knowledge of the prior probability of the patient's having the disease before the test was administered is also needed (Conklin & Froelicher, 1979). This is the foundation of Bayes' Theorem. Essentially, Bayes' Theorem states that the odds of the patient having the disease after a test are the product of the odds before the test and the odds that the test result was a true one (Wilson et al., 1981).

Table 16.4 Performance of a Test With a 70% Sensitivity and a 90% Specificity in a Population With a 1% Prevalence of Disease.

Population	No. with abnormal test	No. with normal test
100 diseased	70 (TP)	30 (FN)
9,900 Nondiseased	990 (FP)	8,910 (TN)
Total	1,060	8,940

Predictive value of an abnormal test $= \dfrac{TP}{TP + FP} = \dfrac{70}{1,060} = 6.6\%$

False positive rate $\qquad\qquad = 100 - 6.6 \quad = 93.4\%$

Relative risk $\qquad\qquad\qquad = 19.4x$

Note. From "Applications of Exercise Testing" by P.K. Wilson et al., 1981, in P.K. Wilson, P.S. Fardy, and V.F. Froelicher (Eds.), *Cardiac Rehabilitation, Adult Fitness and Exercise Testing* (p. 315), Philadelphia: Lea and Febiger. Copyright 1981 by Lea and Febiger. Adapted by permission.

Table 16.5   Performance of a Test With a 70% Sensitivity and a 90% Specificity in a Population With a 50% Prevalence of Disease.

Population	No. with abnormal test	No. with normal test
5,000 Diseased	3,500 (TP)	1,500 (FN)
5,000 Nondiseased	500 (RP)	4,500 (TN)
Total	4,000	6,000

Predictive value of an abnormal test $= \dfrac{TP}{TP + FP} = \dfrac{3,500}{4,000} = 87.5\%$

False positive rate $= 100 - 87.5 = 12.5\%$

Relative risk $= 3.5x$

Note. From ''Applications of Exercise Testing'' by P.K. Wilson et al., 1981, in P.K. Wilson, P.S. Fardy, and V.F. Froelicher (Eds.), *Cardiac Rehabilitation, Adult Fitness and Exercise Testing,* Philadelphia: Lea and Febiger. Copyright 1981 by Lea and Febiger. Adapted by permission.

The odds of the test result being true are known as the likelihood ratio. It is the ratio of true results to false results. In the case of an abnormal test result, the positive likelihood ratio equals

$$\frac{\text{percent with disease with abnormal test}}{\text{percent without disease with abnormal test}} \quad \text{or} \quad \frac{\text{sensitivity}}{1 - \text{specificity}}$$

The conventional analysis of ST-segment depression yields a sensitivity of approximately 70% and a specificity of 90% in maximal or near maximal exercise testing. Therefore, translated mathematically, the likelihood ratio for an abnormal test result equals

$$\text{positive likelihood ratio} = \frac{0.7}{1 - 0.9} = 7.0$$

In the case of normal test results the negative likelihood ratio equals

$$\frac{\text{percent without disease with normal test}}{\text{percent with disease with normal test}} \quad \text{or} \quad \frac{\text{specificity}}{1 - \text{sensitivity}}$$

The mathematical expression follows:

$$\text{negative likelihood ratio} = \frac{0.9}{1 - 0.7} = 3.0$$

Bayes' Theorem is expressed accordingly:

$$\begin{matrix} \text{Posttest odds} \\ \text{of disease} \end{matrix} = \begin{matrix} \text{Pretest odds} \\ \text{of disease} \end{matrix} \times \begin{matrix} \text{Likelihood ratio of} \\ \text{the test results} \end{matrix}$$

The calculation of Bayes' theorem is oftentimes made intuitively. For example, the clinician may suspect the abnormal exercise test response of a 28-year-old woman with chest pain (low probability) to be false. The same abnormal response, however, would be accepted as a true result in a 62-year-old man with angina who had a previous myocardial infarction (high probability) (Wilson et al., 1981).

Application of Bayes' Theorem in a Symptomatic Population

Coronary angiographic studies (Compeau, Bourassa, & Bois, 1968; Friesinger & Smith, 1972; McConahay, McCallister, & Smith, 1972; Proudfit, Shirey, & Stones, 1966) have been used to establish the prevalence of significant coronary artery disease in patients with different chest pain syndromes. Chest pain is a predominant presenting factor in a majority of individuals referred for a diagnostic exercise test. Therefore, the nature of the chest pain would seem to be a practical basis for estimating the prior probability of coronary artery disease.

It has been found that approximately 90% of the patients with true angina pectoris have significant angiographic coronary disease. In patients presenting with atypical angina pectoris, approximately 50% have been found to have significant angiographic coronary disease. *Atypical* is defined as pain that has an unusual location, prolonged duration, inconstant precipitating factors, or does not respond to nitroglycerin (Wilson et al., 1981). Table 16.6 demonstrates the calculation of the probability of coronary artery disease in such patients presenting with chest pain.

Close observation of Table 16.6 demonstrates that the patient with typical angina pectoris has a 90% chance (9:1) of having significant coronary artery disease. An abnormal exercise test increases the odds from 9:1 to 63:1. Such a dramatic change in odds represents a relatively small increase in the probability of disease from 90 to 98%. Because such a patient still has a 75% probability of disease after a negative test, coronary angiography may still be required to rule out definitely coronary disease. The most impressive diagnostic impact is with patients with atypical angina. An abnormal exercise test result would increase the odds from 1:1 to 7:1 and yield a probability of 88%. For all practical purposes this would establish the diagnosis. The probability of coronary artery disease would be reduced to 25% with a normal test result (Wilson et al., 1981).

Table 16.6 Calculation of the Probability of a Patient's Having Coronary Artery Disease (Depending on Clinical Presentation) Given the Results of Exercise Testing.

Pretest odds	Likelihood ratio	Posttest odds	Posttest probability
Typical 9:1	Abnormal test (x7)	63:1	(63/64) = 98%
	Normal test (x3)	9:3	(9/12) = 75%
Atypical 1:1	Abnormal test (x7)	7:1	(7/8) = 88%
	Normal test (x3)	1:3	(1/4) = 25%
Nonanginal 1:9	Abnormal test (7x)	7:9	(7/16) = 44%
	Normal test (3x)	1:27	(1/28) = 4%
Asymptomatic 1:19	Abnormal test (7x)	7:19	(7/26) = 27%
	Normal test (3x)	1:57	(1/58) = 2%

Note. From "Applications of Exercise Testing" by P.K. Wilson et al., 1981, in P.K. Wilson, P.S. Fardy, and V.F. Froelicher (Eds.), *Cardiac Rehabilitation, Adult Fitness and Exercise Testing* (p. 317), Philadelphia: Lea and Febiger. Copyright 1981 by Lea and Febiger. Adapted by permission.

Application of Bayes' Theorem in an Asymptomatic Population

The *Coronary Risk Handbook* (American Heart Association [AHA], 1973), which is based on the results of the Framingham Study (Kannel & Gordon, 1968), provides estimates of the risk of coronary artery disease in asymptomatic patients. These estimates were determined from blood pressures, serum cholesterol values, smoking histories, glucose intolerances, and resting electrocardiograms. Although incidence and prevalence are not interchangeable, Diamond and Forrester (1979) have demonstrated that through appropriate conversion procedures the incidence data from the *Coronary Risk Handbook* can be used to estimate the pretest likelihood of disease in asymptomatic patients. A linear correlation exists between the age-related prevalence estimated from pooled autopsy data and the 6-year incidence reported in the Framingham Study (Diamond & Forrester, 1979). This correlation is displayed in Figure 16.3.

Although estimating risk of coronary heart disease in asymptomatic patients is oftentimes made intuitively, the *Coronary Risk Handbook* provides a scientific method of estimating the probability (per 100) of developing the disease in 6 years according to specified characteristics. In addition it provides average values of associated risk factors with coronary heart disease and average probability values based on the Framingham report. The risk factor profile can be applied to the appropriate tables in the handbook to determine the incidence rate for coronary heart disease in 6 years. This incident rate can then be multiplied by the known constant to develop the prevalence (pretest probability) of disease. This process (see Figure 16.4) represents a mathematical formalization of the intuition used by physicians when they review the literature or when they use past experience to assess asymptomatic patients' pretest likelihood of disease (Diamond & Forrester, 1979).

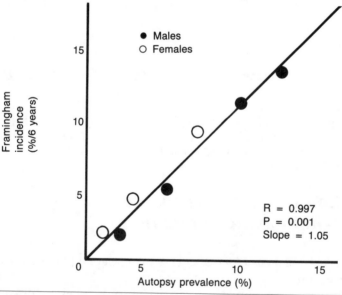

Figure 16.3. Relation of the prevalence of coronary artery disease (derived from autopsy data of 23,996 persons) and the incidence of ischemic heart disease (from the Framingham study). *Note.* From ''Analysis of Probability as an Aid in the Clinical Diagnosis of Coronary Artery Disease'' by G.H. Diamond and J.S. Forrester, 1979, *New England Journal of Medicine,* **300,** p.1353. Copyright 1979 by *New England Journal of Medicine.* Adapted by permission.

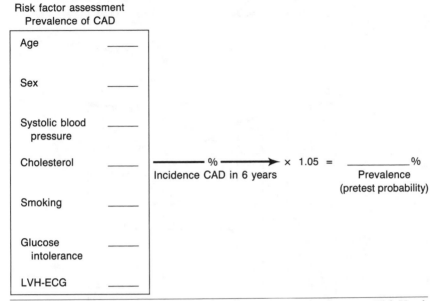

Risk factor assessment
Prevalence of CAD

Age ____

Sex ____

Systolic blood ____
  pressure

Cholesterol ____ _____ % _____→ × 1.05 = _____ %
              Incidence CAD in 6 years   Prevalence
                                          (pretest probability)

Smoking ____

Glucose ____
  intolerance

LVH-ECG ____

Figure 16.4. Establishing prevalence of CAD. *Note.* From *Coronary Risk Handbook* (p. 35) by the American Heart Association. Copyright by the American Heart Association. Adapted by permission.

Figure 16.5 is a graphical representation of Bayes' Theorem based on the definition. Assuming a sensitivity of 70% and a specificity of 90% the predictive value of a positive test result (Curve A) and the predictive value of negative test result (Curve B) can be plotted. These curves are based on a given study population (Kannel & Gordon, 1968; Rifkin & Hood, 1977). The pretest probability (prevalence rate established from the *Coronary Risk Handbook*) can be plotted against Curve A or Curve B to yield the posttest probability of diease (AHA, 1973; Kannel & Gordon, 1968; G. Porter, personal communication).

An example may further clarify use of this information. The following risk factors can be applied to the appropriate table in the *Coronary Risk Handbook* to determine the incidence of coronary artery disease in 6 years based on Framingham results:

- Age—55 years
- Sex—male
- Systolic blood pressure—150
- Cholesterol—235
- Smoking—yes
- Glucose intolerance—negative
- Left ventricular hypertrophy by ECG—negative

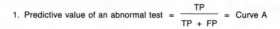

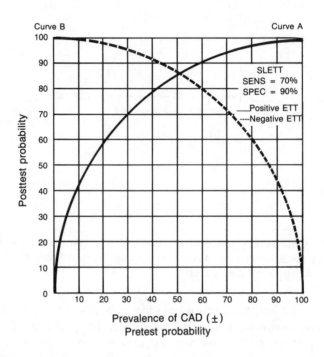

Figure 16.5. Establishing posttest probability of disease from graphical representation of Bayes' Theorem based on the definition. *Note.* From "Bayesian Analysis of Electrocardiographic Exercise Stress Testing" by R.D. Rifkin and W.B. Hodd, 1977, *New England Journal of Medicine,* **297**, pp. 681-682. Copyright 1977 by *New England Journal of Medicine.* Adapted by permission.

Methods of measuring each of the aforementioned characteristics are explained in the *Coronary Risk Handbook* (AHA, 1973). Use of the appropriate tables in the handbook (see Table 16.7) shows a 12.4% chance of this individual developing coronary heart disease within the next 6 years. Prevalence is established by multiplying this value (12.4%) by the constant 1.05. This calculation gives a prevalence or pretest probability for disease of 13.02%. This value can be rounded off and plotted on the x-axis in Figure 16.5. Once the results of the symptom-limited exercise test are known, the posttest probability of disease can be determined. Assuming a positive test result, the 13% prevalence can be matched with Curve A to produce approximately a 50% posttest probability of disease. With this result, the clinician may feel that further diagnostic information is needed. Based on the same risk factor information, if the exercise test result had been negative (Curve B), the posttest probability that the individual did not have disease would have been approximately 97%. In this instance further diagnostic information would probably not be needed. This technique allows for a more scientific approach in establishing diagnosis (AHA, 1973; Kannel & Gordon; G. Porter, personal communication).

Clinical Application of Serial-Likelihood Analysis

Diamond and Forrester (1979) reviewed the literature to estimate the pretest likelihood of coronary artery disease (defined by age, sex, and symptoms) and the sensitivity and specificity of four diagnostic tests: exercise electrocardiography, cardiokymography, thallium scintigraphy, and cardiac fluoroscopy. Each test was selected on the assumption that it detects a different, potentially independent marker of the disease—electrophysiologic (depression of ST-segment), anatomic (coronary artery calcification), mechanical (segmental dysfunction), and perfusive (thallium maldistribution). This assumption of independence is critical to serial analysis of likelihood according to Bayes' Theorem (Patton, 1978).

Table 16.7 Probability (per 100) of Developing Coronary Heart Disease in 6 Years According to Specified Characteristics

55-year-old-man

Smokes cigarettes and LVH—ECG Negative

Systolic blood pressure Chol	105	120	135	150	165	180	195
185	5.7	6.8	8.1	9.6	11.3	13.4	15.7
210	6.5	7.8	9.2	10.9	12.9	15.1	17.6
235	7.5	8.9	10.5	12.4	14.5	17.0	19.8
260	8.5	10.1	11.9	14.0	16.4	19.1	22.2
285	9.7	11.5	13.5	15.8	18.5	21.4	24.7
310	11.0	13.0	15.2	17.8	20.7	23.9	27.5
335	12.5	14.7	17.2	20.0	23.1	26.6	30.4

Note. From *Coronary Risk Handbook* (p. 27) by the American Heart Association. Copyright by the American Heart Association. Reprinted by permission.

Table 16.8   Cumulative Analysis of Likelihood in a 50-Year-Old Asymptomatic Man in Whom the Pretest Likelihood Was 9.7 ± 0.4%.

Test	Result	Posttest likelihood (%)
Electrocardiographic stress	2.0-mm depression of ST-segment	
Cardiokymographic stress	Midsystolic outward motion	99.3 ± 0.8
Fluoroscopy	Right-coronary-artery calcification	
Thallium stress scintigraphy	if normal if abnormal	96.1 ± 4.3 99.1 ± 0.1
Coronary angiography	Coronary-artery disease of three vessels	

Note. From "Analysis of Probability as an Aid in the Clinical Diagnosis of Coronary Artery Disease" by G.H. Diamond and J.S. Forrester, 1979, *New England Journal of Medicine*, **300**, p. 1353. Copyright 1979 by *New England Journal of Medicine*. Adapted by permission.

The practical application of the various tests is illustrated in Table 16.8. This table lists each factor used in analysis of pretest likelihood after the aforementioned tests were performed (Diamond & Forrester, 1979).

For example, assume that an asymptomatic 50-year-old had a pretest likelihood of 9.7% based on risk factor analysis. After an exercise tolerance test (exercise electrocardiogram), the posttest likelihood was 54.3 ± 17.1% (based on literature review of Diamond and Forrester, 1979). This posttest likelihood is an intermediate value for which the use of further diagnostic tests would be useful. A cardiokymographic stress test and cardiac fluoroscopy were therefore performed. The observed abnormalities increased the overall likelihood for coronary disease to 99.3 ± .08%. At this point, a thallium stress test would not appreciably alter this high diagnostic likelihood. A positive perfusion result would increase the likelihood from 99.3 to 99.9%, whereas a negative result would decrease the likelihood to only 96.1%. In this particular patient, the thallium scintigraphy would appear to add little information concerning the likelihood of disease, but it would substantially increase the cost of estimation. Therefore, the physician can not only analyze the cumulative effect of many possible discordant test results but also evaluate the cost-effectiveness of other tests before using them (Diamond & Forrester, 1979). The usefulness of likelihood analysis depends upon how accurately the results correlate with the prevalence of coronary disease as demonstrated through coronary angiography or long-term follow-up studies.

Diagnostic Accuracy of Cardiologists Compared With Probability Calculations Using Bayes' Theorem

In 1982, Hlatky, Botvinick, and Brundage (1982) designed a study to evaluate the diagnostic accuracy of two independent methods of probability calculation with that of cardiologists. Ninety-one cardiologists participated in the study. Each cardiologist evaluated the clinical summaries of eight randomly selected patients. For each patient, the cardiologist assessed the probability of coronary artery disease after reviewing the clinical history, physical examination, laboratory data, and complete results from a treadmill exercise test. This was compared with the probability of disease from two methods employing Bayes' Theorem: (a) a published table of data based on the patient's age, sex, symptoms, and degree of ST-segment change during exercise (Diamond & Forrester, 1979; Diamond, & Hirsh, 1980), and a computer program (CADENZA) using age, sex, risk factors, resting electrocardiogram, and multiple exercise measurements (Diamond & Forrester, 1979). Diagnostic accuracy was assessed on a scale from 0 to 100 with the coronary angiogram as the diagnostic standard. The average diagnostic accuracy on this scale was 80.2 for the cardiologists' estimates, 78.0 for the estimates based on tables (difference from cardiologists' estimates, $p < 0.05$), and 83.1 for the estimates based on computer calculations ($p < 0.01$). The study revealed that probability analysis incorporating sufficient detail can achieve a diagnostic accuracy comparable to that of cardiologists (Hlatlky et al., 1982). Nonetheless, caution is warranted because of recognized limitations of the available data. The standard for comparison of noninvasive tests is coronary angiography, and it is clear that patients coming in for this procedure may not be completely representative of the population in general. Furthermore, the results of several laboratory procedures may not be independent of one another, a requirement for accurate probability calculations employing sequential application of Bayes' Theorem (Hlatky et al., 1982; Patton, 1978). These precautions suggest that probability methods could be improved with the availability of larger, more comprehensive data bases (Hlatky et al., 1982).

Summary

In summary, Bayes' Theorem states that the interpretation or significance of a given test result on a particular patient requires a knowledge of both the sensitivity and specificity of that test for the disease under consideration as well as knowledge of the patient's a priori probability of having that disease before that test is performed. The a priori probability for a disease can be estimated, as in coronary artery disease, by quantitative risk factor analysis or by a knowledge of the prevalence of the disease in the population being tested. The sensitivity and specificity of a test for a disease can only be determined by correlating the criteria for an abnormal test with patients known to have that disease as well as with individuals known not to have the disease. It would appear that Bayes' Theorem has application in just about every diagnostic test performed in medicine (except those rare cases that are both 100% specific and 100% sensitive for a disease process).

Nonetheless, Bayes' Theorem has not been universally accepted. Feinstein (1977) has stated that as clinicians we should answer a question not by estimating probability but by collecting more data. Wagner (1968) suggests an alternative approach:

> Every question that the physician asks in obtaining a medical history, every maneuver that he performs in the physical examination and every subsequent laboratory procedure that he orders should be selected because of the likelihood that the new fact will alter the estimate of the probability that the patient has a particular disease or diseases.

> An essential feature of the diagnostic process is its statistical or probabilistic nature. Rarely can a diagnosis be made with absolute certainty, even by pathologists looking at histological sections. We in medicine have a tendency to assume erroneously that the best test is perfect. It almost never is, a fact revealed when a better test comes along. (p. 877)

Wagner (1982) reports that Diamond (through personal communication) has stated that

> We may be standing at the threshold of a perceptual upheaval in medicine, based on the use of the microcomputer to apply Bayes' Theorem in the cardiologist's office or even at the bedside. In my judgment, within 10 years the computer is likely to join the stethoscope as a symbol of the cardiologist. (p. 877)

It should be emphasized that in applying Bayes' Theorem to clinical diagnostic procedures, the role of the physician is not diminished but enhanced. The approach of Bayes' Theorem of conditional probability aids, but does not replace, the physician's judgment and may assist in decisions of cost-effectiveness of tests.

References

American Heart Association. (1973). *Coronary risk handbook*. New York: American Heart Association.

Compeau, L. (1968). Clinical significance of selective coronary cinearteriography. *Canadian Medical Association Journal, 99*, 1063.

Conklin, J., & Froelicher, V.F. (1979). Value of the exercise ECG test for screening asymptomatic subjects for latent coronary artery disease. In E.K. Chung (Ed.), *Exercise electrocardiography practical approach*. Baltimore: Williams and Wilkins.

Diamond, G.H., & Forrester, J.S. (1979a). Analysis of probability as an aid in the clinical diagnosis of coronary artery disease. *New England Journal of Medicine, 300*, 1350-1358.

Diamond, G.H., & Forrester, J.S. (1979b). *Cadenza II: Computor-assisted diagnosis and evaluation of coronary artery disease*. Seattle: Cardiokinetics.

Diamond, G.H. (1980). Applications of conditional probability analysis to the clinical diagnosis of coronary artery disease. *Journal of Clinical Investigations, 65*, 1210-1221.

Epstein, S.A. (1978). Value and limitations of the electrocardiographic response to exercise in the assessment of patients with coronary heart disease. *American Journal of Cardiology, 42*, 668.

Feinstein, A.R. (1977). Clinical biostatistics. 39. The haze of Bayes, the aerial palaces of decision analysis, and the computerized Ouija board. *Clinical Pharmacology and Therapeutics, 21*, 482-495.

Friesinger, G.C., & Smith, P.F. (1972). Correlation of electrocardiographic studies and arteriographic findings with angina pectoris. *Circulation, 46*, 1173.

Hlatky, M., Botvinick, E., & Brundage, B. (1982). Diagnostic accuracy of cardiologists compared with probability calculations using Bayes' rule. *American Journal of Cardiology, 49*, 1927-1931.

Kannel, W.B., & Gordon, T. (1968). *The Framingham study: An epidemiological investigation of cardiovascular disease*. Bethesda, MD: National Heart, Lung and Blood Institute.

Ledley, R.F., & Lusted, L.B. (1959). Reasoning foundations of medical diagnosis. *Science, 130*, 9-13.

McConahay, D.R., McCallister, B.D., & Smith, R.E. (1972). Post-exercise electrocardiography: Correlation with coronary arteriography and left ventricular hemodynamics. *American Journal of Cardiology, 28*, 1.

Patton, D.D. (1978). Introduction to clinical decision making. *Seminar in Nuclear Medicine, 8*, 273-282.

Proudfit, W.L., Shirey, E.K., & Stones, F.M. (1966). Selective cine coronary angiography: Correlation with clinical findings in 1000 patients. *Circulation, 33*, 901.

Rifkin, R.D., & Hood, W.B. (1977). Bayesian analysis of electrocardiographic exercise stress testing. *New England Journal of Medicine, 297*, 681-686.

Wagner, H.N. (1968). *Principles of nuclear medicine. The diagnostic process.* Philadelphia: W.B. Saunders.

Wagner, H.N. (1982). Bayes' Theorem: An idea whose time has come? *The American Journal of Cardiology, 49*, 875-877.

Wilson, P.K., Fardy, P.S., & Froelicher, V.F. (1981). Applications of exercise testing. In P.K. Wilson, P.S. Fardy, & V.F. Froelicher (Eds.), *Cardiac rehabilitation, adult fitness, and exercise testing* (pp. 313-318). Philadelphia: Lea and Febiger.

Part IV

Drug and Nondrug Treatments of CAD

Chapter 17

Nonpharmacologic and Pharmacologic Treatment of Hypertension

Charles P. Lucas

Life insurance statistics justify the concern of the public and medical communities about the danger of elevated blood pressure. Table 17.1 lists mortality ratios for men, calculated by the Society of Actuaries (1980) in the Blood Pressure Study of 1979. In this study, over 4.2 million insured individuals were observed from 1950 to 1972 for an average length of follow-up of 6.6 years. The total number of policies terminated by death was nearly 106,000. In Table 17.1, a ratio of 100 signifies the average mortality for this insured population, shown here for men ages 40–49. With numbers less than 100 indicating greater longevity, numbers over 100 predict a greater than average likelihood of death. It is apparent from these data that at any level of diastolic blood pressure a higher systolic blood pressure indicates the probability of increased mortality. Similarly, at any level of systolic blood pressure, higher diastolic blood pressure is also associated with a greater likelihood of death.

A major concern about elevated blood pressure stems from the fact that it is such a common problem. Figure 17.1 illustrates the prevalence of hypertension in the United States, as derived from the Health Examination Survey of 1962 (Kaplan, 1973). Hypertension is our most common disease affecting 15-20% of our population: Blood pressure rises progressively with age, so that by age 70, one-third of the population has a blood pressure greater than 160/95.

Even though the risk of death or morbidity from blood pressure is continuous, being low at low levels of blood pressure and higher with increasing levels, it is customary to use only an arbitrary dividing line between normotension and hypertension. Thus mild hypertension has been defined as a diastolic blood pressure of 90-104, moderate hypertension as 105-114 and severe hypertension as 115 mm Hg and above. These definitions are based upon studies showing that the treatment of blood pressure at these levels is associated with decreased morbidity and mortality (see Table 17.2).

Table 17.1 Ratio (Percent) of Actual to Expected Mortality According to the Levels of Blood Pressure (Males Ages 40-69)

(mm Hg) blood pressure (mm Hg)	Under 68	68–72	73–77	78–82	83–87	88–92	93–97	98–102	103–107
98–107	71	72	65	73	—	—	—	—	—
108–117	76	73	73	76	76	—	—	—	—
118–127	91	82	85	89	90	102	—	—	—
128–137	107	103	106	108	116	123	114	—	—
138–147	135	102	137	125	134	143	173	186	—
148–157	—	159	160	153	148	174	184	183	238

Note. From *Blood Pressure Study* by Society of Actuaries, 1980, Chicago: Author. Copyright 1980 by Society of Actuaries. Reprinted by permission.

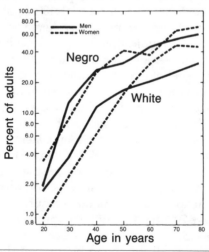

Figure 17.1.   Prevalence of hypertension in the U.S. Health Examination Survey of 1962. *Note.* From "Treatment of Mild Hypertension: Results of a Ten-Year Intervention Trial" by U.S. Public Health Service, 1977, *Circulation Research,* **40**(Suppl. 1), p. 98. Copyright 1977 by *Circulation Research.* Reprinted by permission.

Table 17.2 Therapeutic Trials in Mild-Moderate Hypertension

Deaths from cerebrovascular disease	Percentage decrease in mortality from treatment
Veterans Administration Cooperative Study (1970)	− 74
United States Public Health Service Study (1977)	− 84
Oslo Study (Helgeland, 1980)	− 100
Australian Therapeutic Trial (1980)	− 45
Hypertension Detection and Follow-up Program (1979)	− 58

Deaths from cardiovascular disease	Percentage decrease in mortality from treatment
Veterans Administration Cooperative Study (1970)	− 12
United States Public Health Service Study (1977)	− 15
Oslo Study (Helgeland, 1980)	+ 44
Australian Therapeutic Trial (1980)	− 11
Hypertension Detection and Follow-up Program (1979)	− 26

The Veteran's Administration Cooperative Study (1970) was the first placebo-controlled trial demonstrating that antihypertension drug therapy could reduce cardiovascular complications in patients with diastolic blood pressure between 90 and 114 mm Hg. Two subsequent trials on hypertension, the U.S. Public Health Service study (1977) and the Oslo trial (Helgeland, 1980), failed to demonstrate a significant effect on mortality with treatment, probably because of the small number of participants. The Hypertension Detection and Followup Program (HDFP) study (1979) also investigated the effect of treatment in mild and moderate hypertension. Over 10,000 subjects were randomized into special care (SC) and referred care (RC) groups. The SC group was treated aggressively in special centers, whereas RC patients were referred to their personal physicians with information that they had high blood pressure. This 5-year study found greater blood pressure reduction and a significant (20.3%) decrease in mortality in the SC group, most of it from heart attacks and strokes. This study, probably because of its large and sufficient size, was the first to show that individuals with mild hypertension (90-104 mm Hg) might benefit from antihypertensive therapy. Surprisingly, and for unexplained reasons, mortality from both noncardiovascular- and cardiovascular-related causes was substantially reduced in the SC group. The Australian therapeutic trial (Australian National Blood Pressure Study Management Committee, 1980), in contrast to the HDFP, included a placebo (control) group and dealt with subjects with diastolic blood pressures between 95 and 109 mm Hg. Drug-treated individuals had significantly lower mortality and fewer strokes (45%); but unlike the HDFP, a nonsignificant decrease of 11% in the incidence of heart attacks was observed. Interestingly, placebo-treated patients, whose blood pressure decreased to below 100 mm Hg during the trial, had lower mortality rates than those treated with drugs.

One of the controversies in current hypertension management concerns a study that was a multiple risk factor intervention trial (MRFIT) for patients who were in the upper 10% of risk because of a combination of hypercholesterolemia, cigarette smoking, and hypertension (Multiple Risk Factor, 1982). The MRFIT compared the effect of multiple intervention therapy on patients treated, as in the HDFP, in special clinics (SC) whereas the control group patients (RC) were referred to their own physicians. Impressive reductions in smoking were achieved in the SC group through behavior modification, with minor decreases as a result of intervention in serum cholesterol. Blood pressure was also effectively lowered, more so in the SC group than in the RC group. Disappointingly, the SC group did not have significantly fewer cardiovascular deaths and other related morbid events than the RC group. In fact, in a special subgroup of patients in the SC group, whose pretreatment diastolic blood pressure was less than 100 mm Hg, who had electrocardiographic (ECG) abnormalities at the onset of the trial, and who, in addition, were treated with antihypertensive drug therapy, the mortality rate was higher than in the corresponding RC group.

These studies in their totality led to the conclusion that drug therapy is indicated for individuals whose diastolic blood pressure is 90 mm Hg and above. Yet, if put into practice, this recommendation has major implications. The most recent estimate of the prevalence of hypertension in the United States is 60 million persons, at least 40 million of whom have diastolic blood pressure between 90 and 99 mm Hg, measured on one visit.

In a consideration of drug treatment for such a large segment of the population, any disadvantages must be weighed against the advantages. Drug treatment, as the MRFIT study implied, could have disturbing side effects, an observation that has spawned speculation regarding the cause of this possible drug-related problem. One concern is that diuretic-induced potassium depletion may have caused fatal cardiac arrhythmias in some susceptible patients in this trial. The diuretic associated with increased mortality in the MRFIT study was hydrochlorothiazide. Evidence for cardiac arrhythmias due to diuretic-induced hypokalemia has been presented by Holland, Nixon, and Kuhnert (1981). Although these criticisms of aggressive drug therapy of hypertension have been noted, Gifford et al. (1983) have pointed out the "severe methodological problems inherent in subgroup analyses of the results of a clinical trial like MRFIT in which the sample size and statistical power of the study have been based exclusively on the primary end points (i.e., death caused by coronary heart disease among the total population enrolled in the study)." Moreover, when the HDFP study was exposed to the same subgroup analysis as that conducted in MRFIT, the SC participants with mild hypertension and ECG abnormalities at entry showed no adverse side effects from the therapy that this group received, as compared to that in the RC group.

Although these arguments would tend to blunt some of the concerns expressed in opposition of aggressive antihypertensive therapy for all individuals with mild hypertension, there is still data from the Australian trial (Kaplan, 1973) showing that placebo-treated individuals whose blood pressure declined spontaneously to below 100 mm Hg during the trial had lower mortality than those whose blood pressure response was similar but with the aid of drug therapy. When one adds the fact that certain antihypertensive therapy can produce adverse effects on lipids and lipoproteins, and that even small increases in lipids could have adverse effects on cardiovascular morbidity and mortality, this cause for caution regarding unrestricted antihypertensive therapy seems justified.

Such concern has come from a number of sources (Chobanian, 1983; Freis, 1982; Gifford et al., 1983; Ram, 1983). Freis has criticized both the HDFP and the Australian Trial with respect to the overall effectiveness of treatment of hypertension in those with blood pressure less than 100 mm Hg. As for the effect on myocardial infarction, only the HDFP study showed an overall decrease in mortality (nonfatal myocardial infarction not reported). Because of the design of this project, Freis (1982) stated that very little could be concluded regarding the effect of treatment on this parameter, and that, because of these uncertainties, we may be doing more harm than good by giving lifelong drug treatment to patients with mild hypertension. A recommended compromise would be to begin treatment in those with mild hypertension and additional risk factors and to observe an extended waiting period prior to initiating drug therapy, because of the spontaneous fall in blood pressure observed in a large percentage (about 80%) of placebo-treated patients in the Australian Trial. However, one can also make an equally strong argument to aggressively treat other risk factors independent of the treatment of hypertension.

Oftentimes, the treatment for hyperlipidemia, hyperglycemia, and hypertension are one and the same, namely, exercise, caloric restriction, and a low-fat diet.

In sum, therapy for patients with mild hypertension should be started whenever the diagnosis is established utilizing multiple blood pressure readings over time. Drug therapy for moderate hypertension (average diastolic blood pressure equals 105-114 mm Hg) should, in most cases, be initiated as soon as the diagnosis is firmly established. In those with mild hypertension (average diastolic blood pressure equals 90-104 mm Hg) a reasonable trial period of about 6 months should be adopted during which nonpharmacologic therapy alone is utilized, because a large percent-age of such patients will show a decrease in blood pressure over time. A persistent elevation in diastolic blood pressure above 90 mm Hg that does not respond to these nonpharmacologic treatments should then be treated with drugs that lower pressure and cause the least amount of adverse metabolic disturbances. The following sections will deal with the details of nonpharmacologic and pharmacologic therapies of hypertension.

Nonpharmacologic Therapy

There is increasing interest in treating patients with mild, moderate, and severe hypertension by nonpharmacologic means to avoid the cost, side effects, and mortality associated with drugs. A number of approaches merit review and considerations: sodium restriction, weight reduction, fat restriction, exercise, behavioral training, and potassium administration.

Sodium Restriction

Severe sodium restriction (10 meq/day) was shown to lower blood pressure of patients with malignant hypertension over 40 years ago (Kempner, 1955). A more modest reduction of sodium intake to about 100 meq/day also appears to lower blood pressure (Morgan et al., 1978; Parijs, Joossens, Van der Linden, Verstekeen, & Amery, 1977). Although these reports have been justly criticized, a double-blind, randomized, crossover study by MacGregor et al. (1978) has clearly shown the importance of sodium restriction alone in blood pressure control (see Figure 17.2). This study indicated that a sodium-restricted diet lowered blood pressure by 13/5 mm Hg, a fall that remained when placebo sodium tablets were added to the regimen over a 4-week period. This was followed by an increase in blood pressure of 10/8 mm Hg when 70-80 meq of Na was added to the low-salt dietary regimen (MacGregor et al., 1978). This experiment demonstrates the effect of a sodium-restricted diet of slightly less than 100 meq of sodium per day (from 191 meq) on blood pressure. Furthermore, its double-blind design, controlling for a variety of other variables, makes criticism of the study's conclusion difficult.

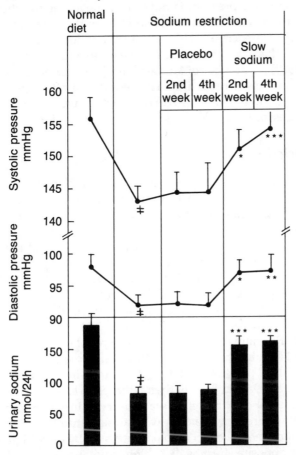

Figure 17.2. Average systolic and diastolic blood pressure and urinary sodium excretion on normal diet, two weeks after dietary sodium restriction, and at biweekly intervals during the randomized crossover trial of slow sodium b. placebo. ***p < 0.001; **p < 0.01; *p < 0.05 comparing equivalent measurement on slow sodium to placebo. ‡p < 0.001 comparing measurement on normal diet to two weeks of dietary sodium restriction. *Note.* From "Double-Blind Randomized Cross-Over Trial of Moderate Sodium Restriction in Essential Hypertension" by G.A. MacGregor et al., 1982, *Lancet,* **1**, p. 351. Copyright 1982 by *Lancet.* Reprinted by permission.

Weight Reduction

In the Framingham study it has been shown that a 1% increase or decrease in weight is followed by a corresponding 1% increase or decrease in blood pressure (Kannel, Brand, Skinner, et al., 1967). That this effect of weight on blood pressure is not due to the artifactual effect on blood pressure of too small a cuff is apparent from the observations of many that obesity is associated with a higher morbidity from hypertension-related sequelae such as strokes and heart attacks (Chiang, Perlman, & Epstein, 1969). A number of studies have been conducted to quantitate this effect of weight reduction. The recent and often quoted study by Reisen, Abel, Modan, et al. (1978) reported an average 26/20 mm Hg fall in blood pressure for a 20-lb decrease in body weight.

Fat Restriction

Epidemiological studies have suggested a small blood pressure lowering effect of vegetarian diets, which are reportedly low in saturated fat (S) and high in polyunsaturated fat (P), fiber, and potassium (Rouse, Armstrong, & Beilin, 1983; Sacks, Rosner, & Kass, 1974). A carefully controlled study of the effect of fat itself on blood pressure was carried out by Pruska, Iacono, Nissinen, Korhonen, and Vartiainen (1983). They studied 57 couples living in two communities in North Karelia, Finland. The couples were randomly allocated to one of three groups: (a) a regular Finnish diet (114 g of fat, P/S ratio 0.2); (b) a regular Finnish diet but low in sodium (77 meq/24 h); and (c) a special diet low in fat but not sodium-restricted (51 g of fat, P/S ratio 0.98). These diets were followed for 6 weeks, after which the 114 subjects reverted to their usual diets. Results are seen in Table 17.3. Blood pressure declined significantly in the fat-restricted group by an average of 9.7 mm Hg but then returned to baseline with the group's return to a usual diet; no effect was observed in the other two groups. These findings are in agreement with animal studies that have demonstrated an incremental effect on blood pressure by diets high in saturated fat, and the opposite effect by diets high in polyunsaturated fats (Dusing, Scherhag, Glanzer, Budde, & Kramer, 1983).

Exercise

In general, people who are physically fit have lower blood pressure than those who are not (Cooper, Pollack, Martin, et al., 1976). This effect, however, could be due to the fact that such individuals have less adipose tissue. In this regard, Franklin, Buskirk, Hodgson, et al. (1979) have shown that an exercise regimen administered to a group of obese middle-aged women caused both weight loss and a fall in blood pressure. In another study (Choquette & Ferguson, 1973) of patients with hyperkinetic circulations, a 6-month conditioning program was associated with a 15/8-mm Hg fall in blood pressure. The blood pressure changes, however, were not related to changes in body weight. Similar effects on blood pressure were obtained by Boyer and Kasch (1970) who, using a 6-month conditioning program, observed a fall in blood pressure of 13/12 mm Hg. There was an average weight loss of only 2.5 lb. Roman, Camuzzi, Villalon, and Klenner (1981), in a study of 30 hypertensive patients whose medication had been discontinued, observed an impressive fall in blood pressure of 21/16 mm Hg after 3 months of intensive physical training at 70% of aerobic capacity. They also observed a return of blood pressure to baseline levels during 3 months of deconditioning. In a study of over 14,000 college alumni, Paffenbarger, Wing, Hyde, and Jung (1983) obtained blood pressure data on individuals 16-50 years after college graduation. Whereas participation in sports in college had no effect on the subsequent development of hypertension, those alumni who were engaged in vigorous sports as adults had a 35% less chance of developing hypertension. In addition to the lack of strenuous exercise, higher levels of body mass index, weight gain since college, and history of parental hypertension all predicted increased risk of hypertension.

Table 17.3 Effect of a High Polyunsaturated Low-Fat Diet on Blood Pressure

Group	Content of diet	Change in BP
Low-fat	51g fat*, 172 meq Na⁺	−7/4
Low-salt	114g fat, 77 meq Na⁺	0/1
Control	107g fat, 192 meq Na⁺	1/1

*P/S changed from 0.27 to 0.98. *Note.* From "Controlled, Randomized Trial of the Effect of Dietary Fat on Blood Pressure" by Pruska et al., January 1983, *Lancet.* Copyright 1983 by *Lancet.* Reprinted by permission.

Behavioral Training

Two behavioral methods for treating hypertension have received the most recent attention. These are biofeedback and relaxation training. Neither can be regarded, however, as a substitute for medication in everyday management of hypertensive patients. In order for biofeedback to be effective, it needs to be administered at frequent (biweekly) intervals and for long periods of time before changes are observed. In one study (Krisst & Engel, 1975) an 18/8-mm Hg fall in blood pressure was obtained. Other reports have been disappointing (Frankel, Patel, Horwitz, et al., 1978). As for relaxation training, impressive results have been obtained, although placebo effects are not always easy to control (Shapiro, Schwartz, Ferguson, et al., 1977).

Potassium Administration

Studies in animals have shown that potassium administration blunts the rise in blood pressure associated with sodium loadings (Dahl, Leith, & Heine, 1972; Louis, Tobei, & Spector, 1971); and from epidemiologic studies in man, it has been observed that low-sodium and high-potassium intakes are associated with lower blood pressure (Denton, 1982; Gleibermann, 1973; Meneely & Battabee, 1976). Within communities, for example, there is a direct relationship between potassium excretion, the sodium/potassium ratio in urine, and blood pressure. Plasma potassium also has been found to be inversely related to blood pressure (Davies et al., 1979) and potassium administration to normotensive subjects for 1 month was associated with a small but significant fall in blood pressure (Khaw & Thom, 1982).

There are only two controlled studies of potassium supplementation in hypertensives (potassium intake was approximately doubled), and both studies showed a small but significant fall in blood pressure (Iimura, Kijima, Kituchi, et al., 1981; MacGregor, Smith, Markandu, Banks, & Sagnella, 1982). The question arises: How should physicians attempt to increase potassium intake in patients with high blood pressure? Is it desirable to prescribe potassium medication and to promote the sale of over-the-counter potassium, in view of the potential cardiac hazard of hyperkalemia? At the present time the answer is no. More appropriately, an increase in potassium intake should be encouraged through diet. In more recent times, we have witnessed the reduction in fruit and vegetable consumption and an increase in the consumption of more processed foods, accounting for a decrease over the past century in our intake of potassium from an estimated 100-250 meq/day to the current intake of 30-80 meq/day (MacGregor, 1983).

Other Factors

Increased dietary fiber has also been suggested as a factor that reduces blood pressure. Such studies, however, are far from convincing. It has been clearly shown that the excessive intake of alcohol as well as certain sympathomimetic drugs used to treat nasal congestion and obesity may increase blood pressure. Furthermore, there is evidence that nonsteroidal antiinflammatory compounds may also raise blood pressure.

Pharmacologic Treatment of Hypertension

The most popular approach to the drug treatment of hypertension is the stepped-care method (Moser, Guyther, Rinnerty, et al., 1980), recommended by the Joint National Committee for the Detection and Treatment of Hypertension (see Table 17.4). With this approach therapy begins with a diuretic. If blood pressure remains uncontrolled on this regimen, nondiuretic drugs are added, most commonly sympatholytic agents such as reserpine, methyldopa, clonidine, and beta-blockers. If blood pressure still remains elevated, vasodilators and other agents can be added as well. Using the stepped-care method, Moser points out that close to 90% of his patients experienced control of their blood pressure.

An alternative approach to the therapy of hypertension has recently received much attention in view of some of the problems believed related to drug therapy, namely, the higher mortality attributed to diuretic-induced hypokalemia, and the metabolic aberrations produced by diuretics and other hypertensive agents on carbohydrate and lipid metabolism (Ames, 1983; Cutler, 1983). In Table 17.5 is a list of antihypertensive drugs found to have adverse effects on serum lipids. These include diuretics such as hydrochlorothiazide and chlorthalidone as well as sympatholytic agents such as alphamethyl dopa and beta-blockers, excluding pindolol. With the exception of HDL cholesterol, the primary effect of these agents is to increase total and/or LDL cholesterol. Fortunately, some antihypertensive agents seem to have a beneficial effect on serum lipids (see Table 17.6). These include prazosin and pindolol, which increase HDL cholesterol; captopril, which blunts the adverse effects of diuretics on total serum cholesterol; clonidine and prazosin, which lower total serum cholesterol and blunt the effect of the diuretic-induced increase; and spironolactone and amiloride, which, unlike thiazide diuretics, have no adverse effect on serum cholesterol. Because of the failure of the potassium-sparing spironolactone and amiloride to raise serum cholesterol, coupled with a similar effect of captopril, also a potassium-sparing drug, it is tempting to speculate that potassium depletion may contribute to the hyperlipidemic effect of thiazide diuretics. The effects of sympatholytic agents on cholesterol would appear to be unrelated to potassium depletion, although catecholamines have been noted to have effects on potassium transport across cell membranes (Epstein & Rosa, 1983).

Table 17.4 Stepped-Care Therapy for Hypertension

Step	Drug

1.	Diuretic (in majority of cases):
	   Thiazide and thiazide derivatives
	   Potassium-sparing agents, if indicated*
	      Amiloride (Midamore)
	      Spironoclactone (Aldactone)
	      Triamterene (Dyrenium)

2.	Andrenergic-inhibiting agent:
	   Clonide (Catapres)
	   Guanabenz (Wytensin)
	   Methyldopa (Aldomet)
	   Rauwolfia alkaloid (reserpine)
	   Beta-adrenergic blocking agents
	      Atenolol (Tenormin)
	      Metoprolol (Lopressor)
	      Nadolol (Corgard)
	      Pindolol (Viskin)
	      Propanolol (Inderal)
	      Timolol (Blocadren)
	   Guanadrel sulphate (Hylorel)
	   Captopril (Capoten)⁺

3.	Hydralazine (Apresoline) Prazosin (Minipress) Captopril (Capoten)⁺
4.	Guanethidine (Ismelin) Minoxidil (Loniten) Captopril⁺

*Usually given in combination with a thiazide
⁺May be used as a step 2, 3, or 4 agent.

In view of these and other possible effects of antihypertensive drugs, it is recommended that the following principles be adopted when treating patients with hypertension:

1. Use diuretic therapy regularly for blacks and older hypertensives (> 50 years of age), because such individuals are more salt sensitive and thus will not respond to regimens that exclude diuretics.

2. Limit the dose of diuretic therapy (50 mg of hydrochlorothiazide or 25 mg of chlorthalidone should be the maximum dose, at which point Step 2 and 3 drugs should be added if the stepped-care method is followed.
3. Prevent hypokalemia by the use of a high-potassium diet that includes fruits, vegetables, and salt substitutes that contain potassium; preference should be given to k-sparing diuretics wherever possible.
4. Encourage the use of nonpharmacologic therapy (exercise and a low-fat, high-potassium diet) to minimize or even eliminate the need for large doses of medication.
5. Try monotherapy with clonidine, prazosin, and beta-blockers such as pindolol first for younger hypertensives (> 40 years of age); failure to respond to these agents should prompt the use of a diuretic as outlined above.
6. Make sure that Step 2 therapy, when added to diuretics, favors drugs such as pindolol, clonidine, prazosin, and captopril because of their more benign effect on serum lipids.

Finally, the goal of therapy should not be forgotten. The important thing is to decrease blood pressure to as low a level as possible without producing harm, metabolic aberrations, or troublesome side effects. In addition, it is important to the level of both systolic and diastolic blood pressure. At the same time, other risk factors should be treated separately and aggressively; they are equally important, especially hyperglycemia, hypercholesterolemia, obesity, and low levels of HDL cholesterol.

Table 17.5   Antihypertensive Drugs That Have Adverse Effects on Serum Lipids

Drug	Serum lipid effect	References
Hydrochlorothiazide Polythiazide Chorthalidone	Increase T cholesterol, LDL cholesterol, and triglycerides	Ames & Hill, 1976; Gluck et al., 1980; Goldman et al., 1980; Grim et al., 1981; Johnson et al., 1974; Schoenfield & Goldberger, 1964.
Alphamethyl dopa	Lowers HDL cholesterol	Ames & Hill, 1982
Beta-blockers*	Lower HDL cholesterol	Cutler, 1983

*excluding pindolol

Table 17.6 Antihypertensive Drugs That Have a Beneficial or No Adverse Effect on Serum Lipids

Drug	Serum lipid effect	References
Prazosin	Lowers triglycerides, LDL cholesterol; increases ratio of HDL cholesterol to T cholesterol; lowers T cholesterol	Leren et al., 1978 Kirkendall et al., 1978
Clonidine	Lowers T cholesterol	Kirkendall et al., 1978
Pindolol	Increased HDL cholesterol	Cutler, 1983
Captopril	Blunts elevation in cholesterol produced by hydrochlorothiazide	Weinberger, 1982, 1983
Spironolactone	None	Ramsay et al., 1980
Amiloride	None	Ramsay et al., 1980

References

Ames, R.P. (1983). Negative effects of diuretic drugs on metabolic risk factors for coronary heart disease: Possible alternative drug therapies. *American Journal of Cardiology, 51*(4), 632-643.

Ames, R.P., & Hill, P. (1976). Increase in serum lipids during treatment of hypertension with chlorthalidone. *Lancet, 1,* 721.

Ames, R.P., & Hill, P. (1982). Antihypertensive therapy and the risk of coronary heart disease. *Journal of Cardiovascular Pharmacology, 4*(Suppl. 2), S206-S212.

Australian National Blood Pressure Study Management Committee. (1980). The Australian therapeutic trial in mild hypertension. *Lancet, 1,* 1261-1267.

Boyer, J.L., & Kasch, F.W. (1970). Exercise therapy in hypertensive men. *Journal of the American Medical Association, 211*(10), 1668-1670.

Chiang, B.N., Perlman, L.V., & Epstein, F.E. (1969). Overweight and hypertension: A review. *Circulation, 39,* 403.

Chobanian, A.V. (1983, August). Treatment of mild hypertension: The debate intensifies. *Journal of Cardiovascular Medicine.*

Choquette, G., & Ferguson, R.J. (1973). Blood pressure reduction in "borderline" hypertensives following physical training. *Canadian Medical Association Journal, 108,* 699.

Cooper, K.H., Pollack, M.H., & Martin, R.P. (1976). Physical fitness levels vs. selected coronary risk factors: A cross-sectional study. *Journal of the American Medical Association, 236*, 166.

Cutler, R. (1983). Effect of antihypertensive agents on lipid metabolism. *American Journal of Cardiology, 51*(4), 628-631.

Dahl, L.K., Leith, G., & Heine, M. (1972). Influence of dietary potassium and sodium/potassium molar ratios on the development of salt hypertension. *Journal of Experimental Medicine, 136*, 318-330.

Davies, D.L., McElroy, K., Atkinson, A.B., Brown, J.J., & Cimming, A.M.M. (1979). Relationship between exchangeable sodium and blood pressure in different forms of hypertension in man. *Clinical Science, 57*, 69s-75s.

Denton, D. (1982). *The hunger for salt: An anthropological, physiological and medical analysis.* New York: Springer-Verlag.

Dusing, R., Scherhag, R., Glanzer, K., Budde, U., & Kramer, H.J. (1983). Effect on changes in dietary prostaglandin precursor fatty acids on arterial blood pressure and vascular prostacyclin synthesis. *Advances in Prostaglandin, Thromboxane, and Leukotrien Research, 12*, 209-215.

Epstein, R.H., & Rosa, R.M. (1983). Adrenergic control of serum potassium. *New England Journal of Medicine, 309*(23), 1450-1451.

Frankel, B.L., Patel, D.J., & Horwitz, D. (1978). Treatment of hypertension with biofeedback and relaxation techniques. *Psychosomatic, 40*, 276.

Franklin, B., Buskirk, E., & Hodgson, J. (1979). Effects of physical conditioning on cardiorespiratory function, body composition and serum lipids in relatively normal-weight and obese middle-aged women. *International Journal of Obesity, 3*, 97.

Freis, E.D. (1982). Sounding board: Should mild hypertension be treated? *New England Journal of Medicine, 307*(5), 306-310.

Gifford, R.W., Jr., Borhani, N., Krishan, I., Moser, M., Levy, R., & Schoenberger, J.A. (1983). The dilemma of 'mild' hypertension: Another viewpoint of treatment. *Journal of the American Medical Association, 250*(23), 3171-3173.

Gleibermann, L. (1973). Blood pressure and dietary salt in human populations. *The Ecology of Food and Nutrition, 2*, 143-155.

Gluck, Z., Weidmann, P., Mordasini, R., Bachman, C., Riesen, W., Peheim, E., Keusch, G., & Meier, A. (1980). Increased serum low-density lipoprotein cholesterol in men treated short-term with the diuretic chlorthalidone. *Metabolism, 29*, 240.

Goldman, A.I., Steele, B.W., Schnaper, H.W., Fitz, A.E., Froclich, E.D., & Perry, H.M., Jr. (1980). Serum lipoprotein levels during chlorthalidone therapy. *Journal of the American Medical Association, 244*, 1691.

Grimm, R.H., Jr., Leon, A.S., Hunninghake, D.B., Lenz, K., Hannan, P., & Blackburn, H. (1981). Effects of thiazide diuretics on plasma lipids and lipoproteins in midly hypertensive patients: A double-blind controlled trial. *Annals of Internal Medicine, 94*, 7.

Helgeland, (1980). Treatment of mild hypertension: A five-year controlled drug trial. The Oslo Study. *American Journal of Medicine*, 725-732.

Holland, O.B., Nixon, J.V., & Kuhnert, L. (1981). Diurectic-induced ventricular ectopic activity. *American Journal of Medicine, 70*, 762-768.

Hypertension Detection and Follow-up Program Cooperative Group. (1979). Five-year findings of the hypertension detection and follow-up program: II. Mortality by race, sex and age. *Journal of the American Medical Association, 242*, 2572-2576.

Iimura, O., Kijima, T., & Kituchi, K. (1981). Studies on the hypotensive effect of high potassium intake in patients with essential hypertension. *Clinical Science, 61*, 77s-80s.

Johnson, B., Bye, C., Labrooy, I., Munro-Faure, D., & Slack, J. (1974). The relation of antihypertensive treatment to plasma lipids and other vasular risk factors in hypertension. *Clinical Science and Molecular Medicine, 47*, 9.

Kannel, W.B., Brand, N., & Skinner, J.J. (1967). Overweight and hypertension: The Framingham study. *Annals of Internal Medicine, 67*, 48.

Kaplan, N. (1973). *Clinical hypertension*. New York: Medcom Press.

Kaplan, N. Mild hypertension: When and how to treat. *Archives of Internal Medicine, 143*, 255-259.

Kempner, W. (1955). Treatment of kidney disease and hypertensive vascular disease with rice diet. *North Carolina Medical Journal, 5*, 125-133.

Khaw, K.T., & Thom, S. (1982). Randomized double-blind cross-over trial of potassium on blood pressure in normal subjects. *Lancet, 2*, 1127-1129.

Kirkendall, W.M., Hammond, J.J., & Thomas, J.C. (1978). Prazosin and clonidine for moderately severe hypertension. *Journal of the American Medical Association, 240*(23), 2553.

Krisst, D.A., & Engel, B.T. (1975). Learned control of blood pressure inpatients with high blood pressure. *Circulation, 51*, 370.

Leren, P., Foss, P.O., Helgeland, A., Hjermann, I., Holme, I., & Lund-Larsen, P.G. (1980). Effect of propranolol and prazosin on blood lipids: The Oslo study. *Lancet, 2*, 4-6.

Louis, W.J., Tobei, R., & Spector, S. (1971). Effects of sodium intake on inherited hypertension in the rat. *Lancet, 2*, 1283-1286.

MacGregor, G.A. (1982, April). Dietary sodium and potassium intake and blood pressure. *Lancet*, 750-753.

MacGregor, G.A., Best, F.E., Can, J.M., Makandic, N.D., Elder, D.M., Sagnella, S.A., & Squires, M. (1982). Double-blind randomized cross-over trial of moderate sodium restriction in essential hypertension. *Lancet, 1*, 351.

MacGregor, G.A., Smith, S.J., Markandu, N.D., Banks, R.A., & Sagnella, G.A. (1982). Moderate potassium supplementation in essential hypertension. *Lancet, 2,* 567-570.

Meneely, G.R., & Battabee, H.D. (1976). High sodium-low potassium environment and hypertension. *American Journal of Cardiology, 38,* 768-785.

Morgan, T., Gillies, A., Morgan, G., Adam, W., Wilson, M., & Carney, S. (1978). Hypertension treated by salt restriction. *Lancet, 1,* 227.

Moser, M., Guyther, J.R., & Rinnerty, F. (1980). Report of the joint national committee on detection, evaluation and treatment of high blood pressure. *Archives of Internal Medicine, 140,* 1280-1285.

Multiple Risk Factor Intervention Trial. (1982). Risk factor changes and mortality results. *Journal of the American Medical Association, 248,* 1465-1477.

Paffenbarger, R.S., Wing, S.L., Hyde, R.T., & Jung, D.L. (1983). Physical activity and incidence of hypertension in college alumni. *American Journal of Epidemiology, 117*(3), 245-257.

Parjs, J., Joossens, J.V., Van der Linden, L., Versteken, G., & Amery, A. (1977). Moderate sodium restriction and diurectics in the treatment of hypertension. *American Heart Journal, 85,* 22.

Pruska, P., Iacono, J.M., Nissinen, A., Korhonen, H.J., & Vartianen, E. (1983, January). Controlled, randomized trial of the effect of dietary fat on blood pressure. *Lancet,* 1-5.

Ram, C.V. (1983) Should mild hypertension be treated? *Annals of Internal Medicine, 99,* 403-405.

Ramsay, L.E., Hettiarachchi, J., Fraser, R., & Morton, J.J. (1980). Amiloride, spironolactone, and potassium chloride in thiazide-treated hypertensive patients. *Clinical Pharmacology Therapy,* 533-543.

Reisin, E., Abel, R., & Modan, M. (1978). Effect of weight loss without salt restriction on the reduction of blood pressure in overweight hypertensive patients. *New England Journal of Medicine, 298,* 1.

Roman, O., Camuzzi, A.L., Villalon, E., & Klenner, C. (1981). Physical training program in arterial hypertension: A long-term prospective follow-up. *Cardiology, 67,* 230-243.

Rouse, I.L., Armstrong, B.K., & Beilin, L.J. (1983). The relationship of blood pressure to diet and lifestyle in two religious populations. *Journal of Hypertension, 1,* 65-71.

Sacks, F.M., Rosner, B., & Kass, E.H. (1974). Blood pressure in vegetarians. *American Journal of Epidemiology, 100,* 390-398.

Shoenfeld, M.R., & Goldberger, E. (1964). Hypercholesterolemia induced by thiazides: A pilot study. *Current Therapy Research, 6,* 180.

Shapiro, A.P., Schwartz, G.E., & Ferguson, D.C.E. (1977). Behavioral methods in treatment of hypertension: A review of their clinical status. *Annals of Medicine, 86,* 626.

Society of Actuaries and Association of Life Insurance Medical Directors of America. (1980). *Build and blood pressure study, 1979.* Chicago: Author.

United States Public Health Service Hospitals Cooperative Study Group. (1977). Treatment of mild hypertension: Results of a ten-year intervention trial. *Circulation Research, 40* (Suppl. 1), 98-105.

Veterans Administration Cooperative Study Group on Antihypertensive Agents. (1970). Effects of treatment on morbidity in hypertension: II. Results in patients with diastolic blood pressure averaging 90-114 mm Hg. *Journal of the American Medical Association, 213,* 1143-1152.

Weinberger, M.H. (1982). Comparison of captopril and hydrochlorothiazide alone and in combination in mild to moderate essential hypertension. *British Journal Clinical Pharmacology, 14,* 127S-131S.

Weinberger, M.H. (1983). Influence of an angiotensin converti-g-enzyme inhibitor on diuretic-induced metabolic effects in hypertension. *Hypertension, 5.*

The author wishes to acknowledge the contribution of Cheryl Duffy for her secretarial expertise.

Chapter 18

Pharmacologic and Nonpharmacologic Intervention for Dyslipidemias

Patrick McBride
Steven N. Blair

In this chapter we review evidence for the efficacy of various pharmacologic and nonpharmacologic interventions on elevated lipids and lipoproteins. A recent NIH consensus conference (National Institutes of Health Consensus Conference, 1985) has stated that beyond any reasonable doubt elevated serum cholesterol is a major risk factor for the development of CAD and that reduction of CAD risk can be achieved by lowering elevated serum cholesterol. Most clinicians probably now support drug treatment for individuals with clearly elevated plasma cholesterol. There is much less agreement over the desirability of intervention for the majority of individuals with lipids in the *normal* range (frequently defined as values within the mean ± 2 s.d.). Our view is that the mass hyperlipidemia of Western society and the resultant epidemic of coronary heart disease (CHD) are due to imprudent living habits, not to some basic metabolic defect requiring high technology medical intervention.

Henry Blackburn (1980) has written about the academic, clinical, and public health viewpoints of atherosclerosis. Academicians are primarily concerned with basic mechanisms of disease at the molecular and cellular level. Clinicians try to diagnose precisely the causes for each patient's atherosclerosis and to devise a proper treatment. The public health view attempts to recognize the cause of disease in large populations, considers the problem or how to manage atherosclerosis outside the traditional medical model, and places a strong emphasis on prevention. We espouse this last position (as does Blackburn). Atherosclerosis in the population is not likely to be managed successfully by medical approaches, although the medical model will continue to be effective in treating known cases of disease. The problems of mass pharmacologic intervention for hyperlipidemia are numerous. Depending on the definition of an optimal cholesterol level, tens of millions of Americans might be considered to be candidates for cholesterol lowering. The expense, logistic problems, and potential side effects make it clear that nonpharmacologic intervention is preferred, except in relatively rare clinical decisions. There is considerable evidence that weight loss and prevention of obesity are causally related to blood lipids. We will review the evidence for this association and for other nonpharmacologic treatments for hyperlipidemia. As public health professionals we have a strong preventive orientation and therefore prefer hygienic measures for treatment of hyperlipidemia. We view pharmacologic intervention as a method of last resort, after nonpharmacologic attempts have failed.

Biochemistry of Lipids

Lipids are critically important components to the human organism. Lipids are found in a variety of types and locations in the human body. They perform a number of essential functions in the body, including the transport and storage of body fuel, hormone production, and cell membrane formation, to name just a few.

Lipids are water-insoluble components of cells that can be extracted by nonpolar solvents (such as ether or benzene). Long chains of hydrocarbons characterize their structure. Complete discussions and illustrations of their structures can be found in any major biochemistry text (Lehninger, 1978). We will attempt to clarify here the information most important and practical to understanding the problems of hyperlipidemia.

Structure, Function, and Measurement of Lipoproteins

Dietary fats are absorbed in the small intestine through small lymphatic channels and converted in intestinal cells into hybrids of lipid and protein called lipoproteins. This aids in their transport through the bloodstream as they form structures that, by their change in polarity, are stable.

Human plasma lipoproteins are divided into classes based on their density and particle size. There are subclasses of these groups based on size and composition of the proteins in their structure (see Table 18.1).

Table 18.1   Subclasses of Plasma Lipoprotein

Characteristic	Chylomicrons	VLDL	LDL	HDL
Particle Size (nm)	75–1000	30–50	20–22	7.5–1.0
Density	< 0.94	0.94–1.006	1.006–1.063	1.063–1.21
% cholesterol	3–7	15	45	18
% triglyceride	80–95	55–65	10	3
% protein	1–2	10	25	45–55

Note. From *Biochemistry* by A.L. Lehninger, 1978, New York: Worth. Copyright 1978 by Worth. Adapted by permission.

Apoproteins.   Apoproteins are proteins associated with specific lipoprotein classes. Seven apoproteins have been identified and all are present in chylomicrons. The role of apoproteins in identifying persons at risk for heart disease has become increasingly clear and it is suggested that apoproteins may be better predictors of coronary disease than the lipoproteins. While apoproteins are not advocated for routine screening and are not available in most clinical situations, they may be useful in the near future. It is important to know at this time for research purposes, at least, which apoproteins are associated with which lipoproteins. Apoprotein A-I and A-II are associated with the HDLs and chylomicrons. Apoprotein B is associated with the VLDL and LDL lipoproteins. Apoproteins C-I, C-II, and C-III are associated with the VLDL, LDLD, and chylomicron classes. Apoprotein E has been associated with the chylomicrons, VLDL, and HDL. Several specific disorders have been identified in individual patients with relatively normal cholesterol levels but abnormal apoproteins, which appears to be a significant risk factor for CAD.

Chylomicrons.   Chylomicrons contain triglycerides (TG). TG are three fatty acid molecules attached to the three hydroxyl groups of glycerol through esterification. Adipose and muscle cells utilize fats by a membrane-bound enzyme system mediated by lipoprotein lipase, which hydrolyzes the free fatty acids from the glycerol. Chylomicrons are at their highest concentration in plasma 2-4 hr after a meal and are cleared from the bloodstream in 10-12 hr.

Cholesterol.   Cholesterol is compounded from the chemical class called sterols and is converted into steroid hormones, bile acids, and cellular membranes. Cholesterol is formed in the liver and small intestine. Dietary cholesterol is also an important source of body cholesterol. If dietary cholesterol is high, liver synthesis of cholesterol decreases. If intake of fats (especially saturated fat) is high, the liver produces more cholesterol. Most of the total body cholesterol is found in cells, with less than 10% located in the plasma.

VLDL. VLDL (predominantly TG) are synthesized in the liver and are produced in larger amounts when excess calories are consumed. Other factors that may increase VLDL in some individuals are high-simple carbohydrate diets, increased ethonol intake, and ingestion of medium-chain triglycerides.

LDL. LDL is a breakdown product of VLDL after cleavage by lipoprotein lipase. LDL and LDL receptors are synthesized in the liver and both are responsible for cholesterol's entering into cells. LDL contains most of the cholesterol found in the serum.

IDL. IDL is a breakdown product of VLDL or chylomicrons. Elevation of IDL appears to be caused by a genetic lack of apoprotein E-III (Miller et al., 1981). This type of lipoprotein is found primarily in Type III hyperlipidemia.

HDL. HDL has received more recent attention in both scientific and lay literature than the other lipoprotein classes. HDL contains much less TG and cholesterol than LDL and probably acts to remove lipids from the bloodstream and perhaps the arterial wall, and returns them to the liver for degradation and excretion. HDL levels appear to be directly related to atherogenic protection. Three fractions of HDL are known and HDL_2 appears to be the primary antiatherogenic subfraction (Miller et al., 1981).

Dyslipidemia Classification

Measurement and classification of serum lipoproteins are based on serum measurements, lipoprotein electrophoresis, ultracentrifugation, and examination of refrigerated plasma. Electrophoresis and ultracentrifugation are commonly used to discern rare types of dyslipidemias. A simplified classification of the various types of dyslipidemias is shown in Table 18.2. Most information necessary to diagnose the type of dyslipidemia is available with measurement of serum triglyceride and cholesterol levels and by examining a serum sample after 12-14 hr of refrigeration. Diffuse cloudiness of refrigerated serum represents VLDL-C. If a creamy ring of fat is on top, chylomicrons are present in excess. If cholesterol is elevated but the serum remains clear, LDL-C is elevated. These techniques allow diagnosis of Type I, IIa, and V (Gotto, 1983; Sloan, 1983). Classification of dyslipidemias may be helpful in assessing risk and determining therapy for the individual. However, reduction in dietary fat is indicated on a population basis in countries consuming the usual Western society diet.

Type I.   Type I dyslipidemia is characterized by fasting chylomicronemia. Both lipoprotein lipase and its activator, apoprotein C-II, are absent. Common associated physical findings are abdominal pain, pancreatitis, and eruptive xanthomas. Atherogenesis is not commonly found here.

Type II.   Type II dyslipidemias are characterized by elevated LDL-C but are subclassified into Types II-a and II-b as VLDL-C are also high in Type II-b. These types are relatively common, and the risk for coronary artery disease is quite high. Tendon xanthomas, xanthelasma, and corneal arcus are frequent physical findings associated with these disorders.

Type III.   This phenotype is rare, characterized by elevation of IDL-C. Total cholesterol and TG are also elevated. Ultracentrifugation is necessary for confirmation if this disorder is suspected. The uncommon physical finding of palmar xanthomas strongly supports the diagnosis of Type III dyslipidemia.

Type IV.   This dyslipidemia pattern is the most common lipid disorder. VLDL is elevated, with a corresponding increase in TG. This disorder is frequently associated with diabetes mellitus, hyperuricemia, and hypertension possibly due to a secondary association with obesity. There is a major risk of accelerated atherosclerosis.

Type V.   This disorder is uncommon and is diagnosed by elevation of both VLDL and chylomicrons. TG and cholesterol are elevated. Insulin may positively affect this disorder as it is an important cofactor in the lipoprotein lipase system. Lipoprotein lipase may be insufficient or defective in those with this phenotype. Abdominal pain, pancreatitis, hepatomegaly, and eruptive xanthomas are physical findings often associated with this disorder. A common pattern of dyslipidemia recently recognized and considered high risk characterizes those individuals with a very low HDL cholesterol. Many people with a low HDL cholesterol have modest elevations of total cholesterol and triglyceride which would otherwise seem to place them at only modest risk. However, the combination of a modestly elevated cholesterol and a very low HDL cholesterol causes a very high total cholesterol/HDL cholesterol level. High ratios of totals to HDL cholesterol have been noted in the Framingham Study to place persons at very high risk for the development of premature CAD (Miller et al., 1977).

Table 18.2 Simplified Classification of Hyperlipidemias

Phenotype	Elevated lipoprotein(s)	Elevated lipids
Type I	Chylomicrons	Triglycerides
Type IIa	LDL	Cholesterol
Type IIb	LDL VLDL	Cholesterol Triglycerides
Type IV	VLDL	Triglycerides
Type V	Chylomicrons VLDL	Triglycerides

It is important to remember that several diseases are associated with dyslipidemia and elevated cholesterol. These must be considered as causes of, or associated with, the above disorders. Secondary causes include diabetes mellitus, hypothyroidism, nephrotic syndrome, obstructive jaundice, and glycogen storage disease, among others.

Associations Between Lipoproteins and Atherosclerosis

Epidemiologic Studies

There is general agreement that the atherosclerotic disease epidemic in twentieth century Western society has multiple causes. Mass clinical disease has not arisen, however, unless a given population group follows the rich—high-fat, high-calorie, and high-cholesterol—diet typically seen in the United States. These populations also demonstrate mass hyperlipidemia with elevated total cholesterol and LDL-C. Thus hyperlipidemia appears to be a *sine qua non* for the development of atherosclerosis. Several excellent reviews on this topic are available (Blackburn, 1979; Keys, 1970; Stamler, 1979, 1980), so we will only comment on a few of the more important epidemiologic studies.

The seven countries' study by Keys (1970) demonstrates that around the world CHD is a major problem only in countries where the population levels of cholesterol are high. In this prospective cross-cultural study the correlation of baseline cholesterol to CHD death was $r = .65$. Countries with high CHD death rates (3/1,000 to 7/1,000/year) all had median cholesterol levels greater than 235 mg/dl. Countries with CHD death rates from .5/1,000 to 1.5/1,000/year had median cholesterol values of 200 mg/dl or lower. A 14-fold range in CHD death rate occurred in comparing Eastern Finland (median cholesterol = 265 mg/dl) and Ushibuka, Japan (median cholesterol = 141 mg/dl).

The investigators from five U.S. longitudinal studies on CHD (the Albany Civil Servant, Chicago Peoples Gas Company, Chicago Western Electric Company, Framingham Community, and Tecumseh Community studies) pooled their findings (The Pooling Project Research Group, 1978). Analysis of this very large data set showed a strong gradient of CHD risk by quintiles of baseline cholesterol. CHD risk was 18%, 96%, and 139% higher in quintiles III-V compared to quintiles I and II combined (cholesterol < 218 mg/dl).

The association of lipoprotein fractions and CHD has also been studied. In Framingham, low HDL-C was associated with increased risk of CHD in both men and women (Gordon, Castelli, Hjortland, Kannel, & Dawber, 1977). Furthermore, HDL-C was associated with CHD at older ages, although total cholesterol is not predictive of CHD in the later years. The results from Framingham are supported by other studies (Goldbourt & Medalie, 1979; Miller, Forde, Thelle, & Mjos, 1977). Elevated LDL-C in Framingham was also associated with increased risk of CHD (Gordon, Kannel, Castelli, & Dawber, 1981).

Epidemiologic studies on lipoproteins and CHD strongly support a causal inference. More than 30 prospective studies have been reported from around the world, and nearly all of them (> 85%) show that elevated baseline cholesterol is significantly associated with increased CHD risk. The associates are strong, show a dose-response relationship, are independent of other risk factors, and have predictive capacity. Predictive ability can likely be improved with current knowledge of the impact of cholesterol fractions. The epidemiologic findings are coherent with results from clinical and experimental lines of medical investigation.

Experimental Animal Studies

Animal studies have demonstrated convincingly that diets high in fats and cholesterol are a major factor in the development of atherogenesis. Even at dietary levels of fat with minimal elevations of serum cholesterol, atherosclerotic lesions developed. Feeding monkeys a usual American diet accelerated atherosclerosis compared to feeding those diets of cultures with lower fat intake (Stamler, 1980).

Other risk factors, such as hypertension and cigarette smoking, have been shown to be synergistic in the development of atherogenesis. In fact, hypercholesterolemia appears to be the primary factor in the development of atherosclerosis, whereas other factors are mainly adjuvants in its development. This is likely due to arterial injury combined with elevated serum cholesterol (Council on Scientific Affairs [CSA], 1983). Dietary therapy, with levels of fat recommended for treatment of hyper-cholesterolemia in humans, has caused regression of atherosclerotic lesions after they have developed in animal models (Gotto, 1981).

Clinical Trials

Definitive clinical trials on diet change and CHD have not been done. Owing to complexity and enormous cost, they may never be done. However, there have been a few clinical studies, and, in general, the results support the causal inference between hyperlipidemia and CHD.

A controlled diet intervention trial was conducted in two Finnish mental hospitals (Turpeinen, 1979). Patients in one hospital were given a diet low in saturated fats and cholesterol and the other hospital's patients were kept on the typical rich Western diet. After 6 years a cross-over occurred and the diets in the hospitals were switched. In both hospitals CHD incidence was about half as great when patients were following the prudent diet as compared to when they were on the rich diet.

The most convincing diet intervention trial yet published was conducted in Oslo (Hjerman, Velve Byre, Holme, & Leren, 1981). In this study 1,232 healthy high-risk, but normotensive, men were randomly assigned to intervention and control groups. These men had elevated cholesterol levels (290-380 mg/dl) and 79% smoked cigarettes. Men in the intervention group were given smoking cessation and diet change programs. After 5 years men in the intervention group had cholesterol levels 13% lower than controls. Smoking cessation occurred in both groups with a 25% quit rate in intervention men and 17% in controls. At the end of the 5-year follow-up, total CHD rates were 31/1,000 in the intervention group and 57/1,000 (p = .028) in the control group. Multivariate analyses suggested that the reduction in CHD incidence was influenced more by cholesterol reduction than by smoking cessation.

Two recent diet-heart studies have reinforced the significance of reducing dietary fat in the prevention of CAD. The Leiden Intervention Trial (Arntzenius, Kromhout, Barth, et al., 1985) indicated a vegetarian diet, low in cholesterol and high in polyunsaturated fat appeared to arrest the progress of coronary lesions in 18 of 39 patients with stable angina pectoris. This study showed that an increased consumption of poly-unsaturated fats can reduce ratios of total cholesterol to HDL cholesterol and that lower ratios of total to HDL cholesterol appear to be the limiting factor in the progression of stable coronary lesions.

The Ireland-Boston Diet-Heart Study (Kushi, Lew, Stare, et al., 1985) found a significant association between mortality from coronary artery disease and the composition of the diet. This study indicated that a low intake of saturated fatty acids and cholesterol, and a high intake of poly-unsaturated fatty acids and dietary fiber, appear to have contributed to a reduced coronary mortality among Irish-Bostonians as compared to brothers in Ireland. These studies add new information on the relation-ship of dietary intake to the progression, and mortality, of CAD.

Defining Dyslipidemia

Cardiovascular Risk (i.e., myocardial infarction or coronary death) has been shown to vary directly with plasma cholesterol level (CSA, 1983). This direct correlation shows a linear relation to risk and, therefore, *optimal* levels of plasma cholesterol are not necessarily *average* levels. Average U.S. cholesterol levels are higher than those in societies that have low rates of CHD. Mean total cholesterol levels of 140-180 mg/dl have been correlated to lowest risk of atherosclerosis and CHD. Risk increases proportionately above levels of 200 mg/dl and this value is thus considered to be the highest optimal level allowed before intervention. The decision of what level of cholesterol to treat is a complicated one, and only general guidelines can be given. In general, individuals with total cholesterol levels above 200 mg/dl should be advised to make appropriate hygienic lifestyle changes (low-fat diet, weight loss, increased physical activity, smoking cessation) in order to achieve more optimal blood lipid levels. If these hygienic measures are ineffective (after a 3- to 6-month trial), and the patient's total cholesterol remains above the 90th percentile for age and sex (approximately 250 mg/dl), pharmacologic therapy should be considered as an addition to nonpharmacologic intervention.

Treatment theory is based on levels associated with low risk for disease, cardiovascular or otherwise. These risks should be individualized and based on personal factors of the patient and carefully measured laboratory data. At least two measurements of blood lipid levels should be made due to laboratory imprecision and biologic variation. While total cholesterol levels are generally stable in relationship to meals, other lipoprotein classes are not as stable and need to be measured fasting. Therefore, if screening only for total cholesterol, fasting is not required. Other measurements should be several weeks apart and should be measured after an over-night 12- to 14-hr fast.

Nonpharmacologic Intervention

Several life-style factors are known to effect the lipoprotein profile. These factors include exercise, diet, weight loss, cigarette smoking, and alcohol intake. In this section we briefly review the epidemiological, clinical, and experimental evidence related to lifestyle and lipoproteins.

Exercise

The effect of exercise on blood lipids has been extensively investigated over the last 20-25 years. For most of that time researchers focused on total serum or plasma cholesterol and TG, although a few early papers did mention various cholesterol fractions (for a review see Wood & Haskell, 1979). Many of the early studies on exercise and blood lipids had serious design flaws such as lack of a control group, *very* short training period, inadequate laboratory quality control, samples of young athletes with already very low cholesterol levels, and lack of attention to potentially confounding factors such as diet or weight loss. In 1976, Naito (1976) reviewed more than 100 studies on exercise and cholesterol metabolism. At that time the results of published studies were conflicting, and no very clear effect of exercise could be documented convincingly.

Although some researchers had measured cholesterol fractions in studies going back to the 1950s, most individuals viewed this work as being of only academic interest with no significant practical application. The classic paper of Miller and Miller (1975) brought renewed interest to the study of cholesterol fractions. They reviewed several lines of evidence and suggested that low levels of HDL-C increase risk of CHD. After a possible mechanism was postulated for the clinical significance of low HDL-C levels, the search for factors effecting cholesterol fractions intensified.

Dr. Peter Wood and colleagues (Wood, Haskell, Stein, Lewis, & Perry, 1977) at Stanford University were among the first researchers to popularize the notion that exercise effects the lipoprotein profile. They reported that middle-aged men and women runners who ran an average of 37 and 31 mi/week, respectively, had lower levels of LDL-C and higher levels of HDL-C. These differences appeared to be independent of differences in adiposity or diet. The cross-sectional association between exercise and the lipoprotein profile has been reported in many studies. Hartung, Foreyt, Mitchell, Vlasek, and Gotto (1977) studied middle-aged men who were classified as inactive, joggers (averaged 11 mi/week), and marathoners (had completed a marathon, averaged 40 mi/week). There was a progressive association of lipoproteins by categories with inactive men having lower HDL-C, higher LDL-C, and lower HDL-C/TC ratios compared to marathoners. Joggers had intermediate values. Middle-aged women in the Lipid Research Clinic Prevalence Study who reported being physically active have higher levels of HDL-C than inactive women (Haskell, Taylor, Wood, Schrott, & Heiss, 1980). High levels of physical fitness (determined by maximal treadmill testing) were associated with high HDL-C and lower TC/HDL-C ratios in women at the Cooper Clinic (Gibbons, Blair, Cooper, & Smith, 1983). Total HDL can be further categorized with the analytical ultracentrifuge into HDL_2 and HDL_3; runners may also differ from control on cholesterol subfractions. Current theory holds that the less dense, larger particle size HDL_2 is the antiatherogenic component (Miller et al., 1981). Men and women runners have twice as much HDL_2 as nonrunners, but the groups do not differ on HDL_3 (Krauss et al., 1977).

Physical fitness and blood lipids are also associated in prospective studies. Our group found that middle-aged men who increased their maximal treadmill test time increased their HDL-C and decreased the TC/HDL-C ratio (Blair et al., 1983) (see Figures 18.1 and 18.2).

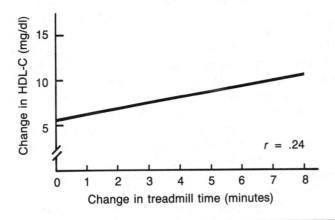

Figure 18.1. Change in treadmill time associated with change in HDL-C; adult men, Cooper Clinic.

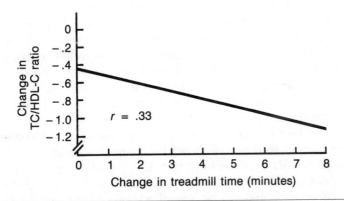

Figure 18.2. Change in treadmill time associated with change in TC/HDL-C ratio; adult men, Cooper Clinic.

It is widely believed that many runners are health nuts and may have diets different from nonrunners, thus at least partially accounting for lipid differences between the groups. We obtained 3-day food records from 61 men and women runners (running at least 15 mi/week) and from 80 randomly selected community controls (Blair et al., 1981). The food records were carefully obtained and coded by a nutritionist and were analyzed using USDA food composition data. We found very few qualitative differences in dietary intake between runners and nonrunners. Runners ate more calories to support their activity, but nutrients thought to effect blood lipids (fat and cholesterol) were the same in the two groups. Thus, we concluded that the large difference between runners and nonrunners in lipoprotein profiles was not likely to be due to diet.

The exercise-lipoprotein association has also been studied experimentally. A study at Stanford by Dr. Wood and co-workers has been reported (Williams, Wood, Haskell, & Uranizan, 1982; Wood, Haskell, Terry, Ho, & Blair, 1982; Wood, Haskell et al., 1983). This study was a one-year randomized clinical trial with 81 initially sedentary middle-aged men. The study had excellent laboratory quality control and extensive control for confounding variables. Results indicated that miles run was highly positively correlated with increases in HDL-C, HDL_2, and HDL-C/ TC ratios. LDL-C was negatively associated with miles run. These findings held after adjustment for weight change. An analysis of diet records indicated that there were no differential changes in the exercise group. A subset of these runners (N = 14) has been followed for 2 years, and the observed changes were maintained over the longer period (Wood et al., 1982). The results of this study suggest a dose-response effect for running. Furthermore, a threshold apparently exists at approximately 10 mi/week (Williams et al., 1982).

The results of epidemiological and cross-sectional laboratory studies in men and women are in agreement on the association between exercise and blood lipids. However, there are some puzzling results from an experimental study with both men and women subjects. Brownell, Bachorik, and Ayerle (1981) reported the expected increase in HDL-C in men subjects, but women in the same study showed a slight decrease in HDL-C. This study was relatively short-term (10 weeks) and perhaps longer followup would show different results. The effect of exercise on blood lipids in women needs further investigation.

In summary, there is congruence between cross-sectional epidemiological and clinical studies supported by changes seen in prospective epidemiological and experimental studies to support the hypothesis that regular physical activity effects the lipoprotein profile. Exercise has a minimal effect on total cholesterol because it appears to reduce LDL-C and increase HDL-C. Furthermore, most of the effect on HDL-C is probably on the apparently antiatherogenic component, HDL$_2$. Although the details are not yet available, tentative steps have been taken towards describing a mechanism by which exercise increases HDL-C (Nikkila, Taskinen, Rehunen, & Harkonen, 1978). Because regular exercise has other beneficial effects on health, it is reasonable to recommend it as a part of a healthy lifestyle, and specifically as a nonpharmacological intervention for hyperlipidemia.

Diet

The association between dietary intake and blood lipids is well established. Evidence for this relationship comes from cross-cultural observations, prospective epidemiological studies, clinical trials, and experiments with several animal species (including humans). There are several excellent reviews of the diet-lipoprotein association (Blackburn, 1980; Glueck, 1979; Keys, 1970), and only the main points will be discussed here.

Keys' (1970) classic studies in seven countries provide evidence that national diet is linked to plasma cholesterol. Populations that habitually consumed diets with 15% or more calories from saturated fat, such as Eastern Finland or the United States, also had elevated total plasma cholesterol (230 mg/dl or greater). A large body of epidemiological evidence supports the hypothesis that the high-calorie, high-fat (especially saturated fat), and high-dietary cholesterol diet of many Western countries is a primary cause of epidemic hyperlipidemia (Keys, 1970; Stamler, 1980).

Shekelle et al. (1981) observed diet and serum cholesterol changes in a prospective epidemiological study. Dietary intake was assessed by standardized interview in 1,900 middle-aged men. Serum cholesterol was also measured. Two examinations were given, one year apart. Changes in diet composition, especially saturated fat and cholesterol, were significantly associated with changes in serum cholesterol.

The National Diet–Heart Study (1968) was a large, randomized, clinical study conducted in the 1960s. In this double-blind study, more than 2,000 middle-aged men were randomly assigned to experimental and control diets. Men receiving the experimental diets were given special foods in which the fat and cholesterol content had been altered. This study was well designed and was conducted with very high standards of quality control in all phases. The results conclusively demonstrated that free-living American men could make major reductions (10-15%) in their serum cholesterol levels by reducing saturated fat intake, increasing polyunsaturated fat intake, and reducing dietary cholesterol.

The Finnish Mental Hospital study (Turpeinen et al., 1979) also clearly showed that experimentally changing the diet of a group of subjects changes their serum cholesterol levels in a predictable way.

Experimental metabolic ward studies confirm the epidemiological studies and clinical trials' results on diet composition and serum cholesterol. As stated by Blackburn (1980), more than 100 well-controlled experimental studies on this issue have been published. These reports indicate that saturated fat intake has about two times the effect in elevating serum cholesterol as polyunsaturated fats have in lowering it. The metabolic ward studies also confirm the cholesterol raising potential of dietary cholesterol.

Much of the early work on the impact of the prudent diet (low saturated fat and cholesterol) was on total cholesterol. It is now clear that most of the effect of the prudent diet on total cholesterol is a result of lowering LDL-C (Gordon, Fisher, Ernst, Rifkind, & Little, 1980). HDL-C is not very responsive to dietary change, with the exception of alcohol intake (Ernst et al., 1980). VLDL-C may be effected by diet change, but is much more responsive to weight loss, however it is achieved.

Weight Control

Several cross-sectional surveys report on the association between body composition and plasma lipoproteins. Body composition has been estimated by various methods, from simple measures of weight to more complex procedures to estimate body fat, but the results are relatively consistent. Total cholesterol, LDL-C, and VLDL-C are directly associated with body fatness (Knuiman, West, & Burema, 1982; Phillips, Havel, & Kane, 1981). HDL-C is inversely associated with body composition (Phillips et al., 1981; Saloren et al., 1983).

We observed decreases in total cholesterol and increases in HDL-C with changes in weight in a prospective study (Blair et al., 1983). In a 1- to 6-year follow-up of 753 middle-aged men who lost an average of 1.7 lb, total cholesterol decreased 2.9 mg/dl and HDL-C increased 1.9 mg/dl. Although the average change was small, it was statistically significant ($p < .01$) and occurred in a population that had relatively favorable lipid values at baseline (total cholesterol = 206, HDL-C = 45). These changes remained after adjustment for age, length of follow-up, and changes in physical fitness.

Perhaps the strongest evidence for the impact of weight change on lipoproteins in a large free-living group is from the Multiple Risk Factor Intervention Trial (MRFIT) (Caggiula et al., 1981). MRFIT was a collaborative study on the prevention of heart disease in which 12,866 high-risk middle-aged men were randomly assigned to special intervention (SI) and referred care (RC) groups (MRFIT Research Group, 1982). SI men were intensively treated in special clinics to lower their risk factors, whereas RC men were simply told they were at risk and referred to their usual source of medical care. SI men were counseled to adopt the prudent diet, and if overweight, weight reduction advice was given (Caggiula et al., 1981). After 4 years the SI men had a mean weight loss of 3.3 lb, and 26% of them lost at least 10 lb. Lipid and lipoprotein changes in SI men over 4 years are shown in Table 18.3 for four weight change categories. Weight reduction was associated with increased HDL-C and decreased LDL-C and triglycerides. These data may be confounded in that the SI men were also receiving dietary counseling to reduce saturated fat and dietary cholesterol. Approximately 50% of the SI men were taking antihypertensive medication by year 4, and the diuretics used in MRFIT are known to increase total cholesterol levels (Grimm et al., 1981). The possible confounding did not vitiate the weight loss findings because additional stratified analyses found consistent lipid and lipoprotein changes in hypertensives and nonhypertensives, and in men who made changes in dietary intake and those who did not.

The MRFIT weight loss data are encouraging in that sizable beneficial changes in lipid and lipoproteins occurred in men who had relatively modest weight loss. Men who only lost 5-9 lb decreased their LDL-C by 6.6% (10 mg/dl) and their triglycerides by 10.6% (21 mg/dl), and increased their HDL-C by 3.3% (1.4 mg/dl). Participants who lost 10 lb or more had even more beneficial lipid and lipoprotein changes. Conversely, even modest increases in body weight were associated with deleterious changes in blood lipids (Caggiula et al., 1981).

Table 18.3   Change in Plasma Lipid and Lipoproteins in MRFIT SI Participants Over 4 Years by Weight Loss Categories

Lipoproteins	All participants baseline values (mg/dl)	Loss ≥ 10 lb	Loss 5-9 lb	Little change	Gain ≥ 5 lb
No. in category		1,391	922	1,899	1,096
LDL-C	162	−8.6%*	−6.6%	−5.8%	−5.1%
HDL-C	42	+4.9%	+3.3%	+0.4%	−2.4%
Triglycerides	203	−19.8%	−10.6%	−0.9%	+17.7%

*Values are % change from baseline. *Note.* From "The Multiple Risk Factor Intervention Trial (MRFIT): IV. Intervention on Blood Lipids" by A.W. Caggiula et al., 1981, *Preventive Medicine*, **10**. Copyright 1981 by *Preventive Medicine*. Reprinted by permission.

Weight Loss and Exercise

From the foregoing review it appears that both weight loss and adoption of vigorous exercise habits produce favorable changes in the lipoprotein profile. Multivariate analyses suggest that the effects of weight loss are independent (Blair et al., 1983; Wood, Haskell et al., 1983). Resolution of the issue, however, is not simple. Exercise is likely to also produce weight loss, but weight loss can also occur in the absence of increasing exercise habits. Williams et al. (1983) recently reported some intriguing analyses from a randomized clinical trial of exercise effects on lipoproteins. Both exercise and weight loss were independently associated with increases in HDL-C and HDL-C$_2$ in this study, as reported earlier (Wood, Haskell, et al., 1983). However, more detailed analyses by Williams et al. (1983) indicated that weight lost by the control group did not necessarily increase HDL-C or HDL-C$_2$. These results suggest the physiologic processes in weight loss produced by exercise may be different than by diet alone. The combined effect of exercise and weight loss is apparently greater than for either alone.

Smoking

Cigarette smoking may have an impact on lipids and lipoproteins. A report from the Framingham study on 4,107 men and women indicated reduction in HDL-C in cigarette smokers (Garrison et al., 1978). After adjusting for alcohol intake and body composition, HDL-C levels were about 6 mg/dl and 4 mg/dl lower in women and men, respectively. Former cigarette smokers who had been abstinent for at least a year and had not switched to cigars or pipes had HDL-C levels similar to nonsmokers.

Willett et al. (1983) report higher TG and total cholesterol and lower HDL-C in smoking compared to nonsmoking women aged 20-40 years. These results held after adjustment for age, height, weight, blood glucose, resting pulse, and oral contraceptive use. The HDL-C in smokers was 7 mg/dl lower, remarkably close to the value reported in the Framingham study.

Although cigarette smoking probably does not have a major impact on lipids and lipoproteins, and possible causal pathways are not well defined, stopping smoking may have a favorable impact, especially on HDL-C. Because there are numerous well-established reasons to stop smoking, we do not need absolute proof of an effect of smoking on lipids to recommend that a person using cigarettes discontinue. It is encouraging that in addition to other health benefits from smoking cessation, a more favorable lipoprotein profile may also result.

Alcohol

There is substantial evidence that alcohol consumption is associated with the lipoprotein profile, particularly the HDL-C fraction. In fact, alcohol ingestion had a greater influence on HDL-C than any other dietary component in the Lipid Research Clinic's Prevalence Study (Ernst et al., 1980). Castelli et al. (1977) also found cross-sectional correlations between alcohol intake and HDL-C in the Cooperative Lipoprotein Phenotyping Study. Correlations between HDL-C and alcohol consumption in several populations are about .20 (Castelli et al., 1977; Ernst et al., 1980). There appears to be a dose response effect, with a range of 10-12 mg/dl difference between nondrinkers and those consuming about 20 oz/week. Individuals who never drink have lower HDL-C levels than individuals who report drinking but who had not consumed any alcohol within the past week. The LRC report indicates that type of alcohol consumed is not important.

Alcohol intake has a modest inverse association with LDL-C and a modest positive association with triglycerides (Castelli et al., 1977). Because alcohol intake may cause beneficial changes in plasma lipoproteins by favorably altering the major factions (HDL-C and LDL-C), it is tempting to recommend moderate alcohol ingestion as a preventive approach for CHD. Most authorities have not done so, however, in view of the serious known side effects of excessive alcohol consumption. Furthermore, in the case of HDL-C, at least, it may be important to examine the subfractions. Alcohol intake is associated with an increase in HDL_3 instead of HDL_2 (Wood, Carnago et al., 1983). Although this is not thought to be harmful, it is also probably not helpful because it is HDL_2 that is reputed to be the antiatherogenic subfraction.

In a retrospective study Willett, Hennekens, Siegel, Adner, and Castelli (1980) found that the effects of alcohol and endurance running were additive. These results were not supported in an experiment by Hartung et al. (1983). In a well-controlled experiment Hartung et al. (1983) found that HDL-C was increased by drinking three cans of beer per day only in inactive men. HDL-C in marathon runners and joggers did not change with changes in alcohol intake. Thus, because exercise increases HDL_2, physical activity is probably a better way to improve the lipoprotein profile than by consuming alcoholic beverages.

Pharmacologic Intervention

The pharmacologic therapy for hyperlipidemia is an area of much controversy. Until recently no prospective study could demonstrate reduced risk of CHD using drugs and diet in a safe manner. The Lipid Research Clinic's Coronary Primary Prevention Trial (Lipid Research Clinic's Program, 1984) tested cholestyramine in middle-aged men and demonstrated 19% lower incidence in coronary heart disease in the treated group. This study, which may not necessarily be extrapolated to other age groups of patients or other drugs, provides strong evidence supporting the lipid hypothesis and for the necessity of reducing elevated total cholesterol and LDL-C. In this trial there were few serious side effects. Nonetheless, side effects of long-term therapy may have more risk than elevated blood lipid levels, as in the case of clofibrate (Coronary Drug Project Research Group, 1975).

In certain patterns of hyperlipidemia and in individuals who have exhausted other means of reducing lipid levels, treatment with medication(s) may be necessary. Therapy should be carefully selected based on the abnormal pattern of blood lipids, and decisions to initiate therapy should weigh possible long-term risk-benefit ratios.

Pharmacologic therapy should be instituted only after appropriate education, diet treatment, and other interventions have been attempted for 3 to 6 months. Baseline lipid and lipoprotein values must be clearly established before therapy begins. Other factors such as associated risk factors, age of patients, and so on will obviously affect the decision to treat with medicines. Periodic checks on compliance with diet are as important as measuring the effects of the drug. Patients must understand that medication does not replace dietary adjustments. Treatment goals should include changes in total cholesterol, HDL-C, and LDL-C levels, and measurements should be made regularly.

Currently approved drugs for hyperlipidemia are cholestyramine (Questran), colestipol (Colestid), nicotinic acid, probucol (Lorelco), dextrothyroxine (Choloxin), clofibrate (Atomid-5) and gemifibrozil (Lopid). Effects of each medication on the lipid fractions and drug side effects are quite different, and therefore medication must be individualized. New medications, including the HMB-Co-A-reductase inhibitors and others, will add to the ability to alter serum cholesterol levels if they prove to be safe for long-term use. Costs of medication vary widely with newer agents being considerably more costly than older agents in general (Sloan, 1983).

Recommended Drugs

Bile Acid Sequesterants. Cholestyramine and colestipol are the two available bile acid sequesterants. They decrease total cholesterol and LDL-C by interrupting enterohepatic circulation of bile acids. Bile acids, produced in the liver, are excreted into the small intestine to enhance digestion and emulsification of fat. The majority of bile acids are re-absorbed and recycled. The bile acid sequesterants, by binding to these acids, increase cholesterol excretion into the stool and force the liver to metabolize additional cholesterol for bile acid synthesis. The range of reduction of serum cholesterol is usually 20–30%.

Side effects of these agents are minimal as they are not absorbed by the gastrointestinal tract. These agents have an unpleasant taste and quality, being gritty in consistency. Colestipol is somewhat more pleasant to take and can be taken in smaller volumes. Most side effects are in the gastrointestinal tract; constipation, abdominal distention, indigestion, nausea, and diarrhea are the usual side effects associated with these drugs. In addition, in some patients the TG level may rise as LDL-C decreases. These agents may interfere with the absorption of thiazides, warfarin, digoxin, thyroxine, and other anionic agents. The loss of bile acids may interfere with the absorption of fat-soluble vitamins (A, D, and K) as well. Dosage range is 12-24 daily, usually given in two doses. These drugs are usually mixed in liquids before being taken by mouth. They are quite costly in comparison to other lipid-lowering drugs.

Nicotinic Acid (Niacin).   Nicotinic acid is a B vitamin that has a marked effect on serum lipid levels. It is inexpensive and has been in use for many years. Nicotinic acid inhibits lipoprotein synthesis and therefore decreases TG, total cholesterol, and LDL-C. It may increase HDL-C levels by as much as 10-15 mg/dl.

Side effects with nicotinic acid include cutaneous flushing, nausea, abnormal liver function tests, hyperuricemia, and hyperglycemia. Although most of these effects are mild, the flushing associated with this compound can be disconcerting to the patient. This flushing is a prostoglandin-mediated dilation of superficial cutaneous capillaries and can be blocked by aspirin or other prostaglandin inhibitors. Tolerance develops to this side effect, and therefore niacin is usually started in low dose and increased gradually. Sustained release preparations are also available. One aspirin given 1/2 hr before a niacin dose is usually sufficient to minimize flushing.

Niacin is effective in many lipid disorders, but is more effective in combination with bile-acid sequesterants. This combination has been shown to lower LDL-C levels by 50%, lower VLDL-C and triglyceride levels by 33%, and increase HDL-C level by 37% (LeRosa, 1983). Compliance is difficult with this combination, however, due to the patient's discomforting side effects and the large amount of medication required.

Dosage of nicotinic acid is usually started at 100 mg three times daily and gradually increased to a total daily dose of 2-6 g per day. Nicotinic acid is available in 100, 250, and 500 mg tablets.

Probucol.   Probucol is a relatively new lipid-lowering agent that inhibits hepatic cholesterol biosynthesis and enhances bile acid synthesis and excretion. Probucol lowers LDL-C levels 10–15%, but can decrease HDL-C levels 20–25%. Probucol has, in one report, impacted favorably on coronary artery disease (Hunninghake, 1983).

Probucol, therefore, has the disadvantage of mixed effects on the lipid profile. In addition, the drug is highly fat soluble and has a prolonged half-life. In fact, the accumulation of probucol over time has led to detectable serum levels 6 months after discontinuing the drug. TG levels may also increase. Other side effects are usually gastrointestinal, especially diarrhea, but are generally mild. The usual dose is 500 mg twice daily.

Clofibrate.   Clofibrate has been a popular agent in the past, but has recently been shown to have major long-term side effects, which have drastically curtailed its use. It remains, however, the drug of choice for Type III hyperlipidemia. It dramatically reduces intermediate and very low-density lipoproteins in this disorder. Clofibrate has only a modest effect on LDL-C and HDL-C. The mechanism of action of this drug is unknown.

Other possible side effects include cardiac arrhythmias, abnormal liver function tests, nausea, myalgias, and displacement of warfarin from albumin in serum. Due to the above serious effects, this drug's usefulness has become considerably limited.

Gemfibrozil.   Gemfibrozil is a newly released homolog of clofibrate, which has received much recent favorable response. It is thought to decrease VLDL synthesis, though the exact mechanism of action is not known. Gemfibrozil is effective in lowering triglyceride levels and VLDL-C, while increasing HDL-C levels, all in significant amounts (Kaukola, Manninen, Malkonen, & Ehnholm, 1981). The effect on lipid levels is quite different than that of clofibrate.

The clinical relationship of gemfibrozil to clofibrate has cast doubt on its long-term safety. Clinical experience with gemfibrozil is not as extensive as other agents yet, but it appears at this time that side effects are mild and low in number. Gemfibrozil does increase the lithogenicity of bile, though apparently less so than clofibrate. Other side effects include gastrointestinal disturbance, skin rash, dizziness, myalgias, elevated liver function tests, and hyperglycemia. Gemfibrozil can displace warfarin from serum proteins.

Gemfibrozil is currently under long-term study in Helsinki (Manninen, 1983). It is available in 300 mg capsules, and the usual daily dose is 1200 mg in two divided doses before meals.

Dextrothyroxine.   This drug lowers both total and LDL-C cholesterol levels but has been shown to have a possible higher mortality rate associated with its use (Coronary Drug Project Research Group, 1975). It should not be used in patients with known atherosclerotic heart disease. Dosage averages 3 mg per day. This drug suppresses the hypothalmic pituitary axis.

Treatment of Hyperlipidemias

Drug therapy for hyperlipidemia should only be considered if all other nondrug interventions fail or the patient is at usually high risk. The patient must be made aware that diet remains the treatment of choice even while on drug therapy. Secondary causes should be looked for and adequately treated. Hyperlipidemia patterns can and should be treated for reasons other than the development of coronary heart disease. For example, both Type I and Type V patterns are associated with very high occurrences of pancreatitis or may be cosmetically unacceptable. Therapy should be specific for each lipoprotein phenotype. The drugs most appropriate for each type of hyperlipidemia are discussed below.

Type I.   The high level of TG, associated with excessive chylomicrons, make gemfibrozil the treatment of choice of most authors. Niacin and clofibrate would be alternative choices but also have many side effects.

Type IIa.   Bile acid sequesterants are generally employed first, and the recent LRC results underscore their value, with niacin and probucol used in combination with the sequesterants or as backup therapy (LeRosa, 1983).

Type IIb.   Niacin and the bile-acid sequesterants are the treatments of choice and are effective alone, or in combination.

Type III.   This disorder is, fortunately, quite rare. Due to its high rate of associated atherosclerosis, treatment is important. Niacin or clofibrate (despite its side effects) may be used in this disorder. These may be substituted for each other depending on an individual's response to treatment or contraindications to their use.

Type IV.   This type of hyperlipidemia is frequently associated with obesity and excessive intake of alcohol or simple carbohydrates. Initial therapeutic steps should include correction of these secondary causes. If the patient does not respond, triglyceride levels should then be treated with niacin as the primary agent, gemfibrozil or clofibrate as secondary choices.

Type V.   This type is rare and not highly associated with atherosclerosis. Niacin, clofibrate, and gemfibrozil are recommended for treatment if indicated.

Conclusion

Mass hyperlipidemia is one of the major health problems of the United States. Elevated cholesterol (and particularly LDL-C) is the primary cause of atherosclerosis, which is the leading cause of death in developed countries. These conclusions are based on extensive evidence from the four major lines of medical research— epidemiological, clinical, pathological, and experimental. Control of atherosclerosis requires sustaining lower levels of blood lipids in the population. The recent success of the Lipid Research Clinic's Primary Prevention Trial (1984) conclusively demonstrates that lowering cholesterol will decrease morbidity and mortality from atherosclerotic disease.

Favorable lipoprotein changes may be accomplished by pharmacologic or nonpharmacologic means, but we believe that nonpharmacologic attempts should be tried first. Several hygienic measures such as dietary change, exercise, and weight loss are safe and effective interventions. Overweight is clearly a significant health hazard and contributes directly and indirectly to risk of CHD. Given the extensive prevalence of overweight in the United States, vigorous public health efforts to prevent and control this problem should be implemented. Weight reduction is a safe and effective way of preventing and managing hyperlipidemia. Physicians and other clinicians should be diligent in identifying and treating overweight individuals. If serious efforts using weight reduction and other life-style interventions fail, pharmacologic intervention should be attempted for patients with hyperlipidemia.

References

Arntzenius, A.C., Kromhout, D., Barth, J.D., et al. (1985). Diet, lipoproteins, and the progression of coronary atherosclerosis: The Leiden intervention trial. *New England Journal of Medicine, 312,* 805-811.

Blackburn, H. (1979). Conference on the health effects of blood lipids: Optimal distributions for populations. Workshop report: Epidemiological section. *Preventive Medicine, 8,* 612-678.

Blackburn, H. (1980). The public health view of diet and mass hyperlipidemia: Part I. *Cardiovascular Reviews and Reports, 1,* 361-369.

Blair, S.N., Cooper, K.H., Gibbons, L.W., Gettman, L.R., Lewis, S., & Goodyear, N. (1983). Changes in coronary heart disease risk factors associated with increased treadmill time in 753 men. *American Journal of Epidemiology, 118*(3), 352-359.

Blair, S.N., Ellsworth, N.M., Haskell, W.L., Stern, M.P., Farquhar, J.W., & Wood, P.D. (1981). Comparison of nutrient intake in middle-aged men and women runners and controls. *Medicine and Science in Sports and Exercise*, **13**, 310-315.

Brownell, K.D., Bachorik, P.S., & Ayerle, R.S. (1981). Changes in plasma lipid and lipoprotein levels in men and women after a program of moderate exercise. *Circulation*, **65**, 477-484.

Caggiula, A.W., Christakis, G., Farrand, M., Hulley, S.B., Johnson, R., Lasser, N.L., Stamler, J., & Widdowson, G. (1981). The multiple risk factor intervention trial (MRFIT): IV. Intervention on blood lipids. *Preventive Medicine*, **10**, 443-475.

Castelli, W.P., Gordon, T., Hjortland, M.C., Kagan, A., Doyle, J.T., Hames, C.G., Hulley, S.B., & Zukel, W.J. (1977). Alcohol and blood lipids: The cooperative lipoprotein phenotyping study. *Lancet*, **2**, 153-155.

Coronary Drug Project Research Group. (1975). Clofibrate and niacin in coronary heart disease. *Journal of the American Medical Association*, **231**, 360-381.

Council on Scientific Affairs. (1983). Dietary and pharmacologic therapy for the lipid risk factors. *Journal of the American Medical Association*, **250**(14), 1873-1879.

Ernst, N., Fisher, M., Smith, W., Gordon, T., Rifkind, B.M., Little, J.A., Mishkel, M.A., & Williams, O.D. (1980). The association of plasma high-density lipoprotein cholesterol with dietary intake and alcohol consumption. *Circulation*, **62**(4), 41-52.

Garrison, R.J., Kannel, W.B., Feinleib, M., Castelli, W.P., McNamara, P.M., & Padgett, S.J. (1978). Cigarette smoking and HDL cholesterol. *Atherosclerosis*, **30**, 17-25.

Gibbons, L.W., Blair, S.N., Cooper, K.H., & Smith, M. (1983). Association between coronary heart disease risk factors and physical fitness in healthy adult women. *Circulation*, **67**, 977-983.

Glueck, C.J. (1979). Dietary fat and atherosclerosis. *American Journal of Clinical Nutrition*, **32**, 2703-2711.

Goldbourt, U., & Medalie, J.H. (1979). High density lipoprotein cholesterol and incidence of coronary heart disease: The Israeli ischemic heart disease study. *American Journal of Epidemiology*, **109**, 296-308.

Gordon, T., Castelli, W.P., Hjortland, M.C., Kannel, W.B., & Dawber, T.R. (1977). High density lipoprotein as a protective factor against coronary heart disease: The Framingham study. *American Journal of Medicine*, **62**, 707-714.

Gordon, T., Kannel, W.B., Castelli, W.P., & Dawber, T.R. (1981). Lipoproteins, cardiovascular disease, and death: The Framingham study. *Archives of Internal Medicine*, **141**, 1128-1131.

Gordon, T., Fisher, M., Ernst, N., & Rifkind, B.M. (1982). Relation of diet to LDL cholesterol, VLDL cholesterol, and plasma total cholesterol and triglycerides in white adults. *Arteriosclerosis*, **2**, 502-512.

Gotto, A.M., Jr. (1981). Regression of atherosclerosis. *American Journal of Medicine*, **70**, 989-991.

Gotto, A.M. (1983). Clinical diagnosis of hyperlipoproteinemia. *American Journal of Medicine*, **74**, 5-9.

Grimm, R.H., Leon, A.S., Hunninghake, D.B., Lenz, K., Hannan, P., & Blackburn, H. (1981). Effects of thiazide diuretics on plasma lipids and lipoproteins in mildly hypertensive patients: A double-blind controlled trial. *Annals of Internal Medicine*, **94**, 7-11.

Hartung, G.H., Foreyt, J.P., Mitchell, R.E., Mitchell, J.G., Reaves, R.S., & Gotto, A.M. (1983). Effect of alcohol intake on high-density lipoprotein cholesterol levels in runners and inactive men. *Journal of the American Medical Association*, **249**, 747-750.

Hartung, G.H., Foreyt, J.P., Mitchell, R.E., Vlasek, I., & Gotto, A.M. (1980). Relation of diet to high-density-lipoprotein cholesterol in middle-aged marathon runners, joggers, and inactive men. *New England Journal of Medicine*, **302**, 357-361.

Haskell, W.L., Taylor, H.L., Wood, P.D., Schrott, H., & Heiss, G. (1980). Strenuous physical activity, treadmill exercise test performance and plasma high-density lipoprotein cholesterol. *Circulation*, **62**(Suppl. IV), IV53-IV61.

Hjermann, I., Velve Byre, K., Holme, I., & Leren, P. (1981). Effect of diet and smoking intervention on the incidence of coronary heart disease. *Lancet*, **2**, 1303-1310.

Hunninghake, D.B. (1983). Pharmacologic therapy for the hyperlipidemic patient. *American Journal of Medicine*, **74**, 19-22.

Kaukola, S., Manninen, V., Malkonen, M., & Ehnholm, C. (1981). Gemfibrozil in the treatment of dislipoproteinemias in middle-aged survivors of myocardial infarction. *Acta Medica Scandinavica*, **209**, 69-73.

Keys, A. (Ed.). (1970). Coronary heart disease in seven countries. *Circulation*, **41**(Suppl. 1).

Knuiman, J.T., West, C.E., & Burema, J. (1982). Serum total and high density lipoprotein cholesterol concentrations and body mass index in adult men from 13 countries. *American Journal of Epidemiology*, **116**, 631-642.

Krauss, R.M., Lindgren, F.T., Wood, P.D., Haskell, W.L., Albers, J.J., & Cheung, M.C. (1977). Differential increases in plasma high-density lipoprotein subfractions and apolipoproteins in runners (abstract). *Circulation*, **56**, III4.

Kushi, L.H., Lew, R.A., Stare, F.J., et al. (1985). Diet and 20-year mortality from coronary heart disease: The Ireland-Boston diet-heart study. *New England Journal of Medicine*, **312**, 811-818.

Lehninger, A.L. (1978). *Biochemistry* (2nd ed.). New York: Worth.

LeRosa, J.C. (1983). Lipid-lowering drug combinations. *Drug Therapy, 8,* 66-72.

Lipid Research Clinic's Program. (1984). The lipid research coronary primary prevention trial results: I. Reduction in incidence of coronary heart disease. *Journal of the American Medical Association, 251,* 351-364.

Manninen, V. (1983). Clinical results with gemfibrozil and background to the Helsinki heart study. *American Journal of Cardiology, 52,* 35B-38B.

Miller, G.J., & Miller, M.E. (1975). Plasma-high-density-lipoprotein concentration and development of ischaemic heart disease. *Lancet, 1,* 16-19.

Miller, N.E., Forde, O.H., Thelle, D.S., & Mjos, O.O. (1977). The Tromso heart study. High density lipoprotein and coronary heart disease: A prospective case control study. *Lancet, 1,* 965-968.

Miller, N.E., Hammett, F., Saltissi, S., Rao, S., Van Zeller, H., Coltart, J., & Lewis, B. (1981). Relation of angiographically defined coronary artery disease to plasma lipoprotein subfractions and apolipoproteins. *British Medical Journal, 282,* 1741-1744.

Multiple Risk Factor Intervention Trial Research Group. (1982). Multiple risk factor intervention trial. *Journal of the American Medical Association, 248,* 1465-1477.

Naito, H.K. (1976). Effects of physical activity on serum cholesterol metabolism. *Cleveland Clinician's Quarterly, 43,* 21-49.

National Diet-Heart Study Research Group. (1968). *The national diet-heart study final report* (American Heart Association Monograph No. 18). Dallas: American Heart Association.

National Institutes of Health Consensus Conference. (1985). Lowering blood cholesterol to prevent heart disease. *Journal of the American Medical Association, 253,* 2080-2086.

Nikkila, E.A., Taskinen, M.R., Rehunen, S., & Harkonen, M. (1978). Lipoprotein lipase activity in adipose tissue and skeletal muscle of runners: Relation to serum lipoproteins. *Metabolism, 27,* 1661-1671.

Phillips, H.R., Havel, R.J., & Kane, J.P. (1981). Levels and interrelationships of serum and lipoprotein cholesterol and triglycerides: Association with adiposity and the consumption of ethanol, tobacco, and beverages containing caffeine. *Arteriosclerosis, 1,* 13-24.

The Pooling Project Research Group. (1978). Relationship of blood pressure, serum cholesterol, smoking habit, relative weight and ECG abnormalities to incidence of major coronary events: Final report of the Pooling Project. *Journal of Chronic Diseases, 31,* 210-306.

Salonen, J.T., Puska, P., Tanskanen, A., Virtamo, J., Tuomilehto, J., & Huttunen, J.K. (1983). Serum HDL cholesterol in a high coronary risk population in eastern Finland. *Acta Medica Scandinavica, 213,* 255-261.

Shekelle, R.B., Shryock, A.M., Paul, O., Lepper, M., Stamler, J., Liu, S., & Raynor, W.J., Jr. (1981). Diet, serum cholesterol, and death from coronary heart disease. *New England Journal of Medicine, 304*, 65-70.

Sloan, R.W. (1983). Hyperlipidemia. *American Family Physician, 28*, 171-182.

Stamler, J. (1979). Population studies. In R.I. Levy, B.M. Rifkind, B.H. Dennis, & N.D. Ernst (Eds.), *Nutrition, lipids, and coronary heart disease.* New York: Raven Press.

Stamler, J. (1980). The established relationship among diet, serum cholesterol and coronary heart disease. *Acta Medica Scandinavica, 207*, 433-466.

Turpeinen, O., Karvonen, M.J., Pekkarinen, M., Miettinen, M., Elosuo, R., & Paavilainen, E. (1979). Dietary prevention of coronary heart disease: The Finnish mental hospital study. *International Journal of Epidemiology, 8*, 99-118.

Williams, P.T., Wood, P.D., Haskell, W.L., & Vranizan, K. (1982). The effects of running mileage and duration on plasma lipoprotein levels. *Journal of the American Medical Association, 247*, 2674-2679.

Williams, P.T., Wood, P.D., Krauss, R.M., Haskell, W.L., Vranizan, K.M., Blair, S.N., Terry, R., & Farquhar, J.W. (1983). Does weight loss cause the exercise-induced increase in plasma high density lipoproteins? *Atherosclerosis, 47*, 173-185.

Willett, W., Hennekens, C.H., Castelli, W., Rosner, B., Evans, D., Taylor, J., & Kass, E.H. (1983). Effects of cigarette smoking on fasting triglyceride, total cholesterol, and HDL-cholesterol in women. *American Heart Journal, 105*, 417-421.

Willett, W., Hennekens, C.H., Siegel, A.J., Adner, M.M., & Castelli, W.P. (1980). Alcohol consumption and high-density lipoprotein cholesterol in marathon runners. *New England Journal of Medicine, 303*, 1159-1161.

Wood, P.D., Camargo, C.A., Jr., Haskell, W.L., Williams, P.T., Krauss, R.M., & Lindgren, F.T. (1983). Effect of cessation and resumption of alcohol intake on serum high-density lipoprotein subfractions: A controlled study (abstract). *Arteriosclerosis, 3*, 508a.

Wood, P.D., & Haskell, W.L. (1979). The effect of exercise on plasma high density lipoproteins. *Lipids, 14*, 417-427.

Wood, P.D., Haskell, W.L., Blair, S.N., Williams, P.T., Krauss, R.M., Lindgren, F.T., Albers, J.J., Ho, P.H., & Farquhar, J.W. (1983). Increased exercise level and plasma lipoprotein concentrations: A one year, randomized, controlled study in sedentary, middle-aged men. *Metabolism, 32*, 31-39.

Wood, P.D., Haskell, W.L., Stern, M.P., Lewis, S., & Perry, C. (1977). Plasma lipoprotein distributions in male and female runners. *Annals of the New York Academy of Science, 301*, 748-763.

Wood, P.D., Haskell, W.L., Terry, R.B., Ho, P.H., & Blair, S.N. (1982). Effects of a two-year running program on plasma lipoproteins, body fat, and dietary intake in initially sedentary men (abstract). *Medicine and Science in Sports and Exercise,* **14**, 104.

We thank Diann Dunkley for typing the manuscript.